YOGA, TAI CHI
MASSAGE, THERAPIES
& HEALING REMEDIES

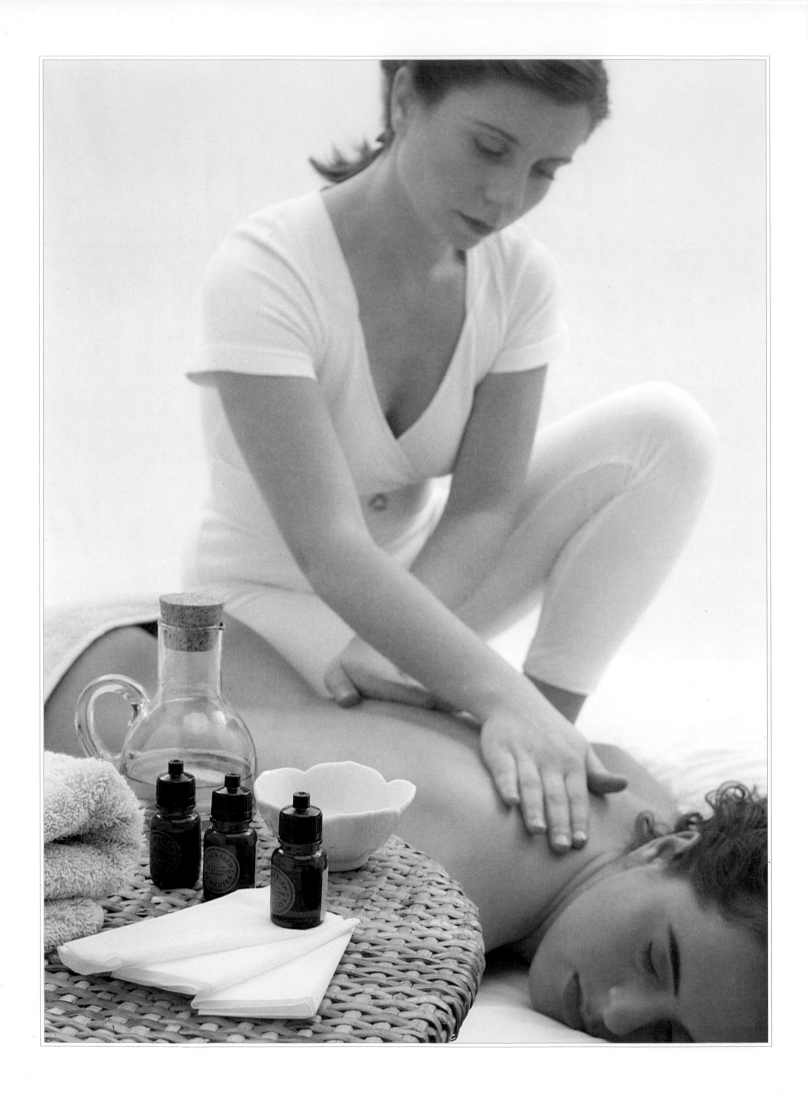

YOGA, TAI CHI
MASSAGE, THERAPIES
& NATURAL REMEDIES

natural ways to health, relaxation and vitality:
a complete practical guide

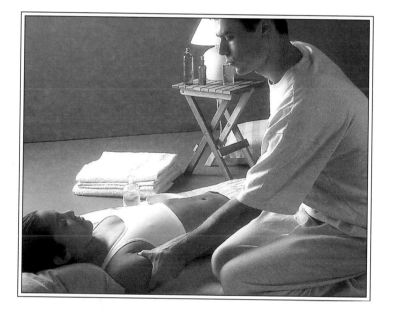

MARK EVANS B Phil., FNIMH

HERMES
HOUSE

This edition is published by Hermes House

Hermes House is an imprint of Anness Publishing Ltd
Hermes House, 88–89 Blackfriars Road, London SE1 8HA
tel. 020 7401 2077; fax 020 7633 9499; info@anness.com

© Anness Publishing Ltd 2002

Published in the USA by Hermes House, Anness Publishing Inc.
27 West 20th Street, New York, NY 10011; fax 212 807 6813

A CIP catalogue record for this book is available from the British Library.

Publisher: Joanna Lorenz
Editorial Managers: Helen Sudell, Joanne Rippin
Designer: Nigel Partridge
Photographers: Sue Atkinson, Simon Bottomley, Dave Jordan, Don Last and Lucy Mason,
Other chapters supplied by: John Hudson (Meditation), Michèle MacDonnell (Alexander Technique), Carole McGilvery
(Aromatherapy), Jimi Reed (Massage), Kate Shapland (Fitness and Exercise) and Paul Tucker (T'ai Chi)
Additional text supplied by: Andrew Ackroyd, Felicity Roma Bowers, Karine Butchart, Suzanne Franzen, Anne Gains,
Clare Harris and Paul Harvey
Exercise advisor: Dean Hodgkin

1 3 5 7 9 10 8 6 4 2

The majority of this volume was previously published as: *The Guide to Natural Living*

IMPORTANT NOTICE
The advice given in this book is appropriate in most cases. However, it cannot take into
account specific individuals' reactions. Neither the author nor the publishers
can accept any responsibility for claims arising from the inappropriate
use of any remedy or healing treatment. For further advice, and
before beginning any treatment suggested herein, read page 121 for
information pertaining to certain conditions and herb restrictions.

CONTENTS

NATURAL REMEDIES

ealth is, or should be, the most natural state of being. The origins of the word are linked with those of wholeness and healing, and it is that complete sense of harmony, of being whole, that brings true health. This is also the ultimate aim of the natural healing systems, those that adopt a holistic view rather than the reductionist perspective that is evident in much of conventional modern medicine.

In the last 10 years or so, there has been a great revival of interest in natural therapies, both as a recognition of their tremendous value and also as a move away from some of the side-effects and impersonal approaches of allopathic medicine. In this section of the book, we are looking at how natural therapies can be used at home, as self-help remedies, for a variety of common complaints; it should not be forgotten, however, that in professional practice more complex or chronic conditions can also be treated by alternative or complementary medicine, and if in doubt over any problem do seek qualified advice.

Many traditions of natural medicine extend back over several centuries, with an impressive accumulation of practical knowledge. For this section we have focused on four main therapies, which not only have such an established tradition but also have good standards of training, clinical research data and widespread acceptance. They are aromatherapy, herbalism, homeopathy and naturopathy.

ABOVE: Fresh fruit is an excellent natural source of vitamins.

OPPOSITE: Herbs can be grown successfully in ordinary garden flower beds, giving off wonderful scents as well as providing a useful source of herbal medicines.

AROMATHERAPY

The use of pure essential oils from plants dates back many centuries, and the history of aromatherapy is in many ways part of the history of herbal medicine as a whole. The Arabic countries are credited with first discovering the process of distillation of oils, around a thousand years ago, and since then their use has spread both eastwards through the Indian sub-continent and westwards into Europe. Much modern research has taken place, for example, in France, ranging from perfumery applications to medicinal uses as powerful anti-infective agents.

Essential oils are highly concentrated substances – pure oil of Rose, for instance, may require 5,000 roses to make just 5 ml (1 tsp) of oil! For this reason they should be treated with respect and used sparingly – small is definitely better (and cheaper). In large doses many essential oils can become somewhat irritating to the skin, and a few are quite toxic if not used correctly. See general warning on page 121.

Since a large part of their effect on our moods and emotional states occurs through our sense of smell, it is important not to use any individual oil for too long, as they become tolerated and less useful. As a general rule, do not use an oil on a daily basis for more than 10 days. Similarly, do not inhale

Keep aromatherapy oils in well-stoppered bottles, out of the sun, when not in use.

Essential oils are very concentrated: add a drop at a time and only use the amounts suggested.

or mix too many oils together at one time; the olfactory centre in the brain becomes confused and an excess of essences can cause headaches or even nausea. Three or at the most four oils should be the maximum; two may be better.

A common way to use essential oils for self-treatment is in the bath. Place 6 drops on the surface of the bath water just before entering. The drops quickly form a thin film over the surface which adheres to the skin and is partially absorbed, helped by the warmth of the water. For oils such as Peppermint, which can make the skin tingle if used in large amounts, just add 3-4 drops, whereas with a mild and generally very safe oil such as Lavender, 10 drops can be used. If using a blend, the above suggestions represent the total number of drops to use in the bath. For compresses, use a maximum of 5 drops in a small bowl of hot or cold water as directed in this book (see page 15).

Another important method for using oils is diluted into a base vegetable oil and applied to the skin in massage. For home use a general dilution rate should be 1 per cent; since essential oils are usually sold in dropper bottles, this means a maximum of 20 drops per 100 ml (4 fl oz/½ cup) of base oil. Different cultures over the centuries have favoured various vegetable oils for massage, mostly dependent on local availability. Probably the most versatile oil is that of Sweet Almond; it is absorbed well into the skin and helps to nourish the skin, too. Other good base oils are Grapeseed, Sunflower and Safflower; the lightest oil of all is Coconut, but it may become solid at cool temperatures.

HERBALISM

Herbal medicine is the most widespread of all forms of medicine across the world, both historically and even today. At some time all cultures have used herbalism as the main system of treatment; its origins are essentially the origins of mankind itself. Probably the earliest herbal tradition comes from India. Medical knowledge from there spread into China on the one hand and into the Middle East on the other. The philosophy underlying Ancient Egyptian, and later Graeco-Roman, medicine has many similarities with both the old Ayur-Vedic system from northern India and traditional Chinese medicine.

Modern Western herbal medicine stems from the knowledge of the Greeks, with a strong input from the Native American tradition too. Increasingly, research being carried out today often confirms centuries-old empirical knowledge. Around 80 per cent of the world's population still relies on herbal medicine for their health needs, and even within conventional Western medicine up to 20 per cent of drugs are derived from plants in one way or another.

Herbs are almost certainly the most popular method of self-help in minor complaints, and introduce people to natural medicine. Throughout this book you will find references to how to take herbs internally; the easiest method is to make a tea, using a rough rule of 5 ml (1 tsp) per person plus the same for the teapot (many of the most popular herbs are available in tea bags, simply use one of these). If using fresh herbs, for example Lemon Balm (*Melissa officinalis*) you can use double the above amounts.

For stronger, more medicinal brews, you need to make either an infusion or a decoction (see page 12). For either an infusion or a decoction, the standard dose is 100-150 ml (4-5 fl oz/½-⅔ cup) – approximately a medium-sized teacupful – three times a day.

These infusions and decoctions can also be used to make a compress or poultice (see page 15). Once again, if using fresh herbs you can use more, perhaps 50 per cent more of each herb.

Many of the herbs found in gardens today have been used by herbalists for over two thousand years.

HOMEOPATHY

As a full system of medicine, homeopathy is much more recent in its development. It owes its modern origins to Samuel Hahnemann, a German physician, who formulated homeopathic theories in the late eighteenth century, although the principles were almost certainly known for hundreds of years before. Essentially, symptoms are seen not as negative effects of illness but as the attempts of the person to resist disease. Hahnemann tested a treatment for malaria on himself by taking many doses of quinine; after some time he induced malarial-like symptoms, and came to the conclusion that quinine worked precisely because it created these reactions in a healthy person; it mimicked and supported our own healing responses.

This led to the principle of "like curing like", and hundreds of homeopathic remedies have since been tested by giving them to healthy people and recording the responses. These "remedy pictures" are then applied to see which one fits the symptoms of an ill person. The other major point of difference between homeopathic and conventional medicine is that when a remedy has been identified as being appropriate to encourage the individual's self-healing mechanisms, it is then prescribed in minute amounts. Hahnemann had found that by diluting his remedies in a special way he was able to get a quicker effect, and he understood these dilutions to work on a more subtle level than simply obtaining a physical reaction.

One of the common scales for measuring the dilutions is the centesimal scale – that is, diluting the remedy in the ratio of 1:100. For a liquid this means one part of the remedy is mixed with 99 parts of a diluent, usually either alcohol or water. This is called a 1c dilution; this is then shaken in a special way, or succussed, and one part of this is added to 99 parts of the diluent to make a 2c dilution, and so on. As you can see, levels of extreme dilution are quickly reached,

and so the remedy cannot be said to be acting physically in a conventional way, and indeed an important part of the "remedy picture" is the emotional reactions that are produced. The personality of the patient is a significant factor in choosing a remedy. Paradoxically, the more dilute the remedy, the more effectively it works.

A homeopathic practitioner may well use a very diluted remedy, to address an imbalance in our basic constitution, if there is a very clear picture that matches the individual.

For self-help treatment choose either the 6c or 30c potencies. For mild problems try taking the 6c dilution (normally remedies are available as tablets or pills, with directions for taking them with the container they come in) 3 times a day for up to 5 days. In more acute conditions, take a 30c dilution in the same way.

In short-term, really acute conditions you can take up to 6 doses of either potency at 3-hourly intervals. Continuing to take the remedies for longer, however, may result in an aggravation of symptoms, as you "prove" the remedy in the same way that Hahnemann did. If in any doubt, and in any case if there is no response within this time, always see a professional homeopath.

ACONITE
(Aconitum napellus)

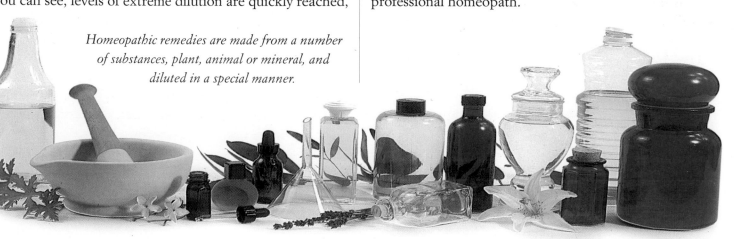

Homeopathic remedies are made from a number of substances, plant, animal or mineral, and diluted in a special manner.

NATUROPATHY

In many respects, naturopathy is really common sense applied to health. The basic principle is that we have tremendous innate healing abilities, and our systems will always attempt to overcome an illness and restore balance. In naturopathy, these attempts are encouraged by utilizing such natural factors as diet, exercise and relaxation, fresh air and the use of water (hydrotherapy). The general thrust of treatment is really to shift responsibility for health back to ourselves as far as possible, and equally to advocate prevention rather than cure.

Increasingly nowadays, ill-health is recognized as arising from environmental factors such as pollution, so an individual can only do so much to keep healthy, and wider measures may well need to be campaigned for. Nevertheless, a lot can be done through self-help action. While fresh, unprocessed foods are the main form of dietary treatment, there are times when this needs to be supplemented in order to raise vitality to a level where self-healing can take place, and so throughout the book there are some suggestions for supplements under different headings.

Exercise is a major form of self-help, obviously within limits of individual comfort. Both posture and correct breathing are an integral part of this, as effort without correct breathing can lead to strain. It is important to ensure that adequate rest or relaxation is taken too (easier to say than do in today's busy world!), and naturopaths would certainly give advice on these areas as part of the treatment.

The application of water by various methods, or hydrotherapy treatment, is another very useful part of naturopathy. The concept of using hot or cold water dates back at least to the Ancient Greeks, and is seen around the world in other old cultures, for example, that of Native Americans. Hydrotherapy treatment had a major revival in

The importance of regular exercise to keep our whole body fit, active and healthy is now well-recognized.

Europe in the nineteenth century, with the Bavarian monk Sebastian Kneipp the most influential figure. To this day, there are many Kneipp centres in Germany, Austria and Switzerland, which still prove very popular with patients. There are also around 120 different hydrotherapy treatments available in German health spas.

One of the simplest methods is to use a compress, or fomentation, made by wringing out a small towel in water and placing over the required area (see page 15). By alternating hot and cold compresses, – normally about 3-5 minutes if hot and up to 1 minute if cold – the local circulation can be strongly stimulated. For people who are considerably overweight it is often better just to use a cool compress, as this is less taxing on the heart. A shower can be used to similar effect by changing the temperature, or cool splashes of water after a warm bath may be used. A specific form of treatment in hydrotherapy clinics is the use of sitz baths, a kind of hip bath, which works on the pelvic and abdominal areas, by sitting firstly in a hot bath then transferring to a cold one for a short time, as indicated above.

As well as these approaches to health and healing, natural therapies range from those that work mainly via the body, such as massage, osteopathy, chiropractic and physiotherapy, through those that deal with energy balance, such as acupuncture, reflexology and shiatsu, to those that approach from the mental or emotional level, such as hypnotherapy, psychotherapy and group work. Each has its own strengths and weaknesses, and each attempts to help to restore balance from its own perspective. Some of them are not so easily applied for self-help, but it is useful to know that if you are unable to sort out your health problems on your own, then there is a wide choice of professional treatments that may help.

MAKING AN INFUSION

An infusion is made by pouring boiling water over an amount of the herb, to extract the properties. It is suitable for leaves and flowers, whose parts are easily extracted.

1 Place the herb in a teapot with a close-fitting lid. Pour in boiling water. Leave to infuse for up to 10 minutes.

2 Strain through a sieve or strainer into a cup. Store the remainder in a jug, preferably in the fridge.

STANDARD QUANTITIES

25 g (1 oz) dried herb or 50 g (2 oz) fresh herb to 500 ml (16 fl oz/2 cups) boiling water.

STANDARD DOSES

One teacup (approximately 150 ml (5 fl oz/⅔ cup)) 3 times a day.

Infusions and decoctions should be stored in tightly-stoppered vessels ideally, and will last for about 3 days in the fridge.

MAKING A DECOCTION

A decoction involves simmering the herb in water to extract its properties, and is suitable for roots or woody parts that do not easily yield their ingredients in a simple infusion. If combining two plants, where one is a root, say Dandelion (*Taraxacum officinale*), and the other a flower, say Chamomile (*Chamomilla recutita*), use the strained decoction of the former for pouring on to the latter to make the infusion.

1 Place the herb in a saucepan and pour on cold water. Bring to the boil and simmer, until the liquid is reduced by a third.

2 Strain through a sieve into a jug, and store in a fridge. It will keep for up to three days.

STANDARD QUANTITIES

25 g (1 oz) dried herb or 50 g (2 oz) fresh herb to 750 ml (1¼ pt/3⅔ cups) water, reduced to 500 ml (16 fl oz/2 cups) after simmering.

STANDARD DOSES

One teacup (150 ml (5 fl oz/⅔ cup)) 3 times a day.

MAKING A HOT OIL INFUSION

Herbs can be infused in oil, to make an extract for use in massage, or in making creams and ointments. Infused oils may keep for a few months, but will be stronger made in small batches for more immediate use. Hot infused oils may be made from herbs such as Comfrey (*Symphytum officinale*), while flowers such as Marigold (*Calendula officinalis*) or St John's Wort (*Hypericum perforatum*) are better as cold infused oils. Any light oil, such as Sunflower, Safflower or Sweet Almond oil, is a suitable medium to use.

MAKING A COLD OIL INFUSION

Some plants contain important medicinal oils which are highly volatile, i.e. they escape with heat, and a cold oil infusion retains their properties much more successfully.

1 Pack a large jar with the herb and cover with oil. Seal and leave in a sunny spot for 2 weeks.

2 Pour slowly through a jelly bag into a clean jug, allowing time for the oil to filter through the fabric.

1 Place the herb and oil in a glass bowl, over a saucepan of simmering water, and heat gently for a couple of hours.

2 Pour through a jelly bag into a clean jug.

3 Squeeze out as much oil as possible through the bag. To make the infused oil even stronger, repeat steps 1, 2 and 3 with the same oil and new amounts of the herb.

4 Pour into clean, dark bottles. Seal and store. Preferably, use small bottles as when opened the oil starts to deteriorate.

3 Squeeze out as much oil as possible through the bag (wear gloves as the oil is hot), to get a really strong extract.

4 Pour into clean, dark bottles. Seal and store. Keep in a cool place and use within 3 months of making.

STANDARD QUANTITIES
250 g (9 oz) dried herb or 500 g (1¼ lb) fresh herb to 500 ml (16 fl oz/2 cups) pure vegetable oil.

STANDARD QUANTITIES
250 g (9 oz) dried herb or 500 g (1¼ lb) fresh herb to 500 ml (16 fl oz/2 cups) pure vegetable oil.

MAKING A TINCTURE

Many herbs contain active ingredients which are not easily extracted by water, or are destroyed by heat, and a tincture solves these problems as well as preserving the extract. A tincture is an extract of a herb in a mixture of alcohol and water, normally 25 per cent alcohol strength. This is one of the most concentrated extracts from a herb, and the alcohol preserves the medicine for 2 years or more. The alcohol used commercially is ethyl alcohol, but a spirit such as brandy or vodka can be used for home tinctures. Do not use industrial alcohol, isopropyl alcohol or methylated spirits, as they are all poisonous.

Because a tincture is such a concentrated extract, only use where recommended, and for short periods of time. Do not be tempted to increase the dosage.

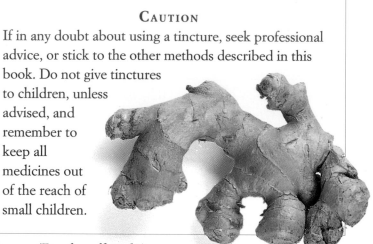

CAUTION
If in any doubt about using a tincture, seek professional advice, or stick to the other methods described in this book. Do not give tinctures to children, unless advised, and remember to keep all medicines out of the reach of small children.

GINGER *(Zingiber officinalis)*

1 Put the herb into a large jar and pour on the alcohol/water mixture. Seal the jar and store in a cool place for two weeks. Shake the jar occasionally.

2 Pour mixture through a jelly bag into a clean jug.

3 Squeeze out the tincture from the bag. Ideally, use a wine press and press the mixture into a clean jug.

4 Pour the strained liquid into clean, dark bottles. Seal and store. Keep in a cool dry place and label.

STANDARD QUANTITIES
200 g (7 oz) dried herb or 40 g (1½ oz) fresh herb to 1 litre (1¾ pt/4 cups) 25 per cent alcohol/water mix (e.g. if using 40 per cent vodka or brandy, add 375 ml (13 fl oz/1½ cups) water to 600 ml (1 pt/2½ cups) spirit to make a 25 per cent strength).

STANDARD DOSES
Up to 5 ml (1 tsp), three times a day. These may be taken diluted in a little water. For concentrated herbs such as Ginger *(Zingiber officinalis),* take up to 10 drops, 3 times a day. Preferably take these with water.

BUCHU *(Barosma betulina)*

WARM AND COLD COMPRESSES

A compress is a way of applying herbal extracts directly to the skin, to reduce the inflammation or promote healing. Usually, an infusion or decoction of the herb is prepared for use in the compress, or simply hot or cold water can be used.

1 Soak a clean cloth or flannel in a hot infusion or hot water.

2 Place on the affected area and hold firmly in place – use a towel or bandage to tie in place if kept on for long. The same procedure applies for cold compresses.

Marigold (Calendula officinalis) *is very soothing for bites and stings.*

POULTICE

A poultice acts in a similar way to a compress, but the herb itself is used, rather than just a liquid extract. Normally poultices are applied hot, and it may be useful to apply a little oil to the skin first, to stop the herb from sticking.

1 Chop up the fresh herb if it is too large, and place sufficient herbs to cover the affected area into a saucepan. Add a little water and simmer for a couple of minutes.

2 Squeeze out any excess moisture and place on the affected area. Cover with a bandage or cotton strips to hold in place.

3 Keep in place for 3-4 hours, replacing every hour with a fresh, hot poultice if necessary.

MAKING AN OINTMENT

An ointment contains oils or fats, but not water, and is useful to form a protective layer over the skin. Petroleum jelly or paraffin wax may be used, but a wonderful natural method is to use vegetable oil, such as Sweet Almond or Sunflower, with beeswax. This is also very easy to make at home.

1 Place the beeswax and oil in a glass bowl over a saucepan of water. Bring the water to the boil and simmer until the wax has melted into the oil. Remove from the heat.

2 Stir continually as the oil/wax mixture cools and stiffens; essential oils may be added at this stage, as recommended, and stirred into the mixture.

3 Pour or spoon into small, clean ointment jars, seal and store. This may keep for a few months under good conditions, but should be made in small amounts as needed.

STANDARD QUANTITIES
25 g (1 oz) beeswax to 100 ml (4 fl oz/½ cup) vegetable oil. If adding essential oils, use 20-30 drops for this amount, but only 10 drops if skin is very sensitive.

MAKING A CREAM

Making an organic cream is very similar to making an ointment, again using beeswax.

1 Place beeswax and oil in a glass bowl in a saucepan of water (see left). Bring water to the boil and simmer until the wax has melted. Place water in another glass bowl, over a saucepan of simmering water. Remove both glass bowls from the heat.

2 Add water to the melted wax/oil mixture, drop by drop, stirring all the time until the cream thickens and cools.

3 At this stage essential oils may be added, as recommended, and gently stirred into the cream.

4 Pour or spoon into small, clean ointment jars, seal and store. Make small amounts as required. This cream may keep for a few months under good conditions.

STANDARD QUANTITIES
25 g (1 oz) beeswax, 25 ml (1½ tbsp) water and 100 ml (4 fl oz/½ cup) vegetable oil. If adding essential oils, use 20-30 drops at the most for this amount of cream.

MIXING ESSENTIAL OILS FOR MASSAGE

When essential oils are used for aromatherapy massage, different oils are combined to increase their therapeutic effect. Light vegetable oils such as Sweet Almond, Grapeseed or Sunflower are the best oils to begin with. For home use the general dilution rate should be 1 per cent (i.e. a maximum of 20 drops per 100 ml (4 fl oz/½ cup) of basc oil). Once you have mixed your oils, store in a cool, dark place and use them immediately, as they are perishable.

2 Gently pour the vegetable oil into your blending bowl.

1 Before you begin, wash and dry your hands and make sure that all your utensils are clean and dry. Have your essential oils at the ready, but leave the lids on the bottles until they are required. Carefully measure out approximately 10 ml (2 tsp) of your chosen vegetable oil.

CAUTION
The essential oil recommendations in this book are extremely safe in the amounts given. If someone has very sensitive skin or lots of allergies then try massaging with just one drop of essential oil per 20 ml (4 tsp) of base oil at first to test for any signs of reaction (rare). If the person is pregnant or may be pregnant, stick to the oils and doses suggested in the chapter on reproduction. If in any doubt, seek medical advice.

3 Add the essential oil, one drop at a time. Mix gently with a clean, dry cocktail stick or toothpick, to blend.

THE NERVOUS SYSTEM

One of the main principles of natural medicine is the holistic approach, taking into account the physical, mental, emotional and indeed spiritual well-being of the person when assessing health; this is most obviously apparent when looking at nervous disorders. Physical symptoms, such as headaches or insomnia, and emotional ones, such as depression, mental strains and stresses, can all weave together to create disease, or simply *dis-ease* – a lack of harmony.

When trying to treat these problems, therefore, it is essential to look at all the reasons for the disorder. One of the first things to do is apply some common sense: is your headache due to an excess of alcohol last night, does your anxiety stem from tomorrow's interview, or your insomnia follow three cups of coffee in the evening? Finding the cause may not solve your immediate problem, but may help you to take preventive steps. In many cases of course, the causes are not so obvious and for persistent or recurring problems professional help should be sought.

Apart from the therapies described in this book, there are many sources of help for nerve-related conditions – since stress is a major factor in much ill-health nowadays, most forms of alternative medicine look at this aspect in their approaches. These might range from counselling and hypnotherapy through to acupuncture and cranial osteopathy. Equally importantly, these should all help to empower *you* to help yourself more effectively, which is the key aim of this book.

ABOVE: Taking time to relax and unwind is important for the overall well-being of our nervous system.

ANXIETY

There are many situations where some level of anxiety is perfectly normal, and a natural response to a stressful situation. It only becomes a problem when the degree of anxiety is out of proportion to the problem, or indeed when there is no objective, external reason for it. Symptoms might include constant feelings of tension, sweating, palpitations, hyper-ventilating and lack of sleep.

ROSE *(Rosa)*

AROMATHERAPY

There are several oils which have a relaxing, calming effect on the nervous system; probably the nicest way to use them is in the bath (see page 17), where the warm water aids relaxation and helps the oils to be absorbed.

CLARY SAGE: a relaxing, warming and almost euphoric effect, especially helpful where anxiety leads to exhaustion.

LAVENDER: calming, helping to balance the mind and emotions, it is one of the gentlest oils to use.

MELISSA: very soothing and, like Lavender, gentle to the skin.

It is useful where anxiety affects the digestion, and also where hormone imbalance creates tension (see Pre-menstrual Problems, page 71).

ROSE: it is wonderfully relaxing and is also considered one of the finest hormone regulators.

YLANG-YLANG: almost sedating, it slows the heart-rate and excessively rapid breathing. Do not overdo it, as large amounts or prolonged usage can result in a headache.

HERBALISM

Herbal remedies are well suited to relieving anxiety, try using one or more of the following herb teas:

CHAMOMILE *(Chamomilla recutita)*: relaxing and good for the digestion; tea bags of it are sold everywhere.

LEMON BALM *(Melissa officinalis)*: this can be safely taken over quite a time for mild anxiety; the fresh herb is much nicer tasting, just gather a few sprigs and take a tea morning and night.

LIME BLOSSOM *(Tilia europaea)*: a very good evening drink, to soothe the mind and calm the digestion and heart-rate.

SKULLCAP *(Scutellaria lateriflora)*: more strongly relaxing, this herb may be easier to find in tablet form.

VALERIAN *(Valeriana officinalis)*: a powerful relaxant, relieving mental and physical tension. Better to take in tablet form, or up to 5 ml (1 tsp) of the tincture, as the tea tastes disgusting!

HOMEOPATHY

As always, long-term problems need professional treatment. In the meantime, a choice of these remedies may help.

ACONITE: for a sudden onset of anxiety or fear, perhaps after a fright, with much restlessness.

ARGENTICUM NITRICUM: for tension giving rise to butterflies in the stomach and indigestion, or a constant craving for sweet things.

ARSENICUM ALBUM: if very restless, fearful, no appetite and very finicky about food.

GELSEMIUM: for nervous apprehension, such as pre-exam nerves or stage fright, with weak trembling knees.

NATUROPATHY

Apart from recommending activities like yoga or meditation to help reduce levels of anxiety in the long term, gentle exercise and warm baths may be helpful to ease tensions and calm down. The addition of a Vitamin B complex supplement in the mornings, and calcium in the evenings will help both to feed the nervous system and restore a more natural rhythm to the energy use through the day – one of the reasons for the popularity of milky drinks as a nightcap is that they are rich in calcium, a natural relaxant.

Lime Blossom tea

DEPRESSION

Just as with anxiety, depression can be due to several reasons, and its symptoms may be quite varied. Conditions like constipation, headaches, insomnia and loss of appetite can all relate to depression and in deep or continuing instances of depression professional help is essential. This is especially so when there is no obvious reason for the feelings, a condition generally labelled endogenous depression.

AROMATHERAPY

Many oils have quite profound effects on mood, and it may be necessary to change the oil used as symptoms vary. The benefits of aromatherapy massage using diluted essential oils (see page 17), with the caring effect of the direct contact, are the most useful way of treating someone with depression, but oils can also be very helpful in the bath (see page 8).

BERGAMOT: this is one of the most uplifting of oils, with a refreshing citrus fragrance which is appealing to both men and women – and gives Earl Grey tea its distinctive aroma.

CLARY SAGE: this is quite relaxing, but with an uplifting, almost euphoric effect as well; good when chronic tension has led to depression or exhaustion.

GERANIUM: this oil actually comes from varieties of scented pelargonium, and has a tonic effect on the adrenal cortex, which helps to regulate stress hormone production.

NEROLI: this oil, from the blossom of the bitter orange, is very concentrated (and also expensive!) so a little can go a long way. It relaxes and soothes, relieving muscle spasm and the irritability which often goes with a depressed state.

HERBALISM

The traditional approach to depression included looking at all the body systems, in particular liver function, and often bitter herbs were prescribed to stimulate digestion and

OATSTRAW (*Avena sativa*)

act as a tonic; a few drops of a tincture (see page 14) of a herb such as Gentian (*Gentiana lutea*) may do the trick in mild cases of depressed spirits. The herbs below can be taken as a tea, or for a stronger effect take as an infusion (see page 12).

BORAGE (*Borago officinalis*): an adrenal stimulant and general tonic, best taken as a tea and for short periods only.

OATSTRAW (*Avena sativa*): an all-round nervous restorative; either use 20 drops of the tincture twice daily, or simply add plenty of oats to the diet, for example, in cereals.

ROSEMARY (*Rosmarinus officinalis*): excellent where nervous exhaustion leads to depression, also good for headaches and sluggish digestion.

VERVAIN (*Verbena officinalis*): a relaxing tonic, very useful for the depression of convalescence from an illness, when everything seems a struggle.

HOMEOPATHY

In the short term, look at these remedies.

AURUM METALLICUM: for deep depression and almost suicidal feelings, perhaps following failure in exams or at work.

IGNATIA: this is especially appropriate for depression following a shock or grief, with pent-up, almost hysterical feelings and a lump in the throat .

KALI PHOS: for nervous exhaustion, leaving a lack of mental or physical energy.

PULSATILLA: generally most useful for mild, gentle people who are prone to weepiness, with a rapid change of mood to feeling miserable – this is often a good remedy for children, but seek medical advice first!

NATUROPATHY

One of the first things to do is overhaul the diet, to make sure there is enough nourishment for the nervous system. Reduce coffee, tea, sugar and alcohol intake. Take plenty of wholefoods, possibly increasing protein intake, if the diet has been poor.

Taking more exercise is a positive move, helping to improve circulation, muscle tone and increase oxygen intake. The main difficulty of course is motivation, so support from an exercise class may be more successful than doing it alone.

Supplement the diet with a good general multi-mineral and vitamin supplement to give a wide spectrum of nutrients.

HEADACHES

Headaches can develop for a number of reasons; usually they can be related to some obvious cause such as nasal congestion or sinusitis, eyestrain, fatigue or tension. The majority of headaches are due to stress or worries, with muscle spasms in the neck leading to head pains. These can be made worse by poor posture, and many jobs create special problems – for instance, computer operators often get eyestrain and stiff, aching shoulders or neck muscles, and consequently headaches.

AROMATHERAPY

Many essential oils have some analgesic properties. A useful way of employing the following for headaches is as a cold compress (see page 15), applied to the temples and forehead – use 5 drops in a small bowl of cold water, wring out a flannel or something similar and place on the area. Alternatively, gently massage a couple of drops directly into the temples.

LAVENDER: relaxing, warming and analgesic, one of the gentlest of oils. Where there is neck tension, apply a hot compress to the neck and upper back at the same time (proportions as above for cold compress).

PEPPERMINT: this is very cooling in its effect, and is also very useful for relieving catarrh and nasal congestion. As it has something of a stimulant action, it could be used in equal amounts with Lavender, as described above, on the temples and forehead.

ROSEMARY: this is even more stimulating to the central nervous system, and is excellent for headaches following

CHAMOMILE
(*Chamomilla
recutita*)

SEVERE HEADACHES

Causes such as very high blood pressure, meningitis or even brain tumours are much rarer; these of course need professional treatment, and severe, unexplained or persistent headaches should be checked out carefully, but most headaches can be identified and cured at home. Where there has been any kind of accident, for instance a whiplash injury, it makes good sense to consult a manipulative therapist such as a chiropractor or an osteopath.

---

mental strain and exhaustion, as well as helping to clear the sinuses.

HERBALISM

At the earliest signs of a headache taking a herbal tea from the choice below can stop it in its tracks; if the headache is more pronounced, or is a repeated problem, try making an infusion (see page 12) for a stronger effect, or else get medical advice.

CHAMOMILE (*Chamomilla recutita*): good for bilious headaches, stemming from over-eating or indigestion, where there is a dull, throbbing pain on top of the head.

LIME BLOSSOM (*Tilia europaea*): soothes the nerves and is very helpful for tension headaches; can be mixed with Peppermint for a more uplifting effect.

PEPPERMINT
(*Mentha piperita*)

PEPPERMINT
(*Mentha piperita*): this works well for digestive or sinus headaches, especially where the head feels hot.

ROSEMARY (*Rosmarinus officinalis*): for headaches related to exhaustion or depression, and also for bilious heavy heads. When the headache is due to a hangover, Rosemary and Peppermint tea can do wonders – but prevention is still better than a cure!

HOMEOPATHY

The choice is large, in part due to the many factors which go to produce the individual symptoms.

For tension headaches, gently massage the temples with small circling movements.

BELLADONNA: for a burning, violent headache with a hot head; the symptoms are worse with any jarring movement of the head, or loud noises.

BRYONIA: for a severe, splitting headache, only relieved by lying very still or with firm, cool pressure across the forehead.

NUX VOMICA: for a sharp headache, either on waking or after food, with nausea or bilious feelings from over-eating; better if taken when lying down, and keeping warm.

PULSATILLA: good for headaches associated with menstruation, also where brought on by too much rich food; relief seems to come from cool applications to the head and being out in the fresh air.

Eating a varied diet of fresh vegetables and wholefoods can ward off many ailments.

NATUROPATHY

In general, the naturopathic approach is to look at prevention, by changing lifestyle to reduce the reasons for headaches. Eating a varied wholefood diet, reducing alcohol, coffee and tea, and getting more exercise and fresh air are all likely to help lower the frequency of headaches for regular sufferers. Drink plenty of fluids, as dehydration can be a factor, especially for people working in hot, stuffy atmospheres and, of course, in hangovers. Avoid dramatic changes in diet, such as crash dieting, which upsets blood sugar levels and can contribute to headaches. Sometimes a Vitamin B complex supplement can be useful in relieving mental exhaustion. For hot, congested headaches use cold compresses to the forehead, perhaps combined with a hot footbath to improve circulation.

BENEFITS OF SELF-HELP

Prevention is better than cure so try to adopt some of the measures outlined in this book to maintain good health rather than just waiting to be ill. If you suffer from several complaints, read all the relevant sections for an overall picture of what you can do to improve your general health and be aware of early signs of trouble.

INSOMNIA

It is important to distinguish between habitual sleeplessness, repeated night after night, and a temporary problem due perhaps to some worry or anxiety. It is also important not to become obsessed with trying to get a certain amount of sleep; not everyone needs an 8-hour quota – quality is more vital than quantity. People generally need less sleep as they get older, or at least less continuously, so if granny has a day-time snooze and sleeps for less time at night, that is perfectly normal.

AROMATHERAPY

Essential oils are a very pleasant and effective means of unwinding and aiding restful sleep – try using them in the bath (see page 8) – or else putting 2-3 drops on to a paper tissue under the pillow at night. Choose from the following, either using a single oil or a blend; do not use the same oil for more than 2 weeks or you will find it becomes less effective.

CHAMOMILE: calming and relaxing in its effects, it is good where indigestion contributes to broken sleep.

CLARY SAGE: this has a sedating and almost euphoric action, *but* do not use if you have had alcohol as you can quickly get drunk, and have nightmares or a hangover feeling later on.

LAVENDER: not only very soothing, but also analgesic, so if any aches or pains contribute to insomnia, this oil is probably the best remedy.

MARJORAM: relaxing and warming, in large amounts it is quite sedating but can leave you feeling a bit thick-headed the next morning, so do not overdo it.

HERBALISM

An infusion (see page 12) of one or more of these relaxing herbs can help a return to a natural sleep pattern if stress has disturbed it. Other ways of using herbs include herb-filled pillows; traditionally hops were used as they are sedating (but not very pleasant-smelling!). Fill a small muslin bag loosely with the appropriate herb and place under your normal pillow.

Another old favourite remedy was cowslip wine; this not only tastes better than the infusion but is certainly very relaxing.

CHAMOMILE: (*Chamomilla recutita*): calms the stomach and the brain, settling the digestion and helping sleep.

HYSSOP (*Hyssopus officinalis*): a gentle relaxant; also helps to ease nasal congestion and colds, which can cause insomnia.

LEMON BALM (*Melissa officinalis*): this helps to restore balance to the nervous system, and can be used safely on children. The fresh herb tastes much nicer, and can be drunk as a tea anytime.

LIME BLOSSOM (*Tilia europaea*): mildly analgesic as well as calming; can soothe headache or other pains.

PASSIONFLOWER (*Passiflora incarnata*): a strong relaxant or sedative, but without any ill-effects. Many commercial herbal tablets for insomnia contain this herb.

HOMEOPATHY

In the short term, look at these remedies:

ACONITE: for restlessness associated with sudden upset or fear, and resulting in tossing and turning in bed.

COFFEA: if the mind is completely awake and the brain will not turn off – just as if you had drunk strong coffee.

Probably the most versatile and useful essential oil is Lavender, distilled from the flowers.

NUX VOMICA: for insomnia due to overwork or excess food or alcohol, waking around 3 or 4 a.m. for several hours, with disturbed dreams.

SULPHUR: for over-excitement, with the mind full of ideas, and easily awakened by the slightest noise.

NATUROPATHY

In order to get the proper rhythm of energy through the day, it is useful to get plenty of exercise and get fresh air in the daytime. It may help to get up fairly early in the morning as well, to restore this balance. Do not sleep in a stuffy room, or drink coffee, tea or cola at night.

At bedtime, a calcium/magnesium supplement such as dolomite tablets can help to relax, especially if taken with a warm herb tea, or perhaps a hot milky drink if you do not suffer from a lot of catarrh.

MIGRAINE

Anyone who has experienced a migraine will know that it is more than a severe headache. Migraines generally involve acute pains, often over one eye, and perhaps disturbed vision or flashing lights. There may also be nausea or vomiting, and sensitivity to bright light.

AROMATHERAPY

Since the sense of smell is altered and often heightened during a migraine, aromatherapy is definitely best used between attacks; use at the earliest stage of a migraine only if the smell is well tolerated.

A central feature of the natural approach to migraines is to distinguish between a "hot" migraine, where the blood vessels are dilated, and a "cold" migraine, where there is excessive constriction of the blood vessels. In the first type, a cold or perhaps just cool compress (see page 15) across the forehead will give relief and oils of Peppermint or Lavender can be used. For "cold" types of migraine, a hot compress on the forehead or back of the neck may help, using Marjoram.

HERBALISM

Catching the migraine early gives the best chance of success (otherwise try to use these infusions regularly, as a preventive). Choose from the following:
CHAMOMILE (*Chamomilla recutita*): for dull, throbbing headache with a feeling of queasiness – add a little Ginger (*Zingiber officinalis*) to relieve more severe nausea.
FEVERFEW (*Chrysanthemum parthenium*): an excellent remedy taken daily to prevent the "cold" type of migraine, where there is a sense of a tight band around the head. This is widely available in tablet form as well.
ROSEMARY (*Rosmarinus officinalis*): good where stress is a trigger for migraines, and where local warmth gives relief.

CAUSES OF MIGRAINE

A migraine can be triggered by all sorts of factors: hormone changes, stress, stuffy atmospheres, noises, smells and certain foods are well-known triggers. Repeated attacks call for professional help; self-help treatments should be largely used as preventive measures.

HOMEOPATHY

During an attack try one of these:
KALI BICH: for an intense headache, preceded by a loss of vision and nausea, made worse in hot weather.
NATRUM MURIATICUM: for a severe, pounding headache with zigzags in front of the eyes, nausea and a pale face. The migraine may also be triggered by menstruation.
SILICA: for pains spreading from the back of the neck over to the eyes, usually right-sided, and often vomiting.

NATUROPATHY

Diet needs to be looked at carefully; try to avoid tea, coffee, alcohol especially red wine, red meat, cheese, chocolate, tomatoes and eggs. Eat plenty of fresh, raw salads and drink lots of fluid, as dehydration can be a factor. Try taking a Vitamin B supplement daily and see if this helps to reduce attacks. In between attacks, exercises to relieve tension in the neck and shoulders can be useful, and also massage of these areas (see left).

NECK MASSAGE FOR MIGRAINE

1 For stiff, aching neck muscles massage the neck with firm circular movements. Try to keep the arms relaxed.

2 Ideally get someone else to massage the neck for you. They can also support your head while they massage.

NEURALGIA

Neuralgia is a sharp pain originating along the course of one or more nerves, and may come about from a variety of causes; both sciatica and shingles (see pages 26 and 27) give rise to forms of neuralgic pain. Facial neuralgia, affecting one of the trigeminal nerves in the face, can give intense pain, and may relate to stress, migraines or dental problems.

AROMATHERAPY

Using warm compresses (see page 15), including analgesic oils, over the affected areas can give much relief. Choose from Chamomile, Lavender, Marjoram or Rosemary oils – alternate the oil used for recurrent pains, or blend them together for greater effect.

HERBALISM

An infusion (see page 12) of Lavender (*Lavandula vera*) flowers, Lime Blossom (*Tilia europaea*) and Rosemary (*Rosmarinus officinalis*) leaves can be very helpful, not only to ease the pains but to ease tension and tone the nervous system. This mixture can also be used as a warm compress directly over the area.

Two other helpful herbs as infusions are:
ST JOHN'S WORT (*Hypericum perforatum*): anti-inflammatory and a nervous restorative. The blood-red oil made by infusing the flowers in pure vegetable oil

VERVAIN
(*Verbena officinalis*)

(see page 13) is an excellent local analgesic and healer.
VERVAIN (*Verbena officinalis*): a relaxant and nervous tonic, very helpful when neuralgia is related to being generally run-down and exhausted.

HOMEOPATHY

In the short term, try the following:
ACTAEA RAC: for facial neuralgia with pains into the cheekbone and as if piercing the eyeball. Pains ease at night.
BELLADONNA: for a hot, burning and flushed face, with mostly right-sided neuralgic pains and twitching muscles.

ROSEMARY (*Rosmarinus officinalis*)

GELSEMIUM: for pains radiating from the neck into the face, possibly with some nausea; migraine-related neuralgia.

NATUROPATHY

Simply using alternating hot and cold compresses, 3-4 minutes hot and a maximum 1 minute cold, repeated a few times, can ease the pains. For chronic sufferers a Vitamin B complex supplement can help to nourish the nervous system. In addition, look at ways of reducing stress such as relaxation or yoga classes.

SCIATICA

Pains along some point of the sciatic nerves, running from the low back down either leg to the foot, are a common form of neuralgia (see page 25). The pains may come about from an injury, and treatment from an osteopath or chiropractor should always be considered as one of the best ways to correct the cause. Poor posture, badly designed chairs or even a full back pocket can all cause pressure and pain in the sciatic nerve.

AROMATHERAPY

Initially, use cold compresses (see page 15) with either Chamomile or Lavender oils included. When the pains are less acute, or in longer-lasting sciatic discomfort, try warm compresses as suggested for Neuralgia (see page 25).

These oils are very helpful, diluted 2 per cent in a base oil and slowly massaged into the affected area.

HERBALISM

Chamomile (*Chamomilla recutita*) or Lavender (*Lavandula vera*) are also two useful herbs to take in infusion (see page 12) to ease muscle spasm and inflammation which add to the pains. For acute muscle spasms in the thigh or legs, try making a strong decoction (see page 12) of Cramp Bark (European Cranberry Bush) (*Viburnum opulus*) and using as a warm compress. A small cupful of this may be taken internally as a powerful relaxant.

CRAMP BARK (EUROPEAN CRANBERRY BUSH)
(*Viburnum opulus*)

IMPROVING YOUR POSTURE

Apart from the suggestions listed on this page, you may want to consider help with improving your posture, learning how to move and hold yourself comfortably. The Alexander Technique and the Feldenkrais Technique are two systems that can help here; there are many qualified teachers of both available. Massage is not generally suitable in an acute phase, but in the longer term it is very helpful (see below for self-massage, or find a good massage therapist for best results).

HOMEOPATHY

ARSEN ALB: for intermittent pains shooting from the thigh down to the knee or even ankle.
IGNATIA: for sharp pains in the lower back and upper thighs, eased by walking around.
RHUS TOX: for severe pains in the hip, radiating down to the knee and causing limping. Generally these pains are worse in damp weather.

NATUROPATHY

Hot and cold compresses, as described for Neuralgia (see page 25), may give relief. Gentle exercise is generally useful, but stop if it becomes too painful. Take a serious look at your posture, how you bend, pick things up and so on. It is important to try to keep your back fairly upright, using your legs

LAVENDER
(*Lavandula 'Nana'*)

to bend or to take the weight.

Look carefully at all the chairs you use. Sit well back on a chair, and use cushions if necessary to get you into a more comfortable position. In general, avoid staying in one position for too long, as the muscles begin to tighten and stiffen. For example, try to have regular breaks on a long car journey, or walk about for a while on the train.

To help ease sciatic pain, massage diluted essential oils, as recommended, into the buttock and upper thigh with slow circular movements.

SHINGLES

This condition is brought about by the same virus, *Herpes zoster*, that causes chickenpox; it can lie dormant in the body for years before triggering an attack, often when you are stressed and exhausted. There is usually some pain in the affected area for a day or so before the very painful blisters appear along the pathway of the affected nerves. Sometimes there is considerable pain around the site for weeks, months or even years after the blisters have gone, and this can be treated in the same way as Neuralgia (see page 25).

AROMATHERAPY

A number of essential oils can act locally very powerfully to reduce the pains, dry up the blisters and as direct anti-viral agents. It may be best to use a combination of two or three of these oils; for small areas of blisters paint the oils on neat, once or twice daily, otherwise use them in the bath or diluted in water as a warm compress (see page 15).

Initially, choose from Bergamot, Eucalyptus or Tea Tree oils; if pains persist, use Lavender for its healing and analgesic properties – good combinations are Bergamot and Tea Tree, Bergamot and Lavender, but all the above are useful.

HERBALISM

Lavender oil (*Lavandula vera*), as described above, is excellent for local use; this can be backed up by taking Lavender flowers as an infusion (see page 12) for their relaxing effect. If there are long-standing pains, after the acute attack has gone (known as post-herpetic syndrome), then a general nerve tonic like Oatstraw (*Avena sativa*) is very helpful – either take 20 drops of the tincture (see page 14) twice daily, or simply include plenty of oats in the diet, for instance as porridge. If depression has set in, an infusion of Rosemary (*Rosmarinus officinalis*) works wonders; drink a cupful in the morning. At the other end of the day, a cup of Lime Blossom (*Tilia europaea*) tea in the evening can help restful sleep.

HOMEOPATHY

Some possibilities are:

APIS MEL: where there is a large amount of blistering, with swelling and a burning sensation. Symptoms are eased by cold applications.

ARSEN ALB: for reddened skin, with the blisters merging together and possibly discharging. Symptoms eased by warm applications.

RHUS TOX: for highly inflamed skin, with small white blisters that are intensely painful and itchy; difficult to keep still due to the irritation and discomfort.

NATUROPATHY

In preventive terms, it is advisable to try to steer clear of someone with chickenpox, especially if you are

LAVENDER (*Lavandula vera*)

feeling very run-down yourself. Since in real life you may be the one looking after your child with chickenpox, this is not so easy! Spraying the sick room with essential oils (see Aromatherapy above for choice), using 10-15 drops in a 600 ml (1 pt/2½ cups) plant spray filled with water, can help too.

If you feel the first signs of irritation, try rubbing the area with a freshly cut lemon. During an attack of shingles a salt bath may give relief and promote healing and drying of the blisters. Take a Vitamin B complex supplement to nourish the nervous system, and look generally at reducing stress and maintaining a healthy lifestyle.

STRESS

Stress is one of those rather vague terms that is very difficult to define. It is also important to say that stress is not in itself harmful, and a certain amount can be necessary to get us motivated and enjoying life; only when the amount of stress is too much for our systems to cope with does it become a problem. People have a marvellous capacity to adapt to and cope with various sources of stress, but when they get overloaded and nervous or adrenal exhaustion sets in, they can become seriously ill.

AROMATHERAPY

Many oils are of value in helping to reduce the impact of stress. The best way of using them is probably diluted in a vegetable oil and used in massage (see page 17), but if you do not have a willing, and trained, partner then use them in the bath (see page 8).

For more uplifting effects choose from Bergamot, Clary Sage, Geranium or Rosemary, while Lavender or Marjoram are more relaxing. Three luxurious, although expensive, oils which have excellent de-stressing properties (and smell wonderful!) are Jasmine, Neroli (or Orange Blossom) and Rose – use sparingly as they are very concentrated. Jasmine is relaxing and almost euphoric, Neroli is an anti-depressant and is refreshing, and Rose is calming and relaxing.

HERBALISM

For the more agitated aspects of being stressed, choose relaxing infusions such as Lavender (*Lavandula*

GERANIUM
(*Pelargonium graveolens*)

SYMPTOMS OF STRESS

Symptoms of stress vary, see also Anxiety and Depression (pages 19 and 20), but if you experience some or all of the following, you may be over-stressed:

❧ Constantly on edge, with a very short fuse and ready to explode for no real reason.
❧ Feeling on the verge of tears much of the time.
❧ Difficulty in concentrating, decision-making or with memory.
❧ Always tired even after a full night's sleep.
❧ Sleep itself is disturbed and unrefreshing.
❧ A feeling of not being able to cope, it's all too much.
❧ Poor appetite, or else nibbling without hunger.
❧ No sense of fun or enjoyment in life.
❧ Mistrustful of everybody, unable to enjoy company.

❧ Inability to relax or unwind even if not working.
❧ Problems in relationships, no interest in sex.
❧ Always fidgeting or having a nervous habit such as biting your nails or chewing your hair.

The first step to improving the situation is to recognize that you are stressed, and to know what your limits are. Taking active steps to reduce the amount of external stress will of course be helpful, as well as looking at the methods below for easing the effects of the stress on your system. Other steps might include trying a class in relaxation techniques, or yoga, T'ai Ch'i and so on, or having professional massage treatments. Getting regular breaks from a stressful lifestyle will help you to cope better and avoid the situation reaching a crisis point.

vera), Lime Blossom (*Tilia europaea*) or Lemon Balm (*Melissa officinalis*), or for acute tensions try Valerian (*Valeriana officinalis*) – since this tastes disgusting, it may be better to buy it in tablet form. When exhaustion has set in, infusions of Rosemary (*Rosmarinus officinalis*), Vervain (*Verbena officinalis*) or Betony (*Stachys betonica*), or a mixture of all three, will act as a tonic. Oats are

helpful to add to the diet, as a nourishment for the nervous system.

HOMEOPATHY

ACONITE: for acute anxiety and mental confusion, with thoughts whizzing round in the head and much restlessness.
CHAMOMILLA: if everything and everybody seems to irritate, and it is

MASSAGE FOR STIFF NECKS

1 Place hands on each shoulder, thumbs on either side of the spine.

2 Rotate thumbs firmly, lifting and squeezing the shoulder muscles. Relax hands and repeat.

BACK MASSAGE TO EASE STRESS

1 To relieve stress and tension, use effleurage, or stroking, on the back. Oil the back and then place hands on lower back with thumbs on either side of the spine.

2 Steadily stroke up the back, allow thumbs to move out at the shoulders to join the fingers, and stroke down the side of the back. Bring thumbs to either side of the spine and repeat several times in a slow, relaxing rhythm. Keep the pressure firm, but not too hard.

NECK AND SHOULDER EXERCISES

1 Lift shoulders, pressing into the neck Relax and then repeat a few times.

2 Roll the shoulders in a circle. Repeat a few times in a backwards circle, then a few times forwards.

---

very easy to get into a temper.

IGNATIA: for mood swings, liable to tears and lots of sighing; may bottle things up and get upset suddenly.

KALI PHOS: for prolonged strain, getting fatigued and rather depressed, very jumpy at the least thing. Tends to withdraw from company, doesn't want to go out very much, generally lacks interest in life.

NATUROPATHY

A good plan is to look at basics; overhaul the diet, cutting out all the stimulants such as coffee, tea or cola drinks which only serve to leave you more exhausted when their effects wear off. Also reduce alcohol; it may help you to relax in small amounts but it easily becomes a dangerous habit and has a depressant action in any quantity.

Try to get some exercise; this not only helps to use up excess adrenalin but builds up physical *and* mental stamina. Deeper breathing will also supply more oxygen to the brain, which is the first essential nourishment it needs. It may be useful to add a multi-vitamin and mineral supplement to the diet for a while, as the body uses up nutrients faster when under stress.

THE RESPIRATORY SYSTEM

In order to prevent respiratory problems, or to help clear them up more quickly, it is essential to take a wider, holistic view of health. If you live in a relatively mild, damp climate, this will make you more prone to respiratory infections and catarrh; coupled with this, the increase in air pollution this century has added significantly to the burden. However, some internal factors, such as diet, exercise and general health, are also important in affecting our resistance to infections, and the more we pay attention to these internal factors, the healthier we will be.

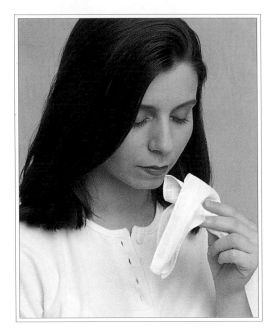

Breathing is one of those bodily functions that normally carry on automatically, but can also be controlled consciously. This is a good illustration of the effect of stress and anxiety on our body, as shallow or over-rapid breathing, nervous coughs and even bronchial spasms can be produced when in an agitated state. Poor posture, lack of exercise or just lack of fresh air, smoking or smoky atmospheres all contribute to an inadequate intake of oxygen and respiratory problems.

ABOVE: The influence of essential oils on our respiratory system can have dramatic effects. Very many essential oils are also extremely pleasing to smell and can help to keep the sinuses clear, for example Lavender (above left), Peppermint and Eucalyptus.

ASTHMA

Asthma is not generally a problem that should simply be tackled at home; it requires professional treatment and attention. Childhood asthma tends to be associated with an allergic response; there may also be hay fever and/or eczema present in the family. In trying to identify the allergens responsible it is often valuable to look further at external factors and also internal ones such as diet, as well as conventional skin testing.

AROMATHERAPY

During an actual attack of asthma, simply sniffing the aroma of a couple of drops of essential oil on a paper tissue may give relief from the spasm of the airways – choose from Lavender, Bergamot, Frankincense or Chamomile. In between attacks, massaging a choice of the above oils, diluted (see page 17), into the chest may help to prevent the spasms and build-up of thick mucus which gives the wheezing symptoms.

Essential oils, diluted in a base oil as recommended, can be massaged into the chest to relax the airways and ease breathing.

HERBALISM

Professional practitioners may use remedies which directly reduce the allergic response, or dilate the bronchial passageways, depending

CHAMOMILE
(Chamomilla recutita)

EYEBRIGHT *(Euphrasia officinalis)*

on specific individual needs. In between asthma attacks, taking an infusion (see page 12) of a mixture of Chamomile *(Chamomilla recutita)*, Eyebright *(Euphrasia officinalis)* and Lavender *(Lavandula vera)* may help to relax the airways, tone up the mucous membranes and reduce inflammation and irritability of the bronchi.

HOMEOPATHY

The professional will similarly look to treat each person individually, so only consider the remedies below in the short term:

ACONITE: at the earliest sign of breathing problems, especially if brought on by a cold, or simply cold weather with strong winds, and where there is much anxiety or fear.

ARSENICUM: when symptoms are worse after midnight, with restlessness and a feeling of exhaustion.

IPECACUANHA: where there is wheezing, with a persistent, rattly cough accompanied by a strong feeling of nausea.

NATUROPATHY

For childhood asthma, or where there is a lot of thick mucus, it is well worth trying a change of diet, to exclude cows' milk products for a while, to decrease sugary baking products and sweets (candy), and to increase fresh vegetables and fruit.

Breathing exercises may be of help, especially for later-onset asthma or when exercise seems to aggravate the condition; a simple method of deepening the breathing pattern is to

A useful breathing exercise for asthma is simply to blow up a couple of balloons a day, to deepen the breath and exercise the diaphragm.

BREATHING EXERCISES

1 Place hands just below the breastbone and take a slow, deep breath. As you breathe in, push out the stomach; this should make the hands move apart a little, as the diaphragm moves.

2 As you breathe out, pull the stomach in. The diaphragm moves back up and the hands come together again. Repeat just 3 or 4 times and then breathe normally.

blow up balloons – for a maximum effect blow them up until they burst! Regular back massage will help release muscle tensions and improve circulation. Using hot and cold compresses (see page 15) on the upper back and/or chest will also stimulate circulation through the lungs and help remove mucus.

FRENCH LAVENDER
(*Lavandula stoechas*)

To stimulate circulation into the back and chest, and loosen phlegm in the lungs, place hands in a cupped shape on the upper back and briskly move them alternately up and down. This should make a hollow sound on the back – slapping is not helpful, or enjoyable! (Be prepared for some coughing if the chest is congested.)

BRONCHITIS

Acute bronchitis, which typically follows an upper respiratory infection such as a heavy cold or influenza, produces a painful dry cough as the infected bronchi become inflamed. This leads to lots of mucus being produced and the cough becoming looser. The condition can recur, and chronic bronchitis is known as the "English disease" due to its frequent occurrence in England.

AROMATHERAPY

Essential oils, used primarily in steam inhalations (see below), are an excellent way to treat bronchitis. In the acute stage using powerfully antiseptic oils such as Lavender, Eucalyptus, Thyme or Tea Tree will be very useful. This can be backed up by gently rubbing a little diluted Lavender oil on to the chest – use 5 drops in 5ml (1 tsp) of olive oil or similar vegetable oil.

For more chronic symptoms choose from one of the following oils which are derived from gums or resins, or simply combine all three in an inhalation.
BENZOIN: is most famous as the ingredient in Friar's Balsam; it has a warming and relaxing effect on the bronchi, and aids expectoration of the thick mucus.

To make an inhalation, choose a bowl large enough to take at least 600 ml (1 pt/2½ cups) of water. Fill it with boiling water and add 2-3 drops of essential oil. As the oils vaporize, inhale the steam as deeply as possible. If you hold a towel over your head this will delay the effects of evaporation. Be careful to place the bowl in a safe position.

SELF-HELP MEASURES
There may not be any infection present in the chronic state; repeated irritation of the lungs produces excess mucus which clogs up the bronchi. Self-help measures include not smoking or being in smoky atmospheres, treating colds and so on promptly, not going out in foggy weather, and using steam inhalations to warm and moisten the airways.

FRANKINCENSE: another expectorant, which slows and deepens the breathing as well as being a good antiseptic agent.
MYRRH: strongly anti-infective, helping to loosen the sticky mucus and shift it off the chest.

HERBALISM

There is a whole treasure chest of herbal medicines for different stages or states of bronchitis; if in doubt do seek professional advice. At the beginning, where there may be a feeling of chill, a tea from fresh Ginger (*Zingiber officinalis*) with perhaps a pinch of Cayenne pepper added will give warmth very quickly. Painful, harsh coughs can be soothed with infusions of Marshmallow leaf (*Althea officinalis*), Hyssop (*Hyssopus officinalis*) and Thyme (*Thymus vulgaris*), or else use White Horehound (*Marrubium vulgare*), an anti-spasmodic and expectorant remedy. A regular intake of garlic, ideally fresh, not only helps to stimulate the removal of excess mucus in chronic bronchitis, but is one of the most powerful anti-infective agents there is, helping to build resistance to all respiratory infections.

HOMEOPATHY

In the acute phase, look at these remedies, but seek qualified treatment if symptoms persist or chest pains set in.
ACONITE: for use in the early stages, with painful, dry cough and much restlessness, with a slight fever.
BRYONIA: for a dry, hacking cough which is made worse by changes in temperature, such as coming into a warm room.
IPECACUANHA: for a spasmodic cough with much rattly mucus on the chest, and a tendency towards vomiting.
PHOSPHORUS: for a hoarse voice, even going altogether, and a dry tickly cough, with a tight feeling like a band around the chest.

NATUROPATHY

Reduce mucus-forming foods: these are primarily dairy products, and also refined carbohydrates such as cakes and pastries. If the weather is damp or foggy, stay indoors, but also avoid rooms being too dry and hot. In chronic cases walking or other exercise in good weather will improve breathing. Hot and cold compresses (see page 15) will really stimulate circulation through the lungs and help breathing.

CATARRH

Irritation of the membranes of the nose and throat will encourage production of mucus; where this becomes excessive or prolonged, for example after a cold, then catarrh is the result. When this occurs lower down the airways, bronchial catarrh follows (see Bronchitis, page 33). Nasal catarrh is even more common in damp climates and the same advice is applicable.

AROMATHERAPY

Where there is a lot of nasal congestion, a steam inhalation with essential oils (see page 33) can be instantly effective in giving relief. In the short term Peppermint is excellent, especially combined with Eucalyptus and/or Tea Tree, to loosen thick, sticky mucus and fight any infection present. For longer term catarrhal problems, try using oil of Pine instead of Peppermint, perhaps with Chamomile, Lavender or Tea Tree.

HERBALISM

Apart from using steam inhalations for temporary relief, either with oils as described above or using a handful each of Peppermint (*Mentha piperita*) leaves, Eucalyptus (*Eucalyptus globulus*) leaves and Chamomile (*Chamomilla*

recutita) flowers to 1 litre (1¾ pt/4 cups) of boiling water, catarrh can often be very successfully treated with infusions (see page 12) of the following:
CATMINT (*Nepeta cataria*): helps to ease nasal congestion and improve the circulation through the nasal passages.
ELDERFLOWER (*Sambucus nigra*): has an anti-inflammatory effect, reducing swelling of the membranes and easing mucus production.
GOLDEN ROD (*Solidago virgaurea*): astringent, toning up the membranes and also reducing excess mucus.
HYSSOP (*Hyssopus officinalis*): loosens up thick phlegm, while calming the breathing; good if there is restlessness and problems with sleeping due to difficulty in breathing.

HOMEOPATHY

Initially think of one of these remedies:
ARSEN ALB: for running, watery catarrh, with a dripping nose.
HYDRASTIS: for a constant post-nasal drip, perhaps associated with blocked Eustachian tubes (connecting to the middle ear), creating a little deafness.
KALI BICH: where there is thick, stringy mucus, which is difficult to shift.
PULSATILLA: in chronic cases, where the catarrh varies at times from clear to a greenish-yellow colour.

Place 25 g (1 oz) dried Chamomile (Chamomilla recutita) *leaves in a teapot and pour on boiling water. Allow to infuse for 5 minutes. Strain and drink a cupful.*

GOLDEN ROD (*Solidago virgaurea*)

NATUROPATHY

Avoid all mucus-forming foods, especially milk and other dairy products, and refined carbohydrates – most breakfasts of cereal and milk fall into this category, as do pastries, cakes and so on. Drinking warm fruit juices can often be helpful. If the catarrh tends to follow on from regular colds, a daily supplement of Vitamin C, up to 500 mg in strength, may need to be taken for a while.

Regular intake of garlic is invaluable in building up resistance to respiratory infections – ideally raw – and since the smell may stop other people coming near you, so colds are harder to catch! Actually, the smelly oil is the most anti-infective part of garlic, and 99 per cent of it is excreted out via the lungs so it works very strongly on the respiratory system. Odourless garlic perles, or capsules, will also work, although not as powerfully as the raw ingredient.

COLDS

Since there are over 200 strains of cold virus, it is not surprising that a cure has not been found. Prevention is better than treatment by far; once a cold has developed, it generally has to run its course. However, treatments can help to relieve symptoms and also stop the cold turning into persistent catarrh or a deeper infection.

AROMATHERAPY

Two methods are most appropriate for using oils to combat cold symptoms and stop complications: steam inhalations (see page 33) and baths. If, in the early stages, the cold is accompanied by a chill, adding 10 drops of Lavender and 5 drops of Cinnamon oil to a warm bath at night will help a lot. More stimulating oils such as Eucalyptus or Tea Tree (10 drops of each) can be used in baths earlier in the day. All the above are valuable in inhalations; a mixture often works better than just one oil.

GINGER (*Zingiber officinalis*)

HERBALISM

One of the herbalists' most traditional standbys for colds is still one of the best: use an infusion (see page 12) of equal amounts of Peppermint (*Mentha piperita*), Elderflower (*Sambucus nigra*) and Yarrow (*Achillea millefolium*). Taken hot just before going to bed, this will induce a sweat, and if the cold is caught early enough, may stop it altogether. Even if too late for this, it will still be

very useful. Other herbs that may be added to the infusion include:
CAYENNE (*Capsicum minimum*): a favourite North American Indian remedy: use 1.25 ml (¼ tsp) of the powder to really stimulate the circulation.
CINNAMON (*Cinnamomum zeylanicum*): use a cinnamon stick, and break it into the mixture of herbs, for a gentle, warming and sweat-inducing effect.
GINGER (*Zingiber officinalis*): grate a small piece of fresh root ginger into the mixture for extra heat.

HOMEOPATHY

ACONITE: for early stages of colds, when starting suddenly, perhaps after exposure to cold winds.
GELSEMIUM: for influenza-like symptoms, feeling chilly and trembling but with a flushed face.
NAT MUR: when there is a lot of sneezing, the nose is sore and inflamed and producing lots of mucus, either watery or like raw egg-white.

Fresh fruit is a natural source of Vitamin C.

CINNAMON (*Cinnamomum zeylanicum*)

NATUROPATHY

Immediately increase Vitamin C intake; at the earliest stages very high doses of a Vitamin C supplement, up to 2,000 mg, may stop the infection alone, but if left too late, this is not needed and may make the bowels too loose. 500 mg is an ample dose to take regularly until the remaining symptoms clear up. Another useful supplement is sucking zinc lozenges, with up to 20 mg zinc gluconate in them, every 3-4 hours initially (taking *tablets* does not have the same effect).

Eat lots of fresh fruit for natural Vitamin A, B and C, and add plenty of raw garlic to food. Cut out sugary, starchy or milky foods. A short cleansing diet of just fresh fruit and salads, and plenty of liquids such as warm fruit juices or herb teas, will encourage the body to throw off the cold more effectively.

COUGHS

A cough is a natural reflex reaction to any irritation, inflammation or blockage in the airways. It often accompanies an infection such as a cold or bronchitis, but may come about through nervousness, with no direct irritation at all. By keeping the bronchial tubes open and clear, coughing can be of vital importance, and treatment should generally be aimed first at making the cough more effective rather than just suppressing it.

AROMATHERAPY

A useful way to help a cough do its job more effectively is by using oils in a steam inhalation (see page 33); oils can be chosen to soothe the lining of the air passages, fight infection if needed, and loosen mucus to make it easier to be removed.

Soothing oils include Benzoin and Lavender. Many essential oils are antiseptic, especially Thyme and Eucalyptus; to increase expectoration choose Frankincense or Marjoram. In fact all the above oils are helpful for tackling coughs. Choose a blend that you like the smell of – and remember that if the cough does not improve within a few days, seek professional help, especially for children.

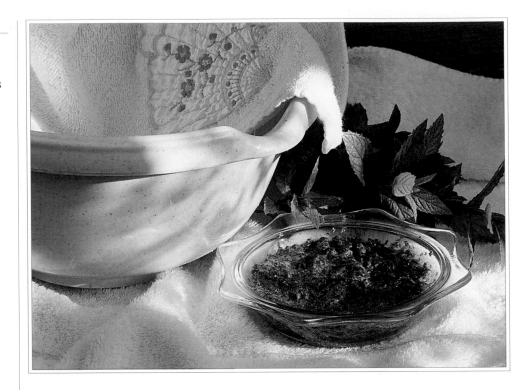

THYME (*Thymus vulgaris*)

HERBALISM

This is an area where herbs are of special benefit; if in doubt get qualified treatment. Choose from one or a mixture of the following, taken as warm infusions (see page 12).

COLTSFOOT (*Tussilago farfara*): one of the best cough remedies, particularly for irritating, spasmodic coughs. It will soothe, loosen mucus and reduce the spasm.

HYSSOP (*Hyssopus officinalis*): a calming and relaxing expectorant, when the cough is

Fresh or dried herbs can be used to make a steam inhalation, to loosen congested mucus and open the airways.

associated with restlessness and irritation.

MARSHMALLOW (*Althea officinalis*): a demulcent remedy, which means it is highly soothing to the inflamed tubes. For a harsh, dry and painful cough always include Marshmallow in a mixture, to ease the soreness.

THYME (*Thymus vulgaris*): powerfully antiseptic, this relieves a dry cough linked with a respiratory infection.

WHITE HOREHOUND (*Marrubium vulgare*): an expectorant, freeing up thick, sticky mucus and helping it to be removed more effectively.

TYPES OF COUGH

It can be useful to divide coughs into two types; when the membranes are hot and dry the cough is painful and non-productive. As mucus is produced, the cough becomes moist, looser and can feel almost choking. The first kind needs soothing, while the latter requires help in removing the excess mucus. Choose the appropriate treatments in each case.

HOMEOPATHY

For short-term treatment of a cough, try a few doses (see page 10) of one of these remedies:

ACONITE: for a dry, short cough which may occur first thing in the morning, or come on after exposure to cold, dry winds.

BRYONIA: for a really spasmodic, dry cough which shakes the whole body and is worse with movement or after eating.

IPECACUANHA: for a moist cough, with some wheezing and a feeling of choking, and often much nausea.

PHOSPHORUS: for a dry, irritating and tickly cough, made worse by changes in temperature.

NATUROPATHY

Initially coughs are often quite dry and painful; taking a little honey from a spoon will help to soothe this. To make the honey much more powerful, try mashing a little chopped raw onion or garlic into it first; it is anti-social but very effective! Cut out all dairy products from the diet, to reduce the catarrh.

Either steam inhalations or a hot compress (see page 15) will encourage expectoration and stimulate the lungs to work better.

Once a cough has been eased, try not to slip back into eating patterns which include a lot of sugar, dairy products, cakes or pastries, as this can lower resistance to infection and help the cough to linger on or even to return in full force.

Fields of commercially-grown lavender.

GARLIC *(Allium sativum)*

For children, and for anybody where the cause is unknown, when the cough persists it is important to seek medical advice, as professional help may be needed. Similarly, if the mucus is bright green or yellow this indicates the presence of an infection, and advice should be sought.

EARACHE

Earaches most often develop through an infection, perhaps following a cold or sinusitis, for instance. Because infections can spread through into the middle or even inner ear, with potentially serious complications, earaches should not be neglected. If an earache is associated with catarrh, this should be treated too. Do *not* put anything into the ear unless it has been examined to ensure that the eardrum is not perforated.

AROMATHERAPY

Use hot compresses (see page 15) over the ear to draw the inflammation outwards, and hopefully help any pus that may be present to come out also. Two very good oils to use are Chamomile and Lavender; a combination of both may be most effective.

HERBALISM

Hot compresses are the most effective home treatment; Chamomile (*Chamomilla recutita*) may be used as an infusion (see page 12) for this purpose too. Taking garlic internally will help to reduce any catarrh and fight infection – if on proper examination the eardrum is not perforated, then a clove of garlic can be crushed into 5 ml (1 tsp) of olive

Aromatherapy oils can be added to warm water to make a soothing compress.

BELLADONNA (*Atropa belladonna*)

oil; this is warmed to blood temperature and a few drops gently inserted into the ear for an excellent local antibiotic.

HOMEOPATHY

As acute remedies only, choose from the following:
BELLADONNA: for throbbing pains, with a flushed face, a lot of heat around the ear and perhaps a high temperature. HEPAR SULPH: for a very painful ear, very tender to touch, and which may be discharging offensive pus – this situation

EARACHE IN CHILDREN
Earaches, especially in children, need to be treated quickly as an infection within the middle ear can be both painful and damaging. Speedy home help can be very useful to avoid these problems, but get medical help if earache worsens or persists.

requires medical attention quite quickly so do not let it go on unchecked. PULSATILLA: if there is a lot of thick, green catarrh present, and the earache and congestion is worse in hot rooms or stuffy atmospheres.

NATUROPATHY

Apart from all the local treatments by compress suggested above, follow the advice given for Catarrh (see page 34), especially if there is a pattern of recurring earaches, as prevention should be the primary aim.

CHAMOMILE (*Chamomilla recutita*)

HAY FEVER

Hay fever is an allergic reaction, which can be triggered not just by grass pollens but in some people by various flower or tree pollens too. It is often seen together with other allergic reactions such as asthma and/or eczema, and if it is not relieved by the suggested self-help approaches, then seek qualified treatment. Practitioners may well start to act preventively before the hay fever season.

AROMATHERAPY

Simply sniffing a drop or two of an essential oil may be the best method; steam inhalations (see page 33) can be used but might be too hot for some people. You may well need to vary the oils used through the hay fever season, as they can become less effective if used for too long. Choose from Chamomile, Tea Tree, Pine, Melissa or Eucalyptus.

HERBALISM

Two herbs are very helpful in reducing the symptoms of hay fever: Chamomile (*Chamomilla recutita*) and Eyebright (*Euphrasia officinalis*).

Make an infusion of Chamomile (Chamomilla recutita), *when cool soak a couple of cotton pads and place on the eyes. Rest for 10 minutes with the pads in place.*

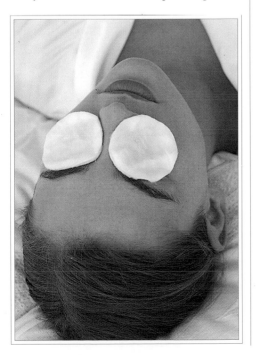

HAYFEVER SYMPTOMS

The membranes lining the nose are most often affected, with either congestion or else a streaming nose and sneezing; frequently the eyes or throat become inflamed too. An all-year-round allergic reaction, or allergic rhinitis, can be set up, with symptoms triggered by mould spores, house dust, fur and car exhaust fumes, for instance.

Slices of cucumber may be used on tired, sore eyes in the same way as herb pads.

They can both be used in two ways: firstly, as a tea taken 2 or 3 times a day (in severe cases try an infusion for stronger effect, see page 12) to reduce the inflammation and excess mucus, and, secondly, by soaking pads of cotton wool in a cooled infusion and placing on the eyelids to soothe sore, irritated eyes.

Where the mucus is very watery, alternative internal infusions to the above, or additions to them are:

GROUND IVY (*Glechoma hederacea*): very astringent, reducing excess mucus and drying out the secretions.

RIBWORT (*Plantago lanceolata*): also anti-catarrhal and astringent, toning up and healing the membranes.

HOMEOPATHY

Sometimes it can be worth using Mixed Pollens themselves in homeopathic dilution, before symptoms have started. Otherwise choose from:

ALLIUM CEPA: for a burning nasal discharge; the eyes will run too (think of your reaction to cutting up onions!).

ARSEN ALB: if the eyes are burning, with tears that feel hot. If the nose runs, that too will feel burning, sneezing gives no relief to the irritation.

EUPHRASIA: if the nose runs profusely, with lots of watery mucus, although it may block at night; the eyes feel sore and gritty, with burning tears.

NATUROPATHY

Reduce mucus production by cutting out dairy products (also see Catarrh, page 34), and when the symptoms are severe, take high levels of Vitamin C (up to 2,000 mg per day, unless diarrhoea occurs) to act as a natural anti-histamine.

Rinse out the eyes with an eyebath, using cool distilled water or a proprietary eyewash, to give temporary relief – you can also ease the nose by sniffing up distilled water to wash out the pollens.

INFLUENZA

Anyone who has had influenza will know that it is a more serious complaint than simply having a bad cold. Different viral strains produce differing symptoms, but generally there is a fever, aching muscles, headache and general weakness. Sometimes there may also be a harsh cough. In older, frail people it can seriously debilitate.

AROMATHERAPY

Several oils have considerable anti-viral activity, and help to boost the immune system. It is important though to use them at the earliest sign of influenza for maximum benefit. Either use them in the bath or as steam inhalations (see pages 8 and 33); it may also be a good idea to fumigate the house with oils at the same time, to help prevent everyone else getting the infection. This is best done by either putting 2-3 drops on a radiator to evaporate or else adding around 10 drops to a small plant spray filled with water, frequently spraying the room.

Dried herbs enable you to enjoy herbal teas all year long and are as effective as fresh herbs.

CINNAMON
(Cinnamomum zeylanicum)

Choose from Tea Tree, Eucalyptus, Lemon or Lavender oils.

HERBALISM

In the early stages of a chilled feeling, use a warming tea such as Cinnamon (*Cinnamomum zeylanicum*) – break a stick into a teapot – perhaps with 2.5 ml (½ tsp) of Cayenne (*Capsicum minimum*) or ground Ginger (*Zingiber officinalis*) added. When feeling more feverish, you can provoke sweating by taking infusions (see page 12) of Catmint (*Nepeta cataria*) and/or Elderflower (*Sambucus nigra*). The deep muscular aching can be relieved by using an infusion of Boneset (*Eupatorium perfoliatum*), either on its own or mixed with either of the above.

To stimulate the immune system, and also ward off complications such as bronchitis, take plenty of garlic, preferably raw – hot garlic bread or toast is a nice way to take it for all the family.

HOMEOPATHY

Choose from these remedies if not able to get professional treatment:
BRYONIA: if feeling very hot and dry, thirsty for cold drinks, aching all over, headache made worse by movement.
GELSEMIUM: for a hot head and face, but with chills that go up and down the back; burning headache but without any real sense of thirst.
NUX VOMICA: for thoroughly chilled feelings, cannot get warm at all, limbs and back are aching, stomach upset.

NATUROPATHY

At an early stage try having a hot bath to which you add 30–60 ml (2–4 tbsp) of Epsom Salts, then go straight to bed.

Generally restrict the diet, drinking fruit juices until the feverish period has passed, and then starting on fruit, vegetables and whole grains at first. If very hot and sweaty, try applying a cool compress to the chest and trunk.

Immediately the symptoms start, it is advisable to take high levels of Vitamin C to boost the immune system, around 3,000-4,000 mg to start with, reducing over 3-4 days to 500 mg until completely better.

INFLUENZA STRAINS
Influenza occurs in bouts of epidemic proportions, with periodic changes in the viral strains responsible. This makes vaccination programmes more difficult and less effective. Influenza can be a real killer, and attention to good health to prevent the onset of serious symptoms is essential, especially for older people in winter.

LARYNGITIS

Laryngitis is an acute inflammation of the larynx and vocal chords, leading to a very sore throat, hoarseness and even loss of voice. It may follow on from a cold or other infection, or be due to overstraining the voice by shouting, severe coughing or irritations such as smoke or dust.

AROMATHERAPY

The best method for treatment is undoubtedly steam inhalation (see page 33); the natural choice of oil is probably Benzoin, but you could also use Sandalwood or Thyme. As the oils vaporize with the steam, they soothe the dry, inflamed membranes and ease the breathing as well as being highly antiseptic.

HERBALISM

Local treatment is by gargle; there are a number of useful herbs for this, they are most effective as tinctures (see page 14), otherwise use cooled infusions (see page 12). Choose from these astringent herbs: Sage (*Salvia officinalis*), Thyme (*Thymus vulgaris*), Agrimony (*Agrimonia eupatoria*) or

Holding a towel over your head will concentrate the herbal vapours and delay the effects of evaporation.

Raspberry Leaf (*Rubus idaeus*), which will help to tone up the puffy membranes. For a very soothing effect, add Marshmallow (*Althea officinalis*) to the gargle, or take 10 ml (2 tsp) of a decoction (see page 12) of the root 3 or 4 times a day.

HOMEOPATHY

One of these remedies should be suitable in the short term:
ACONITE: for sudden laryngitis following exposure to cold, dry winds, with a high temperature and a dry cough.

CAUSTICUM: for a hoarse voice, which may go completely, with a burning, raw throat and irritating cough.
PHOSPHORUS: if you cannot talk louder than a whisper, symptoms may have been brought on by overuse of the voice; with a dry cough and a desire for cold drinks and ice-cream.

NATUROPATHY

Cut out dairy produce to reduce excess catarrh, and take plenty of fruit juices. Try placing a cold compress (see page 15) around the throat, if the problem has been around for a while, it may be an idea to use a hot compress followed by a cold one. Sucking zinc gluconate lozenges not only soothes the throat but directly tackles any infection; in addition to fruit and juices it may be useful to take 500 mg of Vitamin C for a few days, or fresh lemon juice and honey drinks.

MARSHMALLOW
(*Althea officinalis*)

SINUSITIS

The sinus cavities are air spaces in the bones of the skull, behind, above and below the eyes. They act as a kind of sound-box, helping the voice to resonate. Like the nasal passages they are lined with mucous membranes, and an infection in the nose or throat can spread to the sinuses; acute sinusitis can be very painful and needs prompt treatment. Chronic sinusitis may be linked to allergic reactions such as hay fever.

AROMATHERAPY

Steam inhalations (see page 33) are the best way to work directly on the membranes, loosening thick mucus and fighting infection. Choose from oils of Chamomile, Eucalyptus, Lavender, Peppermint, Pine, Thyme or Tea Tree; a combination may be best, or else change around the oils. In acute sinusitis, the inhalations can be taken 4 times a day to ease the pain and relieve the congestion, reducing to once daily as the symptoms ease, until the sinuses have cleared up.

HERBALISM

Apart from steam inhalations as outlined above, using infusions internally (see page 12) can help to reduce the catarrh and inflammation. Look at the following herbs (see also Catarrh, page 34):

Oil of Eucalyptus is very effective used as part of a steam inhalation.

CATMINT (*Nepeta cataria*): reduces nasal congestion and helps to liquefy the thick, sticky mucus.

ELDERFLOWER (*Sambucus nigra*): reduces inflammation by improving circulation through the area, clears long-term catarrh, and eases congestion.

GOLDEN SEAL (*Hydrastis canadensis*): has an astringent effect, cooling and toning up swollen, inflamed membranes. As this herb is quite expensive and difficult to find loose, it may be easier to take in tablet form, up to 500 mg a day.

It is also often very valuable to take plenty of garlic, either raw or as garlic perles, to fight any infection.

HOMEOPATHY

Try to match the remedy to the symptom pattern – look also at suggestions for Catarrh, Colds or Hay Fever (pages 34, 35 and 39).

CATMINT (*Nepeta cataria*)

HEPAR SULPH: for painful swelling of the nasal cavities, tender to the touch, with infected, yellow mucus discharge.

NAT MUR: a profuse, watery discharge, sneezing and a frontal headache are typical symptoms calling for this remedy.

SILICA: for a dry, blocked nose and a severe headache, perhaps with bouts of sneezing; worse with cold and better with warmth.

NATUROPATHY

Immediately cut out all dairy products, and restrict white flour, pastries, cakes and so on. Eat plenty of fresh fruit and vegetables. Avoid smoky atmospheres, and do not fly when nasal passages are acutely inflamed or blocked, as the changes in air pressure can given severe pain and could damage the eardrum.

Use alternating hot and cold light compresses (see page 15) or just splashes of water around the nose; start with hot water for about 3 minutes and then cold for no more than 1 minute, repeating 2 or 3 times. This will reduce congestion and inflammation, and thus ease the pains. Using an inhalation can be a helpful back-up to this.

SORE THROATS

Sore throats are more and more common nowadays, with increased airborne pollution, smoky, dry atmospheres in air-conditioned buildings and so on. The irritation can range from an annoying tickle to a rasping soreness, and may be linked to other infections. Where the throat inflammation, or pharyngitis, also extends down to the larynx, the voice may be affected – see also Laryngitis and Tonsillitis (pages 41 and 44).

MYRRH (*Commiphora molmol*)

AROMATHERAPY

Use steam inhalations (see page 33) with oils such as Benzoin, Lavender or Thyme. One drop *only* of essential oil of Lemon on 2.5 ml (½ tsp) of honey acts as a powerful local antiseptic, as well as being soothing.

HERBALISM

If possible, use the following herbs as tinctures for gargling; if unavailable then use cooled infusions (see page 12): Agrimony (*Agrimonia eupatoria*), Sage (*Salvia officinalis*), and Thyme (*Thymus vulgaris*) are all astringent, toning up the membranes, the latter two also being quite antiseptic. For a more powerful effect try using a tincture (see page 14) of Myrrh (*Commiphora molmol*), together with one or more of the others. If making infusions, add two broken liquorice sticks to give a more soothing

effect, or else use Marshmallow (*Althea officinalis*) leaf in equal amounts with the other herb(s).

HOMEOPATHY

The choice is wide, depending on the causes and the nature of the symptoms. It is advisable to look at other headings in this section too.

APIS MEL: for a red, swollen, burning throat and difficulty in swallowing anything.

KALI BICH: for sharp pains, relieved by swallowing, although there may also be a feeling of a "frog-in-the-throat" which is not relieved. The throat is especially dry and sore first thing in the mornings, with some sticky mucus.

MERC SOL: for a painful and raw throat, with a lot of watery, possibly unpleasant-smelling saliva.

NATUROPATHY

For adults and older children the diet can be restricted to fruit juices only for a day or two at most; younger children and infants will be unlikely to cope with this, so simply reduce the dairy foods and give plenty of fruit juices. If the throat is swollen and feels very hot, try a cold compress (see page 15) around it. If

AGRIMONY

(*Agrimonia eupatoria*)

OCCUPATIONAL HAZARDS
Many occupations involve excessive use of the voice e.g. teaching, and sore throats are commonplace. The regular use of herbal gargles can ease this discomfort, and help to prevent loss of voice or an actual infection. Keeping the throat moist by drinking liquids often, helps too.

available, suck zinc lozenges. Rest the voice and keep in a warm atmosphere.

In modern offices the dry air leads to frequent sore throats. Sip liquids often, and try to make the air more moist if possible, for example with plants.

SAGE (*Salvia officinalis*)

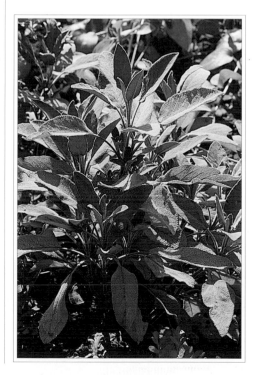

TONSILLITIS

Inflammation and infection of the tonsils most often occurs in children or younger adults; it used to be the fashion to remove the tonsils but unless they become chronically badly infected and act as a focus for other infections, it is now considered better to keep them. They act as an early warning sign of lowered vitality, and if this first line of defence is lost, then more deep-seated conditions can occur in later life.

AROMATHERAPY

Essential oils are not for internal use, unless under qualified treatment, and are rather unpleasant for local treatment. In tonsillitis they are best used as supportive treatment, using steam inhalations (see page 33) of Benzoin, Eucalyptus or Thyme to ease inflammation and fight general infection.

HERBALISM

All the herbs mentioned under Sore Throats (see page 43) for gargling are excellent here too, especially Myrrh (*Commiphora molmol*), Thyme (*Thymus vulgaris*) and Sage (*Salvia officinalis*). For repeated bouts of tonsillitis take garlic daily, either perles/capsules or fresh. Another essential herb to use for chronic

GARLIC (*Allium sativum*)

CONE FLOWER (*Echinacea angustifolia*)

tonsillitis is Cone Flower (*Echinacea angustifolia* or *E. purpurea*); this boosts the immune system and may be taken in tablets or else as a tincture (see page 14), 20 drops twice daily.

HOMEOPATHY

Remedies applicable to tonsillitis include:

ACONITE: for sudden onset of inflammation, with hot, red and burning tonsils and thirst for cold drinks.

HEPAR SULPH: for pain on swallowing, as if something is stuck in the throat, tonsils swollen and discharging a yellow pus.

LYCOPODIUM: for chronic swelling of the tonsils, which look as if they are pitted with small white discharging ulcers; cold drinks make the sensation worse.

NATUROPATHY

The tonsils' actions, in trapping and removing infective bacteria that would otherwise cause deeper problems, means that they are more easily infected themselves. This can produce an infection of the adenoids too, with nasal congestion.

Where these symptoms occur, it is helpful to cut out dairy projects for a while. In any case, take plenty of fluids, especially fruit juices. Freshly-squeezed lemon juice, with a little honey, is a local antiseptic. Repeated attacks of tonsillitis are often a sign of lowered health in general, and may need professional treatment.

THYME (*Thymus vulgaris*)

WHOOPING COUGH

This highly infectious bacterial infection tends to occur in epidemics every few years. Thick, sticky mucus gives rise to a spasmodic cough and the difficulty in inhaling with this gives the characteristic whooping sound. It is mostly seen in children, and in babies it can be serious, so get professional help as soon as possible. Symptoms can linger on for several weeks, so continue to help breathing by the measures listed below.

AROMATHERAPY

Relief for the condition is most dramatic with steam; either use inhalations (see page 33) or with infants simply hold them near steam, such as a basin filled with piping hot water or near a hot bath (make sure they do not touch very hot water). Very good oils to add to the steam are Cypress, Lavender and Tea Tree.

HERBALISM

Start to give herbal teas/infusions at the first sign of coughing – do not wait for the respiratory distress that can set in with the whoop. Use steam to free the mucus, as mentioned above. In young infants and babies, diluted teas

Keep all medicines and aromatherapy oils out of the reach of small children.

should be strong enough; older children may need infusions (see page 12), again diluted (for dosages see page 9). Look at these herbs, and use a blend of the most appropriate:

CHAMOMILE (*Chamomilla recutita*): helps to calm the person down, reduces catarrh and accompanying nausea.
COLTSFOOT (*Tussilago farfara*): one of the best cough remedies, helping to ease the spasmodic nature of the cough.
LAVENDER (*Lavandula vera*): a relaxing expectorant, soothing the cough and breathing and also generally calming.
THYME (*Thymus vulgaris*): highly antiseptic, soothing the dry cough that may herald the start of the problem.
WHITE HOREHOUND (*Marrubium vulgare*): good expectorant, loosening the sticky mucus and reducing spasm.

An alternative treatment that can work wonders is to chop or crush two cloves of garlic into 15 ml (1 tbsp) of honey and leave for a couple of hours, or even overnight. Give up to 5 ml (1 tsp) either neat or diluted in a little warm water, 4 times a day.

HOMEOPATHY

Ideally seek qualified advice for this ailment, but a remedy often used for the characteristic rapid paroxysmal cough is Drosera. Often the bout of coughing can result in vomiting. If children have been in contact with whooping cough, it can be worth trying this remedy as a prophylactic: give 3 doses of 30c dilution (see page 10) in a 24-hour period.

SELF-HELP MEASURES

Anyone who has heard the distinctive whooping sound will always remember whooping cough. Early treatment is most helpful; self-help measures such as steam treatments can speedily relieve symptoms, but babies and tiny infants should ideally be professionally checked as well.

NATUROPATHY

Keep the fluid intake high, especially if there is vomiting with the coughing bouts; also give only small amounts of light food rather than big meals. Avoid dairy products in order to lessen mucus production, and give easily digested foods.

For older children, supplementing diet with 500 mg Vitamin C daily for a couple of weeks will help to boost the immune system – reduce or stop if diarrhoea develops.

Try to keep the diet light, wholesome and low in dairy foods for quite a while after the initial symptoms have eased, as any build-up in mucus can cause more problems for several weeks.

WHITE HOREHOUND (*Marrubium vulgare*)

THE CIRCULATORY SYSTEM

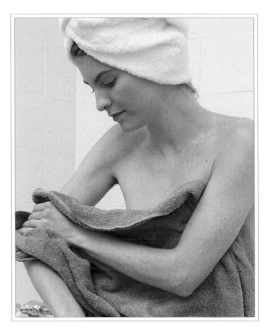

Circulation is absolutely vital for health; the blood transports oxygen and all our other nutrients around the body to all the cells, and carries away the waste materials from cellular activity. Without good circulation we simply do not have the fuel to provide enough energy for health. In cooler climates many people suffer from poor circulation, and lowered immune systems can often follow.

Disorders of circulation can occur in the heart or in the blood vessels; the former are not suitable for self-treatment, and for any prolonged or serious circulatory problems it is best to get professional treatment. For example, angina is a cramping of the heart muscles due to narrowing or obstruction of the coronary arteries. When the supply of oxygen to the cardiac muscles does not meet any extra demand, perhaps when walking uphill, the characteristic cramp and pains of angina occur for a short while. Resting eases the pain after a few minutes. Angina can be relieved by taking infusions of Lime Blossom *(Tilia europaea)*, but full professional treatment needs to look at individual causes as well as the health of the heart.

ABOVE: Alternating hot and cold baths is a useful self-help measure for improving circulation. Herbs such as Marigold (Calendula officinalis) *(above left) and Witch Hazel* (Hamamelis virginiana) *can also help astringe and tone swollen veins.*

CHILBLAINS

For people with poor peripheral circulation, living in cool, damp climates often creates chilblains. When circulation is reduced in cold weather, the oxygen supply to the fingers and toes is restricted to the point that the skin cells are damaged and swelling, redness and itching occurs. Warmer weather improves the condition, but using radiant heat, such as warming by the fire, can tend to aggravate the swelling and burning itchy sensation.

AROMATHERAPY

Only use oils locally if the skin is unbroken; otherwise an inflamed reaction may be set off. Massage the affected areas with warming oils such as Black Pepper, Ginger or Marjoram, using a vegetable oil containing a maximum of 3 per cent essential oil. For longer term treatment during the winter months, add oils of Cypress, Juniper, Pine or Rosemary to baths (see page 8 for dilutions), or use them diluted in a base oil as above for regular brisk massage of the hands and feet.

HERBALISM

Locally, use a footbath to which is added a decoction (see page 12) of fresh Ginger root (*Zingiber officinalis*), using up to 15 g (½ oz) per 750 ml (1¼ pt/ 2⅔ cups) of water, or add a tea made from ground Ginger, or for maximum circulatory-stimulating effect Cayenne (*Capsicum minimum*). Do not use the latter if the skin is broken.

Handbaths, or footbaths, are good ways to improve circulation to the extremities. Place hands in a bowl of hot water, with essential oils added as recommended.

GINGER DECOCTION

Ginger can be made into a tea, but a stronger medicine is made from a decoction.

1 Simmer 15 g (½ oz) chopped rhizome in 750ml (1¼ pt/2⅔ cups) water until the liquid is reduced to about 600 ml (1 pt/2½ cups).

2 Strain through a sieve and store in a jug. Give in doses of 5-20 ml (1 tsp -1½ tbsp), three times a day. It will keep in the fridge for 3 days.

Internally, teas from the above herbs will generally improve circulation. For a gentler effect on the extremities use an infusion (see page 12) of Yarrow (*Achillea millefolium*); this dilates the tiny blood vessels in the hands and feet, helping them to warm.

HOMEOPATHY

Since treatment may be needed for a couple of weeks or so, use low potencies such as 6c (see page 10).
AGARICUS: if the symptoms are worse when cold, and there is itching and burning with redness of the skin.
CALCAREA CARBONICA: if there is relief from cold, the feet in particular feeling damp and cold to the touch.
PETROLEUM: if, as well as burning and itching, there is chapping and cracking of the skin; typically the fingers get splits at the tips.

NATUROPATHY

Use alternating hot and cold foot or handbaths, using warm rather than too hot water, for about 4 minutes, and then cold for up to 1 minute. Make sure the feet or hands are well dried. Repeat for 10-15 minutes, nightly for a week if needed. Giving the hands or feet a brisk friction-rub daily will also help the circulation

Increase Vitamin C in the diet by eating more fresh fruit and potatoes; if you suffer badly from chilblains, take a supplement of Vitamin C, up to 1 mg until better, possibly together with 300–400 iu of Vitamin E to improve the elasticity of the blood vessels.

FEVER

The raising of the body temperature, usually in response to an infection, is something that natural medicine sees as generally a positive healing attempt by the body. Most of our vital processes are stimulated by the higher temperature, and conversely many infective organisms cannot survive as well, so the fever response is one that can be aided rather than instantly suppressed.

AROMATHERAPY

In order to encourage sweating at the stage of resolving the fever, a warm bath with a maximum of 10 drops of one of these oils may help – if bathing is not appropriate, use them at 1 per cent dilution in a little vegetable oil and massage the back or chest. Chamomile, Cypress, Lavender or Tea Tree are good choices. For a more cooling effect use 5 drops of oils of Eucalyptus, Lavender or Peppermint in a small bowl of tepid water and sponge the upper back, neck and chest.

HERBALISM

If at the early, shivery stage of an infection, use a tea with Ginger (*Zingiber officinalis*) – 2.5 ml (½ tsp) ground ginger, or peel and grate a small piece of fresh root – and Cinnamon (*Cinnamomum zeylanicum*) – 2.5 ml

CATMINT (*Nepeta cataria*)

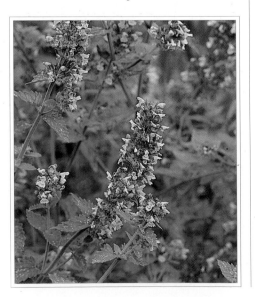

CHECKING THE TEMPERATURE

By taking the temperature, and checking on feelings of heat or cold, the stages of the fever can be noted and treatment given. Initially, our internal thermostat is turned up, making us feel cold and shivery; as circulation is boosted and we reach the higher levels, we can feel more comfortable, although with a raised temperature. If the process goes too high, or the infection is not controlled, the thermostat is reset back to normal and we feel feverish and hot. Sweating reduces the temperature. Body temperatures around 38°C (100-101°F) often give the best results in fighting infection. Children's temperatures often go higher, and so may an adult's; if left for too long this can make us feel very unwell and cooling may then be needed, either by inducing sweating or through sponging with tepid water. If in doubt get professional help.

(½ tsp) ground cinnamon, or half a cinnamon stick.

When the fever makes you hot and restless, sweating can be provoked by taking a hot infusion (see page 12) of Elderflower (*Sambucus nigra*). (At normal temperatures this will not make you sweat.) Other suitable infusions to

ELDERFLOWER (*Sambucus nigra*)

relieve the symptoms are: Boneset (*Eupatorium perfoliatum*), Catmint (*Nepeta cataria*), Peppermint (*Mentha piperita*) and Yarrow (*Achillea millefolium*), while Lime Blossom (*Tilia europaea*) can be added to aid the dilation of the blood vessels and assist general relaxation. Hyssop (*Hyssopus officinalis*) is another excellent herb to calm the system; a tea may be taken frequently while symptoms prevail.

HOMEOPATHY

As with herbalism, there are many homeopathic remedies available and the cause/exact reaction needs to be sorted out first. A few to choose from, in mild feverish states are:

ACONITE: for dry, burning skin and great restlessness and agitation; symptoms may come on quickly.

BELLADONNA: for a high temperature, with a hot, very red face and a racing pulse. In extreme fever cases the person may also be delirious and highly excitable.

EUPATORIUM PERFOLIATUM: for an influenza-type of fever, with chills followed on by heat, aching muscles and maybe sweating.

FERRUM PHOS: for milder fevers, with less obvious causes; a hot, throbbing head and frequent sweating.

NATUROPATHY

Avoid active exercise; take plenty of rest but do not swaddle in heavy bedclothes; keep the room aired.

BONESET
(*Eupatorium perfoliatum*)

Herbs can help combat a fever by either provoking sweating, or by aiding the dilation of the blood vessels.

Drink fruit juices, herb teas or water, and restrict food until the temperature has returned to normal. Sponge the face and chest with tepid water if the temperature is too hot. A cold pack or compress around the trunk will also reduce excessive heat; use something large like a towel wrung out in cold water and wrapped around the body and then wrap in a larger, dry towel or blanket.

Feverish conditions used to be much more common, and traditional practitioners such as herbalists developed quite sophisticated techniques to deal with them. They have become rarer nowadays, but natural measures remain very important in helping to cope with a fever. If the temperature rises to the point where someone becomes delirious or even has a convulsion, get urgent medical aid. Young children can be quite prone to convulsions, but this is rarer as we get older.

HYSSOP
(*Hyssopus officinalis*)

HAEMORRHOIDS

Haemorrhoids, or piles, are swollen veins in the rectum due to a restricted local blood supply and congestion in the pelvic cavity. Occasionally they may protrude externally, and can give rise to bleeding especially with a bowel movement. Piles can occur during pregnancy due to the increased pressure, but are often associated with chronic constipation, when frequent straining to empty the bowels causes extra pressure on the veins.

AROMATHERAPY

Using oils such as Cypress or Juniper in the bath can help to stimulate pelvic circulation; also adding a couple of drops of either to a bowl of cool water and then using this for a compress (see page 15) may help too. Massage of the abdomen (see right) with a 2 per cent dilution of oils of Marjoram or Rosemary can help ease constipation and relieve haemorrhoids.

PILEWORT *(Ranunculus ficaria)*

HERBALISM

Local treatment can help to astringe and tone the swollen veins. Use commercial creams made with extract of Pilewort *(Ranunculus ficaria)*, Horse Chestnut *(Aesculus hippocastanum)* or Marigold *(Calendula officinalis)*, or use a compress of distilled Witch Hazel *(Hamamelis virginiana)*; the tincture (see page 14) is much more astringent, if available use this diluted at the rate of 15 ml (1 tbsp)

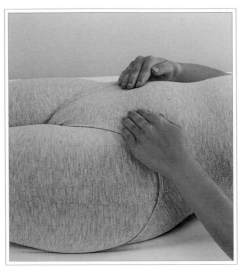

Press fingers steadily into the low abdomen, and massage with small circular movements, to release tension and improve local circulation.

to a small bowl of warm water.

Prolong bleeding from piles can eventually lead to anaemia. Drinking Nettle *(Urtica dioica)* tea may relieve this, but take steps to avoid constipation too.

HOMEOPATHY

Some possible remedies are:
AESCULUS: for a dry itching and stinging sensation, and a tendency for the veins to prolapse and protrude externally.
HAMAMELIS: for a burning soreness, often with bleeding.
SULPHUR: for hot, burning and itching in the anus; the pains are made worse by standing and better when lying.

NATUROPATHY

Practitioners in all of the therapies are likely to give dietary advice, and it is sensible to ensure you eat plenty of fresh vegetables and fruit to give adequate fibre and ease constipation, see also Constipation (page 57). Hot and cold compresses or even hot/cold baths will improve local circulation and reduce congestion; ice packs may be useful to reduce swelling at times. Exercise is also helpful to get the circulation going; ideally get individual advice. Avoid long periods of standing.

WITCH HAZEL *(Hamamelis virginiana)*

POOR CIRCULATION

Poor circulation to the extremities is quite common in cooler climates, and particularly in elderly people or those who do very little exercise. (See also Chilblains, page 47). Poor circulation can lead on to more serious conditions such as phlebitis or thrombosis, so it should not be neglected, and professional medical help should be sought if in any doubt.

HAND MASSAGE

1 Place some base oil in a bowl, with essential oils added as recommended. Massage into palms of hands with a steady circular movement.

2 Squeeze down the fingers to stretch and loosen them, pushing towards the palm. Repeat steps 1 and 2 several times.

FOOT MASSAGE

1 To stretch the feet, place hands with thumbs on top of the foot, keeping a firm grip with both of the hands.

2 Move thumbs outward, as if breaking a piece of bread (be gentle with your partner!); repeat movement several times.

too, and cayenne pepper is the strongest circulatory stimulant, perhaps simply use in cooking for this effect as well as its flavour.

HOMEOPATHY

To improve circulation, the following remedies may be of help in the short term, but if symptoms persist and the fingers and toes become numb, then seek professional medical advice:

SECALE: For cold hands and feet with a burning sensation. The rest of the body also feels cold, and the fingers and

NETTLE
(*Urtica dioica*)

AROMATHERAPY

Massage the hands or feet with diluted oils such as Black Pepper, Lavender, Marjoram or Rosemary. These can be added to a warm footbath for a stronger short-term treatment. Use a maximum of 10 drops in total, and try a blend of 2 or 3 of these oils. Avoid if skin is broken, get advice first.

HERBALISM

Take hot herbal teas regularly to aid peripheral circulation; choose from Elderflower (*Sambucus nigra*), Ginger (*Zingiber officinalis*), Lime Blossom (*Tilia europaea*), Nettle (*Urtica dioica*) or Yarrow (*Achillea millefolium*). Daily intake of garlic stimulates blood flow

Exercise is the best way to help yourself in improving circulation. Regular activities stimulate blood flow, and keep the heart and lungs in good condition. Skipping has become more popular as an exercise, and is an excellent way to keep warm.

THE BLOODSTREAM

Since the circulation transports nourishment, both oxygen and nutrients from food, around the body it is essential for our overall health and vitality. Waste matter from all our cells is carried away in the bloodstream for elimination, and white blood cells form an essential part of our immune system. Keeping circulation flowing well, therefore, should be a priority for everyone.

As we get older, circulation tends to slow down and this is exaggerated if we stop exercising or being active. With increasingly sedentary lifestyles in many countries, it is very important to move as much as possible at work, or in retirement, to combat reduced circulation.

toes can become quite blue or white. Take 6c every 30 minutes for up to 10 doses.

CARBO VEG: For cold hands and feet with a mottling of the skin. The skin feels icy cold to the touch and appears blue,

YARROW (*Achillea millefolium*)

CAYENNE (*Capsicum minimum*)

with prominent veins. Skin can also appear blotchy.

NATUROPATHY

Various substances constrict the peripheral blood vessels, most notably caffeine and nicotine, so reducing or cutting out coffee and tobacco will help greatly. Exercise is another essential, wherever possible, and in colder weather keep the wrists and ankles warm as well as the hands and feet themselves. Additional amounts of Vitamin C (up to 500 mg per day) and Vitamin E (up to 400 iu per day) can boost circulation and aid the elasticity of the blood-vessel walls.

CAUTION

Do not increase the doses from those suggested here: it is likely to do more harm than good.

VARICOSE VEINS

Swollen veins most often occur in the lower legs, but can happen elsewhere, see also Haemorrhoids (page 50). The veins in the legs contain one-way valves that allow blood to flow back up towards the heart. If the calf muscles weaken, for example after prolonged standing, or the valves start to work less efficiently from other causes such as pregnancy, obesity or poor nutrition, then blood collects in the veins, and they swell.

AROMATHERAPY

All the natural therapies are likely to recommend both periods of rest, especially with the feet raised above the level of the thigh to let gravity assist venous return, and exercise to improve muscle tone.

Massage, above the area of varicosed veins and in an upwards direction towards the heart, will reduce the congestion. Essential oils of prime use here are Cypress, Chamomile and perhaps Juniper; use diluted at 2 per cent in vegetable oil.

HERBALISM

Externally, apply tinctures (see page 14) of Marigold (*Calendula officinalis*) or Witch Hazel (*Hamamelis virginiana*), diluted 50:50 with water, 2 or 3 times a day. Internally, a cup daily of an infusion (see page 12) of Lime Blossom (*Tilia europaea*), can help to improve peripheral circulation. Horse Chestnut (*Aesculus hippocastanum*) has a strengthening effect on the blood vessels; it may be taken in tablets as directed, or as the tincture at the rate of 30 drops twice daily.

MARIGOLD (*Calendula officinalis*)

HOMEOPATHY

CARBO VEG: for a sluggish circulation leading to blueness of the skin, cold extremities and painful varicose veins.

HAMAMELIS: for swollen, congested veins with a purplish blotching under the skin and tired, aching legs; may also have piles.

PULSATILLA: for painful veins, blue in colour; may be associated with pregnancy; pains in legs eased with walking about and in cool, fresh air.

Plenty of fresh fruit is essential in any diet.

NATUROPATHY

Use hot and cold bathing of legs, or spray cool water up the legs at the end of a shower. Walk more; also look at yoga and swimming as good forms of exercise. Reduce alcohol intake; if very overweight try to lose weight steadily.

A supplement of Vitamin E (up to 400 iu daily), together with 5 ml (1 tsp) Lecithin granules daily, can ease the swelling and pains by improving the elasticity of the blood vessels; another helpful substance is Vitamin C (up to 500 mg). In the long term just take plenty of fresh fruit and vegetables and keep fats to a lower level.

THE DIGESTIVE SYSTEM

In many respects the digestive system is the most important set of organs in the body, for it is here that we absorb all the nutrients we need in order for all our cells to function and hence for us to survive. The old adage "we are what we eat" has a lot of validity, since poor nutrition can lead not only to problems such as constipation, flatulence or diarrhoea but also to more general ailments like headache, chronic tiredness, poor concentration and memory.

The digestive system is also an integral part of our immune defences, recognizing potentially toxic substances and either breaking them down into safer compounds

or else eliminating them. Western dietary and lifestyle habits have created their own disorders, from gastric ulcers to constipation and irritable bowel syndrome; this last condition has become something of a "waste-basket diagnosis" – if nothing else shows up, then that is what you have! Treatment for this should really be individual, as stress, diet, posture and exercise all play a part in each person's symptoms.

ABOVE: Eating fresh fruit is a good way of increasing dietary fibre intake.

ACIDITY AND HEARTBURN

Many people get occasional bouts of acid dyspepsia, usually related to a temporary problem such as having eaten rich, spicy foods or having eaten too quickly when feeling rushed and stressed. If the symptoms happen very regularly, you may need to look more carefully at what you eat and how fast you eat it. If there is persistent discomfort, seek professional treatment; see also Flatulence and Indigestion (pages 59 and 61).

AROMATHERAPY

Using hot or warm compresses (see page 15) over the abdomen, with up to 10 drops of oils such as Chamomile or Lavender in a small bowl of water, can give relief from the inflammation and spasm that accompany excess acidity. These oils, diluted at 2 per cent in a base oil, can also be gently massaged into the abdomen if the discomfort is not too great.

SLIPPERY ELM (*Ulmus fulva*)

HERBALISM

Digestive disturbances generally respond very well indeed to herbal treatment, and acid dyspepsia can be improved considerably. For a temporary problem choose from the suggested herbs and use as warm teas; for repeated acid/heartburn symptoms use stronger, as infusions (see page 12) or as otherwise directed.

CHAMOMILE (*Chamomilla recutita*): a relaxant and anti-inflammatory remedy that helps the whole digestive tract; if acid symptoms are related to stress and/or over-eating of rich foods, this

---

HEARTBURN SYMPTOMS

When excess acid leaks back up into the gullet, this inflames and irritates the lining of the oesophagus and the feeling of heartburn is produced. Taking antacid tablets regularly may not only mask underlying problems, but can also be counter-productive as the stomach tries to compensate by creating more acid.

---

herb makes an excellent choice.

LEMON BALM (*Melissa officinalis*): another excellent herb where the condition is caused by stress; if available use the fresh leaves for a much finer flavour.

MEADOWSWEET (*Filipendula ulmaria*): although chemically related to aspirin, Meadowsweet is soothing for an inflamed stomach (but may need to be avoided if there is a hypersensitivity to salicylates such as aspirin) and reduces acidity.

SLIPPERY ELM (*Ulmus fulva*): this is highly soothing to the inflamed gullet or stomach, and may be taken before meals, either as tablets or by mixing 5 ml (1 tsp) of the pure powder in a little warm water – it lives up to its name as it goes down, coating and soothing the membranes.

HOMEOPATHY

As usual, individual characteristics will determine proper prescribing of remedies, but initially choose from:

CARBO VEG: for a burning feeling in the stomach, and acid reflux with waterbrash (gas being brought up into the mouth with acidic fluid) and sometimes nausea; symptoms often caused by over-eating or drinking.

LYCOPODIUM: for definite heartburn, much wind and a feeling of fullness after only a little food.

NUX VOMICA: when taken too much rich food, alcohol and coffee leading to nausea and acidity but also an empty, hungry feeling in the stomach.

NATUROPATHY

Often a glass of milk is suggested as a temporary measure, to neutralize the acid. This is not always suitable, and certainly not on a regular basis, as dairy produce can create its own digestive problems. It may be helpful to avoid solids for up to 24 hours after a bad bout of acid heartburn. Using a hot compress over the abdomen can relieve pains. Avoid coffee, alcohol, tobacco, chocolate, pastries or spicy foods for at least a couple of days, and if prone to this complaint, then try to slowly cut them out.

MEADOWSWEET (*Filipendula ulmaria*)

COLIC

Colic is the term used to describe spasmodic bouts of cramping pains, especially in the bowel which often associated with trapped gas; see Flatulence (page 59). Colic is especially common in babies. The symptom may be related to tension generally, but if there are other digestive disturbances, do seek professional advice. It is always a sensible precaution to seek medical advice where babies are concerned.

AROMATHERAPY

Gentle massage of the abdomen, in a clockwise direction, using oils of Chamomile, Fennel or Peppermint will help – dilute the oils at the ratio of 3-4 drops per 5 ml (1 tsp) of base oil.

HERBALISM

For an occasional attack of colic, use hot teas of Catmint *(Nepeta cataria)*, Chamomile *(Chamomilla recutita)*, Fennel *(Foeniculum vulgare)*, Ginger *(Zingiber officinalis)* or Peppermint *(Mentha piperita)*. Using aromatic seeds like Aniseed *(Pimpinella anisum)*, Caraway *(Carum carvi)*, Dill *(Anethum graveolens)* or Fennel *(Foeniculum vulgare)* in food, or simply chewing a few of the seeds after a meal can help a lot if you are prone to colic after eating. If the problem is frequent, get professional treatment.

HOMEOPATHY

BRYONIA: if the spasms are made worse by any movement, or by local heat, better by lying still with bent knees.

FENNEL
(Foeniculum vulgare)

ABDOMEN MASSAGE

1 Starting in the lower right hand corner, steadily but firmly press in with both hands.

2 Slowly move hands in a clockwise direction around the abdomen, using small circles to massage the colon.

CHAMOMILLA: especially good for colicky babies, or teething infants; the bloated abdomen tends to be improved by local warmth, such as a hot water bottle.
MAGNESIA PHOSPHORICA: if warmth, pressure over the abdomen and walking about ease the discomfort, but burping does not.
NUX VOMICA: for colic brought on by over-eating or drinking alcohol; symptoms eased by sitting or lying down, and worse if upright.

NATUROPATHY

In most cases local warmth over the lower abdomen helps; a hot-water bottle is the easiest method. Internally, herbal teas, as detailed above, will give the best relief, as they not only reduce spasm but aid digestion too. It may well be necessary to look at and treat other digestive problems; see also entries for Constipation, Diarrhoea

---

ANISEED
(Pimpinella anisum)

and Gall-Bladder Problems (pages 57, 58 and 60). If frequent colic occurs, do look at how fast you eat, whether you curl up into a comfortable chair after a meal, or if your diet has a lot of fatty, spicy foods or dairy produce. If any of these apply, try to change that pattern and see if the colic improves without needing other treatment; if not get advice. Often it is most helpful simply to eat meals in a more relaxed way, rather than gulping food down while "on the run".

CONSTIPATION

This is a problem that is largely confined to a typical Western diet and lifestyle. Inadequate amounts of dietary fibre, and perhaps a lack of exercise, lead to the slow passage of faeces through the bowel and this in turn allows water to be re-absorbed, leaving hardened, rabbit-like stools. The frequency of bowel movements is less important than the harder consistency; straining can cause piles (see Haemorrhoids, page 50).

AROMATHERAPY

One of the most effective methods of self-help is daily clockwise massage of the lower abdomen (see page 50), and this can be performed using 2 drops of oils of Lavender, Marjoram or Rosemary in 5 ml (1 tsp) of base oil. Lavender and Marjoram are more relaxing, if tension is a factor, while Rosemary has a more tonic effect.

HERBALISM

Always start with gentle laxatives, or aperients, which increase bowel tone without giving griping. One of the best is Dandelion Root *(Taraxacum officinale)*, ideally taken as a decoction (see page 12) – although you may get a gentle action from one of the Dandelion coffee drinks on the market. Another simple herb to use is Liquorice *(Glycyrrhiza glabra)*; either chew one of the liquorice sticks that you can buy from a health food shop or add it to the Dandelion Root for the decoction. If constipation persists, switch to trying another herb that works in quite a different way. Linseed *(Linum usitatissimum)* absorbs liquid and creates a soft bulk internally that aids the peristaltic wave movements that propel faeces through the bowel. Take 10 ml (2 tsp) at breakfast, with at least 300 ml (½ pt/1¼ cups) of water. Ideally soak the Linseed overnight in a little water to start the swelling process. It may look like frog-spawn but it can relieve tense constipation! Make sure you take plenty of liquids however.

TYPES OF CONSTIPATION

There are essentially two types of constipation. Where there is inadequate fibre and a sluggish digestive system, treatment should be aimed at toning up the bowel; when the constipation is linked to high levels of stress and spasm, see Colic (page 56), treatment may need to focus on relaxation and even reducing excessive fibre such as bran. If in doubt seek professional treatment, as the regular use of laxatives may be completely counter-productive.

Given that approaching $500 million are spent in the United States each year on self-prescribed laxatives, there are good reasons to look at more natural ways!

HOMEOPATHY

As usual, try to match the symptom pattern to the person.

BRYONIA: for hard, dry stools with much thirst and a dry mouth too. The stools can look a very dark brown colour.

NUX VOMICA: for a bloated abdomen; after a bowel movement there is a definite feeling that the bowel has not been properly emptied. Often due to a history of over-eating and chronic use of laxatives.

SULPHUR: for dark, hard stools which are moved only with pain and straining and may cause a burning sensation. Sometimes there is a pattern of alternating constipation and looseness.

NATUROPATHY

In most instances, increase dietary fibre by eating more fresh vegetables and fruit, whole grains and beans or pulses. Bran is a somewhat excessive form of fibre when taken on its own rather than as part of a wholefood meal, so take only small amounts of it, if at all. Ensure that you increase exercise, particularly for the abdominal muscles, and regularly do deeper breathing exercises to encourage the diaphragm to move up and down; this acts internally to massage part of the colon and aid peristalsis.

If constipation occurs after antibiotic treatment, the normal intestinal bacteria can be stimulated by taking a Vitamin B complex supplement, and also with *Lactobacillus acidophilus.* This is the bacteria that turns milk into yoghurt. Taking a little plain, *live* yoghurt daily may do the trick; if this is not enough or if sensitive to dairy foods try one of the proprietary acidophilus supplements.

DANDELION ROOT *(Taraxacum officinale)*

DIARRHOEA

Loose, frequent bowel movements can happen as a short-term reaction to infection, inflammation or food poisoning, and as such are quite a positive, cleansing action. A common experience is holiday diarrhoea, and this is usually a response to exposure to unfamiliar bacteria.

AROMATHERAPY

Massage of the abdomen (see page 56) with antiseptic and relaxing oils like Chamomile, Lavender and Neroli can ease diarrhoea caused by minor upsets and also by anxiety and nervousness. Eucalyptus can be used in the same way if an infection is definitely suspected as the cause. Add Fennel or Ginger if there are griping pains with the diarrhoea. For all these oils, dilute to 3 per cent in a base oil.

HERBALISM

If mild food poisoning or infection has upset the bowels, as well as a choice of infusions (see page 12) listed below, try eating garlic as a natural gut disinfectant.

AGRIMONY (*Agrimonia eupatoria*): astringent and healing to the inflamed and swollen membrane lining the gut, helpful in mild gastro-enteritis.

CHAMOMILE (*Chamomilla recutita*): calming and anti-inflammatory, reduces the impact of tension on the digestive tract. This is one of the first herbs to think of in many digestive disorders.

MEADOWSWEET (*Filipendula*

LAVENDER (*Lavandula angustifolia*)

CAUSES OF DIARRHOEA

Some foods have a laxative effect naturally, for instance prunes or figs, so over-indulgence will give temporary diarrhoea. Stress and anxiety often increase peristalsis and hurry bowel contents through. Repeated diarrhoea may indicate more complex digestive problems and should be treated professionally. Prolonged diarrhoea, especially in young children, can be quite serious as it causes dehydration; ensure adequate fluid intake and seek professional advice. A simple yet dramatically effective rehydration drink can be made by dissolving 5 ml (1 tsp) salt and 15 ml (1 tbsp) sugar in 600 ml (1 pt/ 2 ½ cups) of boiled water. Keep in the refrigerator in a screw-topped bottle and give small amounts frequently. Use for a short time only.

ulmaria): this will help to settle an acidic stomach, see Acidity and Heartburn (page 55), as well as being mildly astringent.

RIBWORT (*Plantago lanceolata*): this has excellent toning, soothing and healing properties for use in diarrhoea from many causes, where there is inflammation.

THYME (*Thymus vulgaris*): this will fight infections and improve digestion generally, settling churning, loose bowels and killing harmful bacteria.

HOMEOPATHY

Many homeopathic remedies feature diarrhoea in their symptom "picture"; three generally useful remedies are:

ARSENICUM ALBUM: typically for diarrhoea from food infected with bacteria; the stools tend to be burning to the skin, dark, greenish brown and smelly.

NUX VOMICA: diarrhoea alternating with constipation, due to over-rich foods, alcohol and so on. Worse after a large meal, any discomfort is relieved by bowel movement.

PULSATILLA: rich, fatty meals, or foods like onions, or excessive nervousness are common triggers for the diarrhoea. The stools are very variable. (Pulsatilla people tend to be gentle, shy, pale and prone to being weepy if ill.)

NATUROPATHY

Try not to use treatments to stem diarrhoea for at least 24 hours, to allow any natural cleansing process to take place. Take plenty of fluids, especially mineral water or herb teas if warm drinks are desired. Moving on to easily assimilated foods such as soups, fruit or vegetable juices helps replace lost nutrients, speeds up recovery and lets the inflamed bowel settle. Plain boiled rice is one of the best first solids, or possibly dry toast.

It may be useful to consider a multi-mineral supplement if diarrhoea was intense, to replenish the minerals lost. Fruit and vegetables can soon be returned to the diet as well.

FLATULENCE

The accumulation of gas in the stomach or intestines can occur as an isolated event, for instance after a meal containing particularly wind-producing foods, or can be a constant, chronic sign of a digestive problem. In the latter case, it may indicate a condition such as diverticulitis or irritable bowel syndrome, and these will need to be addressed in order to sort out the causes of the flatulence.

AROMATHERAPY

Many essential oils have a carminative action, which means that they help to shift gas out of the digestive system (up or down, depending where it is!) and also reduce bloating and spasm that can go with the wind. It may be most appropriate, however, to use the aromatic herbs from which the oils are extracted (see Herbalism entry below). Oils such as Caraway, Chamomile, Fennel, Marjoram and Peppermint could also be used as a warm compress (see page 15) over the abdomen to help relieve the symptoms; use up to 5 drops in a small bowl of warm water.

HERBALISM

A number of herbal teas are excellent at relieving flatulence, but do remember that if this is a major problem to get professional herbal treatment. Choose from Catmint (*Nepeta cataria*), Chamomile (*Chamomilla recutita*), Lemon Balm (*Melissa officinalis*) or Peppermint (*Mentha piperita*) if the problem is in the stomach; any of these plus Dill (*Anethum graveolens*) or Fennel (*Foeniculum vulgare*) if the small intestines seem to be affected, and Ginger (*Zingiber officinalis*) or Peppermint (*Mentha piperita*) for bowel flatulence, although there are several others that may be useful depending on the problem (see other entries in this section).

CARAWAY
(*Carum carvi*)

EATING HABITS

A useful starting point for self-treatment of flatulence is to look at eating habits; are you eating very quickly, while tense, or grabbing a bite to eat "on the run"? This is likely to lead to swallowing gas with the food; inadequate digestive enzymes may be produced and the meal can ferment in the intestines rather than be properly digested.

This leads to more gas being created and flatulence gets worse. Also, take care not to do a lot of bending, or sitting curled up on a low sofa, immediately after a meal, as this encourages a gas build-up with bloating and collicky pains.

HOMEOPATHY

Several remedies featured elsewhere in this section may help; try to look beyond the flatulence to deeper causes and seek the remedy for those. Initially, pick from Chamomilla, Carbo veg, Nux vomica or Pulsatilla, for flatulence brought on by eating too rich or too big a meal.

NATUROPATHY

Often flatulence can be caused by eating too heavy a mixture of foods – consider reducing the fat content of your diet, and restricting the combinations of proteins and carbohydrates you eat. If this helps a lot, then you might want to consider exploring the Hay system of eating.

One reason for flatulence can be after administration of antibiotics, as the intestinal bacteria have been decimated; these can be encouraged to multiply by taking plain "live" yoghurt, or possibly more concentrated supplements such as *acidophilus* tablets/powders. A high-fibre, raw-food diet is often recommended for general health; this is in itself likely to give you more gas, especially if you switch over suddenly to this kind of diet. The increase in bacteria needed to cope with the fibre creates a lot of wind. Some flatulence is therefore quite natural, if not exactly sociable! It is often better to change the diet more gradually to ease the problem.

GALL-BLADDER PROBLEMS

Gallstones may steadily grow in size or number with very few symptoms for a long time, except perhaps increased indigestion or flatulence, but may cause acute colic if the gall-bladder gets inflamed. Gallstones need professional treatment, and sometimes surgery, but there is much that can be done to ease the discomfort alongside qualified medical help.

AROMATHERAPY

Not really a first-choice discipline, but warm compresses (see page 15) over the right side of the abdomen, using diluted oils of Lavender, Marjoram or Rosemary, may relieve spasm and colic.

HERBALISM

Start with the most gentle herbs. If gallstones are definitely present, a scan is needed to establish their size before any treatment is prescribed. CHAMOMILE (*Chamomilla recutita*) tea is both anti-inflammatory and anti-spasmodic, and gently stimulates the whole digestive process.
DANDELION ROOT (*Taraxacum officinale*) is an excellent mild liver tonic; ideally

MARJORAM (*Origanum majorana*)

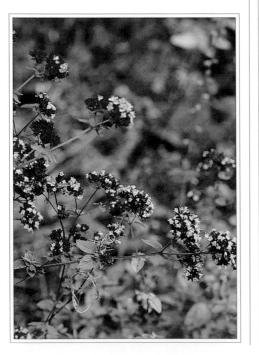

make a decoction (see page 12) and take a small cupful twice a day. Look also at the herbs listed for Colic and for Flatulence (pages 56 and 59); they are

DANDELION DECOCTION

Although dandelion leaves can be made into a tea, a stronger medicine can be made from the roots by making a decoction.

1 Simmer 50 g (2 oz) clean, chopped root in water.

2 Strain through a sieve and store in the fridge. Give in doses of 5-20 ml (1 tsp-1½ tbsp), 3 times a day. It will keep for 3 days.

ROSEMARY (*Rosmarinus officinalis*)

likely in most cases to aid digestion and relieve congestion in the liver and gall-bladder.

HOMEOPATHY

As a short-term measure, try a few doses of either of these before consulting a qualified practitioner:
BRYONIA: where food lies heavily in the stomach, there may be nausea, biliousness and headache.
NUX VOMICA: for feelings of nausea in the mornings, if brought on by rich meals.

NATUROPATHY

Disturbances in the gall-bladder, with or without gallstones, will affect how well fats are digested, so the first step is to restrict animal fats and dairy produce, while increasing vegetables and fruit. To encourage bile production and flow, eat vegetables such as artichokes and bitter salads such as endive and chicory, as well as taking plenty of garlic and fruit to reduce cholesterol (lemon juice is powerful in this respect). Use smaller amounts of light oils such as Olive, Sunflower and Safflower in dressings.

INDIGESTION

Indigestion is a general term for discomfort, often accompanied by bloating, acidity, heartburn, nausea or bowel disturbances (see other entries in this section). Usually it is a temporary problem, brought about by eating too much or the wrong kind of food, excess alcohol or from stress. Longer-term digestive pains may be caused among other reasons by taking aspirin-related drugs, by heavy smoking or other digestive ailments.

AROMATHERAPY

A warm compress (see page 15) including Chamomile or Lavender oils may give some relief, or try gently massaging a 2 per cent dilution of one of them into the abdomen if indigestion is milder.

HERBALISM

Herbal teas in the first place may well sort out the immediate indigestion, choose from:

CHAMOMILE (*Chamomilla recutita*): for the effects of over-eating, also if in a stressed state.

LEMON BALM (*Melissa officinalis*): for nervous indigestion; related to meals or not, settles a churning stomach.

MEADOWSWEET (*Filipendula ulmaria*): for acid indigestion, especially if accompanied by some looseness in the bowels.

LEMON BALM (*Melissa officinalis*)

PEPPERMINT (*Mentha piperita*)

PEPPERMINT (*Mentha piperita*): for indigestion with plenty of flatulence and bloated abdomen, or even nausea. Also think of taking Slippery Elm (*Ulmus fulva*) if indigestion pains are persistent, either 5 ml (1 tsp) of the powder blended in a cupful of water, or the pure tablets, with one or more meals, to soothe the stomach.

HOMEOPATHY

For an occasional bout of indigestion, try a couple of doses (see page 10) of:

ARGENT NIT: where there is a lot of wind, with belching and possibly heartburn, a craving for sweet or fatty foods which tend to upset the digestion and give diarrhoea.

LYCOPODIUM: for pains and wind; if hungry but can only take small amounts of food, worse with cold foods or drink.

NUX VOMICA: useful for the effects of eating and drinking too much, causing pain, heartburn and even vomiting.

NATUROPATHY

If indigestion is quite bad, cut out solid food for 24 hours if possible, taking only herb teas or fruit juices (particularly pineapple which contains digestive enzymes), and reintroduce foods gently, starting with something light like soup or puréed apple. If indigestion is repetitive, try taking a Vitamin B complex supplement as a digestive stimulant, or else look at a digestive enzyme supplement such as Pepsin in the short term, but it may be better to get professional treatment. Avoid drinking lots of fluid at mealtimes, as this will dilute your natural digestive juices.

Chamomile tea is a relaxing aid to the digestive system.

MOUTH ULCERS

These small ulcers, that can occur on the tongue, gums or the lining of the mouth, are sometimes due to local trauma, for instance biting your cheek or wearing ill-fitting dentures, but often they reflect a state of generally being run-down. Recurrent "crops" of mouth ulcers may therefore need more overall treatment; see Stress (pages 28-9) as well as anything directed locally.

AROMATHERAPY

The essential oil of choice for treating mouth ulcers is undoubtedly Myrrh. This is not only astringent and healing but also has an anti-fungal property; one of the reasons for mouth ulcers can be fungal infection, for example *Candida albicans* (the cause of thrush). Myrrh is best used in tincture form (see Herbalism below); you can make your own in small amounts by dissolving the essential oil in alcohol – use 5 drops in 5 ml (1 tsp) of a spirit such as vodka or brandy. This can be applied neat right on to the ulcers, or use 2.5 ml (½ tsp) in a little water as a mouthwash. You can add 1 drop of oil of Fennel to make it taste better, dissolving it thoroughly.

HERBALISM

Local treatment is by means of herbal tinctures (see page 14), to stimulate healing

CONE FLOWER
(*Echinacea angustifolia*)

and reduce the inflammation. The strongest, although worst tasting, is Myrrh (*Commiphora molmol*); others to choose from are Marigold (*Calendula officinalis*), Sage (*Salvia officinalis*) and Thyme (*Thymus vulgaris*). Pay attention to general health, and seek professional treatment if the ulcers are persistent or recurring. Cone Flower (*Echinacea angustifolia* or *E. purpurea*) may be a useful herb to take; it boosts the immune system and is widely obtainable in tablet form, or a tincture of the fresh plant is also available – take 10 drops in water 3 times a day.

HOMEOPATHY

Remedies are more likely to be of benefit if they are chosen for the background causes, but some examples of those remedies that are of value for the ulcers are:

BORAX: for painful small ulcers that feel hot in the mouth and may even bleed, when eating for instance.

MERC SOL: when there is an unpleasant, metallic taste in the mouth, with larger, almost greyish ulcers and perhaps bleeding gums; good for oral thrush.

NAT SULPH: for very painfully sensitive ulcers which may look like blisters, the discomfort is relieved by something cold such as an ice cube.

NATUROPATHY

Recurrent mouth ulcers can often indicate a poor diet, or nutritional deficiencies. Nutrients most likely to be

MYRRH (*Commiphora molmol*)

lacking, and consequently of most benefit in treating the problem, are Vitamin B2, Vitamin C and zinc, and supplements of these may be needed in the short term until the diet can be improved to give sufficient amounts – increase green leafy vegetables, fresh fruit, whole grain bread (including the wheatgerm) and for non-vegetarians eat some meat and fish.

Mouth ulcers most often occur at times of stress or when the immune system is lowered in some way, so it is generally advisable to look at ways of reducing the impact of stress (see pages 28-9) if ulcers are recurring frequently.

For direct local treatment, try applying pure wheatgerm oil, for example by piercing a natural, oil-based Vitamin E capsule, and dabbing a little on to the ulcer. If there are foods, for instance vinegar, that do aggravate the ulcers, obviously leave them out of the diet for a while.

NAUSEA AND VOMITING

There are a great many reasons for feelings of nausea, or actual vomiting. Often this is a temporary reaction, for example to over-eating or drinking, food poisoning, a gastric infection, violent coughing, travel sickness, or associated with a migraine; if nausea or vomiting is persistent, then professional help is essential. Children in particular can easily become dehydrated from repeatedly vomiting.

AROMATHERAPY

Warm compresses (see page 15) over the stomach may be of help. Choose from oils of Chamomile, Lavender or Peppermint, up to 5 drops in a small bowl of water. Taking 1 drop *only* of oil of Cloves or Peppermint, on a sugar lump, may help to directly settle the stomach. A useful oil to spray around the sick room is Lemon, this is not only helpful to allay feelings of nausea but also is much fresher smelling and less sickly than some oils, so will be generally appreciated by the household!

HERBALISM

The remedy of first choice is probably Ginger (*Zingiber officinalis*); either take frequent sips of a weak tea, or of 10 drops of tincture (see page14) in a little water, or chew a small

CRYSTALLIZED GINGER

piece of fresh ginger. Another possibility – say, for travel sickness – is to chew a little crystallized ginger, or drink flat ginger ale.

Other potentially useful herbs to settle the stomach are Chamomile (*Chamomilla recutita*), Lemon Balm (*Melissa officinalis*) and Peppermint (*Mentha piperita*); try weakish herb teas. All these herbs aid digestion generally, and ease flatulence, so can help to sort out the causes of nausea as well as the symptoms themselves.

HOMEOPATHY

As ever, try to establish the causes and the overall pattern. In the meantime, useful remedies include:
ARSENICUM ALBUM: for severe nausea, perhaps associated with diarrhoea, and a great thirst but unable to take more than a few sips at a time.
IPECACUANHA: for sudden and persistent nausea or vomiting, with much watery saliva and frequent belching; symptoms are made worse by cold drinks.
NUX VOMICA: following over-indulgence or excessive drinking, nausea may come on soon after the meal, with waterbrash and food coming back into the mouth.

NATUROPATHY

Obviously keep off solids in the short term, but do keep up fluid intake, either warm or cool drinks depending on preference. When the sickness has subsided, re-introduce light, easily assimilated foods such as clear soup, then slightly more solid dishes like plain whole grain toast, boiled brown rice and cooked vegetables. Gradually return to your normal diet over a couple of days. Smaller meals will be helpful. If anxiety is producing the nausea, then relaxation exercises will help; see Anxiety and Stress (pages 19 and 28-9).

LEMON BALM (*Melissa officinalis*)

CAUSES OF NAUSEA

Nausea or vomiting can usually be linked to a specific situation – eating too much rich food, or drinking too much alcohol, anxiety or travel are common triggers.

Continual feelings of nausea indicate a greater disturbance; again this may be obvious as in morning sickness of pregnancy. Where the cause is not obvious, and if symptoms are not quickly cleared up with self-help, get medical advice as soon as possible.

The Reproductive System

The health of our reproductive system is completely intertwined with our general health. Our creative and reproductive energies derive from our basic vitality, and it is this that herbalism seeks to sustain and enhance. With self-treatment, therefore, it is also sensible to look at overall health. Many books, for instance, link together the reproductive and urinary systems; clearly they have physical links, and treatment for conditions such as an enlarged prostate will affect urine flow directly.

Tension and stress can strongly disturb hormone production, and conversely during hormonal changes, such as the menopause, there is a lowered capacity to cope with stresses. Good nutrition, exercise and posture all affect our reproductive organs. It thus makes sense to give yourself a general overhaul if you have any of the problems discussed below, and do remember that the suggestions made are no substitute for professional treatment.

A word of caution for women who are pregnant or intending to become pregnant. The following aromatherapy oils should be avoided during pregnancy (particularly during the first five months) because of their strong diuretic properties or tendency to induce menstruation: Bay, Basil, Clary Sage, Comfrey, Fennel, Hyssop, Juniper, Marjoram, Melissa, Myrrh, Rosemary, Thyme and Sage. Use all essential oils in half the usual quantity during pregnancy and take extra care when handling them. Ensure that the oils you are using are pure essential oils, as adulterated blends or synthetic oils can sometimes have less predictable effects. Because of their potentially toxic nature and strong abortive qualities, Oreganum, Pennyroyal, St John's Wort, Tansy and Wormwood should only be used by a qualified aromatherapist and must be avoided during pregnancy.

RIGHT: *A healthy diet, with plenty of whole grain foods, is essential to all our body systems.*

IMPOTENCE

The inability of a man to achieve or maintain an erection is a condition that most often results from mental or emotional problems, perhaps anxiety in general or about a particular relationship or sexual situation. The whole area of sex drive is a major subject in its own right (see Reading Suggestions, page 125); there are often physical causes of persistent infertility, but libido can be improved in many ways.

AROMATHERAPY

Due to the subtle yet profound impact that aromatic essential oils can have on our moods and emotions, they can play a very positive part in reducing the effects of stress on libido. One obvious way to use them is in the bath; another may be to get your partner to give you a massage with diluted essential oils (2.5 per cent dilution in a carrier oil), this should be with the aim of creating close contact without the pressure of needing to "perform" – if making love does result that's fine, just don't make it a condition of the massage!

Suitable oils to consider include Sandalwood (which is often liked by men as well as women), Jasmine, Neroli and Ylang Ylang. These are all likely to have a relaxing and uplifting effect. One factor in choosing an oil is because you like the smell; this may seem desirable generally but in this kind of problem it is obviously essential.

HERBALISM

As outlined in the introductory section, the herbal approach should be to look at boosting vitality and better health. Many herbs that may help with problems of impotence are thus tonics; they may have other actions over time, and so only use the suggested herbs for a short period, say 3 weeks, before taking a break or seeking professional advice.

Where tension is a major factor, try using Oatstraw (*Avena sativa*) in tablets

DAMIANA *(Turnera diffusa)*

or up to 2.5 ml (½ tsp) of the tincture (see page 14) twice daily. If exhaustion or depression are more significant, then take teas of either Damiana (*Turnera diffusa*) or Rosemary (*Rosmarinus officinalis*): these are both tonics and Damiana in particular is valuable in toning the male hormonal system. Another possibility is Ginseng, which helps our systems adapt better to excess stress. This is available in tablet or liquid form – there are really three kinds, with varying effects: Asiatic (*Panax schinseng*) which is more stimulating, American (*P. quinquefolium*) which is more relaxing, and Siberian (*Eleutherococcus senticosus*) which is an unrelated plant with similar tonic properties.

Ginseng remedies should generally be avoided by people with very high blood pressure, without first seeking professional herbal advice.

HOMEOPATHY

Undoubtedly the best results will be found by seeing a professional homeopath, since there are so many factors which will determine the best remedy. Some examples are:

ARGENT NIT: a good remedy where there is a lot of apprehension or fear, in this case about a relationship or sexual situation.

KALI PHOS: strengthens the nervous system, when exhaustion or even depression is interfering with general vitality. Good for younger people, who have temporarily exhausted themselves.

SEPIA: for loss of sex drive and lowered interest in your partner and the relationship. Good for slightly older people, or those more chronically run-down, tired and exhausted.

NATUROPATHY

Sexual vitality depends on general health and well-being, and so attention should be paid to diet. Of particular benefit are Vitamins E, B and C, and also zinc (10 mg), and there may be a case in the short term for supplements of these, possibly in a multi-vitamin and mineral tablet.

Exercise, and also adequate rest, are both important, and splashing warm and cold water around the pelvic area will stimulate circulation. For similar reasons, avoid excessively hot baths before intercourse. Finally, don't drink a lot of alcohol as a means of trying to reduce anxiety before intercourse – it doesn't help in maintaining an erection!

MENOPAUSAL PROBLEMS

The change of life, when periods cease, can be a tremendously variable experience; for some women there is very little disturbance to their lives, except for the relief of no longer having monthly bleeding. For others, symptoms such as hot flushes, anxiety, insomnia, heavy periods, depression or severe vaginal dryness make their lives thoroughly miserable for a long time. Each person is different; don't hesitate to get advice.

AROMATHERAPY

During the pre- or peri-menopausal phase, which may last for years leading up to the point when ovulation finally stops, the periods may become quite erratic (see also Menstrual Problems, page 68). Useful oils to think of include Geranium and Rose, both of which seem to have a regulating, balancing effect on the female hormone cycle. Also, uplifting oils such as Bergamot, Neroli or Jasmine can help a great deal with the emotional swings that may occur – other life changes, such as children growing up and leaving home for the first time can often

ROSE *(Rosa species)*

HORMONE REPLACEMENT THERAPY

Conventional treatment has now focused on hormone replacement therapy (HRT), and while this has helped ease the symptoms for a lot of women, others react badly to it and it is very clearly not suitable for everybody. There are other ways of helping the process, some of which are described below.

coincide at this time, so there may be a general sense of upheaval and loss.

For all these oils, either use a few drops in the bath, or dilute to 1 per cent in a base oil and massage into the skin. Try ringing the changes with the oils too, so that you do not use one exclusively for more than a couple of weeks. While it may not seem scientific, if you are drawn towards the scent of a particular essential oil, then it is most often what you need at the time!

HERBALISM

Many herbs have quite powerful hormonal effects – the contraceptive pill itself was originally derived from a species of Mexican Yam – and professional treatment may be needed here. A common herb which can often improve problems such as hot sweats, depression and irritability, is Sage *(Salvia officinalis)*. Not only is this a tonic for the nervous system, and reduces excess sweating, but it has oestrogenic activity and can ease the dramatic drop in hormone levels that upset the whole system. Take 2 small cupfuls of an infusion (see page 12) for a month to see if it is helping.

Another herb with hormonal effects is Chaste Tree *(Vitex agnus castus)*. The berries are used, and act via the pituitary gland to encourage the ovaries, and seem to have a more progesterogenic effect (see also Pre-menstrual Symptoms, page 71). This herb may be taken as a tea or in tablet form (up to 300 mg per day); do not overdo the dosage as this can induce an itching sensation on the skin, and as always if there is no improvement, then seek professional advice. Simple relaxants like Chamomile *(Chamomilla*

CHASTE TREE
(*Vitex agnus castus*)

recutita) and Lime Blossom (*Tilia europaea*) may help to reduce some of the emotional swings that may happen during the menopause.

HOMEOPATHY

The emphasis of all these therapies is to assist the normal changes that occur with the stopping of menstruation, without trying to interfere to any great extent. Homeopathic treatments will similarly aim to encourage the physiological and mental adjustments. On a self-help basis, you may find some relief from excessive symptoms with remedies such as the following:

HRT AND HEART DISEASE
Recent information has suggested that HRT may be helpful in protecting against some kinds of heart disease; this does, however, need to be balanced against an increased risk of some other diseases. An active lifestyle on the other hand can provide good health benefits for the heart and circulation, as well as the bones and muscles, and should be thought of as an essential part of good health during and after the menopause.

PULSATILLA: for hot flushes with a lot of sweating, perhaps giving a musty odour. If cold drinks generally ease symptoms, then this may be a suitable remedy. SEPIA: for sudden hot flushes, with a feeling of faintness, reddened face and probably some sweating. Warmth may actually help to ease the discomfort. May be inclined towards anxiety or irritability.

NATUROPATHY

Keeping to a healthy diet can do wonders for overall vitality, and this in turn helps to give you greater resilience against any problems during

the menopause. Hot flushes may be eased by taking additional Vitamin E, around 100 iu twice a day, while at least 500 mg calcium per day, preferably in a supplement containing a little Vitamin A and D and magnesium, can help to prevent osteoporosis from calcium loss. It is essential to continue to do some exercise, such as walking, cycling or even jogging, which also helps to maintain calcium levels as well as strengthening the heart and lungs.

LIME BLOSSOM (Tilia europaea) is a simple relaxant which may help reduce the emotional swings which are often associated with the menopause.

MENSTRUAL PROBLEMS

Disturbances in the menstrual cycle can be of various kinds, and can be due to a wide number of factors, so it is essential to take a broad, holistic view of health. For persistent problems, or if self-help does not correct matters, do seek professional help.

AROMATHERAPY

In order to get relief from painful periods, with cramping pains, a gentle and slow abdominal massage may be needed. Using oils which aid relaxation of muscle spasm, such as Chamomile, Lavender, Lemon Balm or Marjoram, will help a great deal. If massage cannot be tolerated, try using a few drops of one of these oils in a hot compress over the abdomen. Lemon Balm, often called Melissa oil after its Latin name, also has a generally balancing effect on the menstrual cycle; however, it is highly concentrated, and very expensive (often adulterated) and drinking a tea from the fresh leaves may be more suitable for longer term treatment. Rose oil seems to have regulating effects too, but is also expensive.

Many essential oils have a stimulating effect on the uterine muscles, and need to be avoided in pregnancy, or suspected pregnancy – used as above, they may be useful in scanty or irregular bleeding. Refer to the list on page 64 for a list of oils to avoid in pregnancy, but avoid all essential oils if in doubt that pregnancy is a possible cause and get professional advice and treatment.

HERBALISM

Menstrual disorders are an area where herbal medicine comes into its own for two reasons: firstly, many herbs have quite significant hormonal effects and, secondly, the holistic

TYPES OF MENSTRUAL PROBLEMS

Lack of periods altogether (or amenorrhoea) can happen due to emotional traumas, excessive exercise, sharp swings in weight such as loss brought on by anorexia or physical debility; irregular periods may result from similar causes, and of course both disturbances can happen when going into the menopause. More commonly for many women, periods may become too painful (dysmenorrhoea) – this may be due to a hormonal imbalance (see also Pre-menstrual Symptoms, pages 71-2). Excessively heavy menstrual bleeding (or menorrhagia) may happen without any obvious cause, but can also indicate more complex disorders such as fibroids or pelvic infection. A potential problem with menorrhagia is the risk of becoming anaemic. Finally, don't forget one of the most obvious reasons for lack of periods – pregnancy!

approach of herbalism means treatment can help restore overall balance much better than simply using synthetic hormones.

Painful periods may be relieved

in the first place by taking infusions (see page 12) of either Lemon Balm (*Melissa officinalis*) or Chamomile (*Chamomilla recutita*). More severe cramping can be eased with a decoction (see page 12) of either Cramp Bark (European Cranberry Bush) (*Viburnum opulus*) or Valerian (*Valeriana officinalis*) – both of these taste quite disgusting, so may be better in tablet form (up to 5 g).

Heavy periods may be regulated by infusions of Yarrow (*Achillea millefolium*) or more strongly by Lady's Mantle (*Alchemilla vulgaris*) or White Deadnettle (*Lamium album*) – these are also all useful to drink to reduce leucorrhea, or discharge, between periods; if anaemia is suspected, try drinking ordinary Nettle tea regularly. Some herbal remedies are perhaps best left to professional practice, especially when hormonal imbalances are behind the symptoms.

HOMEOPATHY

The need for professional help in complex cases also applies to homeopathic treatment, but here are a few possible remedies for occasional problems:

ACONITE: for suppressed menstruation due to a sudden shock or from getting

VALERIAN (*Valeriana officinalis*)

LADY'S MANTLE
(*Alchemilla vulgaris*)

thoroughly chilled (getting cold feet, literally or metaphorically).

NAT MUR: for irregular periods, which may be profuse when they do start; associated with feelings of general sadness and when possibly the delay is due to emotional upset.

PULSATILLA: for painful, spasmodic and scanty periods most often linked to tension; can be helpful when periods have failed to start in puberty.

NATUROPATHY

Exercise is beneficial in improving blood flow through the pelvic basin. During a period this may speed up the bleeding but will also probably shorten the length of the bleeding, and reduce muscle spasm. Hot and cold applications to the lower abdomen and back will have similar effects – these can be done by finishing a shower by reducing the temperature for a few seconds, or by splashing with cool water at

the end of a bath, or even using hot/cold compresses (see page 15). A diet high in natural fibre from vegetables, fruit, pulses, beans and whole grains will not only provide nourishment for the reproductive system but will also help to avoid constipation which can accompany painful periods.

Useful supplements may include calcium, preferably with magnesium, to ease painful cramps if taken just prior to and during the period (around 500 mg). Vitamin E, up to 300 iu daily, may be useful during this time of the cycle too, especially if periods are scanty and painful. Both iron and folic acid may be required if there is any sign of anaemia.

Regular exercise improves pelvic circulation and muscle tone, thereby reducing congestion and cramps.

SELF-HELP MEASURES

A major factor for many women in producing disturbances of the menstrual cycle is excessive stress. This can cause irregular, scanty or painful periods for instance. Changes in lifestyle, to include more opportunities for relaxation, perhaps increased exercise and an improved diet, can have a dramatic effect on hormone levels and menstrual patterns.

Another potential cause of irregular periods is sudden and drastic dieting. Excessive dieting is never a good idea, and can result in the temporary loss of periods altogether. If you need to lose weight, do it gradually and under the guidance of a professional dietician or your family doctor. Natural forms of medicine and treatment may be required alongside self-help, but don't neglect the latter.

Oil of Evening Primrose, or a similar supplement such as Starflower oil, may be valuable in helping to regulate the periods. Evening Primrose oil may be taken just for 10 days pre-period, up to 2,000 mg, or throughout the month at half the dosage.

MORNING SICKNESS

At least half of all pregnant women experience nausea or vomiting during the first 12 weeks or so of their pregnancy; only in rare circumstances does this become so severe as to warrant drugs or hospital treatment. There seems to be good reason to link the sickness, which may actually occur at any time of day or night, with a lowered blood sugar level, and it is often very useful to eat regularly to maintain a more even state.

AROMATHERAPY

Essential oils can be of some use in this condition – their concentration and powerful effects, however, mean that caution is needed during pregnancy with all oils (see page 64 for further advice). For nausea, simply try smelling a drop of Ginger or Peppermint oil on a paper tissue.

HERBALISM

The prime remedy for nausea, including morning sickness, is Ginger (*Zingiber officinalis*). This can be taken in various ways; try chewing a piece of crystallized ginger, or even a piece of peeled fresh ginger, or making ginger tea and sipping frequently. A very useful method is to eat biscuits (cookies) made with fresh ginger, nibbling one as and when the need arises – this temporarily raises the body's sugar level as well as providing the effect of the ginger itself. Other useful herbs are Chamomile (*Chamomilla recutita*) and Peppermint (*Mentha piperita*) taken as teas; as a practitioner I have found that in pregnancy the smell of the former often seems to be more off-putting than any benefit from the herb, but see for yourself.

CAUTION
While the suggestions made here are all well-tried and safe, it is not advisable to self-treat during pregnancy. This book is <u>not</u> a substitute for seeking professional or medical advice, this is especially true for ailments during pregnancy.

HOMEOPATHY

There are several remedies in which nausea or vomiting are major indications; try one of these for a few days to see if they give any relief:

IPECACUANHA: for continual nausea, and frequent vomiting, which does not give much relief. The tongue generally seems quite clean in appearance.

NUX VOMICA: for nausea and a lot of retching; it may be more difficult to vomit but it does help ease the nausea. The tongue is coated and may look almost brown.

SEPIA: mostly just for nausea, especially associated with smelling food or getting chilled; or

PEPPERMINT (*Mentha piperita*)

GINGER (*Zingiber officinalis*)

when the symptom is relieved with warm drinks or possibly a warm application to the stomach.

NATUROPATHY

The fact that early morning is a particularly bad time for getting the nausea confirms the importance of the blood-sugar levels; try keeping some whole grain biscuits by the bed to nibble if you feel empty and nauseous on waking. In general avoid greasy or fatty foods and cut down on coffee and alcohol. A diet with plenty of whole grains, pulses and vegetables will help to keep blood-sugar levels more constant, as will eating at regular times during the day.

Eating a piece of fruit when hungry can help keep nausea at bay.

PRE-MENSTRUAL SYMPTOMS

There are a number of symptoms that can occur in the second half of the menstrual cycle, i.e. leading up to the period, due mostly to imbalances in hormone production. These symptoms tend to be lumped together by the medical profession into pre-menstrual syndrome (PMS), but not all women experience them in the same combination or in the same way.

AROMATHERAPY

Essential oils can be helpful in reducing fluid retention; this is most effectively done by using them with lymphatic drainage massage, so do see a professional aromatherapist if this is a major part of your symptoms. Using oils such as Geranium, Grapefruit, Juniper or Rosemary in the bath, and also doing skin-brushing, frequently stroking your limbs up from the extremities towards the heart, are good methods of self-help.

HERBALISM

Probably the most valuable herb for disturbances of the second half of the menstrual cycle is Chaste Tree (*Vitex agnus castus*). The berries are used, and they help to normalize hormone function, particularly in lifting progesterone levels – lowered progesterone is most often the trigger for the symptoms. They can be

COMMON PMS SYMPTOMS

Symptoms include mood changes, with irritability and/or weepiness, headaches and sometimes migraines, fluid retention, tender breasts, and deep aching in the low abdomen or thighs before and at the start of the period. This half of the cycle can also be when creativity and energy, including sexual energy, can be higher so do not automatically assume that the pre-period phase has to be awful.

COUCH GRASS
(*Agropyron repens*)

obtained in tablet form. In very large amounts Chaste Tree can give an irritating sensation under the skin; if this occurs simply stop taking it.

Herbs which have diuretic effects may be useful in giving some relief; try infusions (see page 12) of either Cleavers (*Galium aparine*) or Couch Grass (*Agropyron repens*) – yes, this scourge of gardeners does have important medicinal properties! Two other helpful herbs are Chamomile (*Chamomilla recutita*), both as a diuretic and gentle relaxant, and Lemon Balm (*Melissa officinalis*) which eases the emotional

---

SKIN BRUSHING

1 To improve lymph drainage in the legs and thighs, try daily skin brushing. Lightly and briskly brush the upper legs in an upwards direction a few times, from the knees to the thighs.

2 Then brush the lower legs upwards a few times. Repeat steps 1 and 2, always starting with the upper leg and always brushing upwards towards the heart.

LEMON BALM
(Melissa officinalis)

swings that may happen. In recent times one herb that has gained a high reputation for balancing hormonal swings is Evening Primrose *(Oenothera biennis)*, and it may be worth taking capsules of this in the second half of the period cycle, between 1,000 and 2,000 mg are usually needed. Any improvement in symptoms may take 3-6 months to appear.

HOMEOPATHY

Some possible remedies are:

CALC CARB: for overweight people who feel the cold easily if only during this phase, and have clammy hands and feet; may also experience tension and low abdominal pains.

CALC PHOS: for cold but drier extremities, pains and cramping, with pre-menstrual bloating.

Women for whom either of the above remedies are suited will probably get relief from pre-menstrual discomfort by taking a warm bath or using a hot-water bottle.

LYCOPODIUM: this may be appropriate when there is a good deal of pre-period irritability and tension, which quickly ease when the period starts. Abdominal

STRESS AND PMS

It can be easy to label all physical and emotional upsets as PMS (men tend to this very often), and overlook other causes of problems. Try to keep a check on whether symptoms definitely occur in monthly cycles. A good way of doing this is to keep a diary to keep a record of mood swings and general discomfort. Tension and irritability can be due to over-stress, or genuine relationship problems, which need to be sorted out. Trying to relax can also help if in a stressful situation (see also Stress, pages 28-9).

pain associated with this tension is the major physical symptom.

NATUROPATHY

Both diet and exercise can help tremendously in minimizing pre-menstrual problems. Cut down on alcohol and coffee during this part of the cycle at least, as they both affect fluid balance, and drink plenty of water to encourage kidney

EVENING PRIMROSE
(Oenothera biennis)

function. There has been a lot of evidence that Vitamin B6 can reduce symptoms; this is probably best taken as a supplement (up to 50 mg) as part of a whole Vitamin B complex, maybe with the addition of magnesium (200 mg). Evening Primrose oil has already been discussed earlier; for both this and Vitamin B6 it may be easier to take half the suggested doses throughout the whole of the month.

Regular exercise such as walking, cycling, swimming and running can help reduce the pelvic congestion that may accompany PMS; similarly, splashing hot and cold water around the lower abdomen regularly will improve circulation (see also Menstrual Problems, pages 68-9).

CAUTION

Never mix herbal remedies with homeopathic ones. You should always keep to one system, rather than swapping between the two. Do not increase the dosages suggested here – herbs and plants are very powerful and can produce adverse effects if used without due care and attention.

If in any doubt, consult professional advice.

PROSTATE PROBLEMS

The prostate gland is situated at the base of the bladder, and produces part of the seminal fluid. It surrounds the urethra, but normally causes no problems for urine flow. It is roughly the size of a walnut, but a common condition as men get older is a benign enlargement. This leads the prostate to compress the urethra, and perhaps even the bladder, and urine flow becomes slower to start and/or stop, with some dribbling.

AROMATHERAPY

To be used only as an adjunct to seeking professional treatment. Where there is benign prostate enlargement causing some difficulty in passing urine, placing a hot compress (see page 15) using a few drops of oils of Chamomile, Juniper or Pine over the low abdomen can quickly ease the pressure and get the urine to flow better. If the prostate is inflamed, oil of Chamomile should be included due to its anti-inflammatory effect.

HERBALISM

For an enlarged prostate, an infusion (see page 12) of one or both of the following remedies can help a good deal:

HORSETAIL (*Equisetum arvense*): a strong

SCOTS PINE (*Pinus sylvestris*)

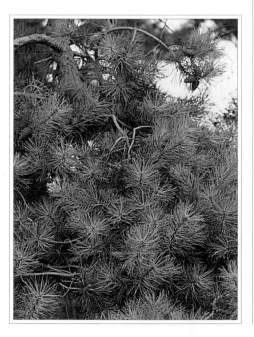

INFLAMMATION OF THE PROSTATE

Another problem can be prostatitis, or inflammation of the prostate, possibly due to a low-grade infection, and this can produce frequent, uncomfortable urination and tenderness of the gland itself. More rarely, although important to bear in mind in older men, prostate cancer can occur. This is, of course, outside the scope of self-treatment; it may be symptomless for some time, until the swollen gland restricts urine flow.

diuretic, increasing urine flow and helping the bladder to empty itself completely – failure to do so can lead to cystitis. It is also astringent and anti-inflammatory, toning the swollen membranes.

WHITE DEADNETTLE (*Lamium album*): another astringent remedy, which seems to have a regulatory effect on blood flow through the pelvic area, and so can reduce excess swelling of the prostate.

These two herbs combined can soothe the membranes and improve urine flow.

Benign prostate enlargement is often associated with lowered testosterone levels, and Saw Palmetto (*Serenoa serrulata*) is a very useful herb in this context. The berries not only have a diuretic and urinary antiseptic effect, but they also have a hormonal action to address the underlying problem. A

decoction (see page 12) is strongest, but the berries could be taken with one or both the other suggested herbs in infusion form.

HOMEOPATHY

Some possible remedies are:

APIS MEL: when there is inflammation, probably with some enlargement, so that there is a frequent desire to pass water, but with only small amounts of stinging, burning urine.

BELLADONNA: when urination is also painful and difficult; the pressure causes some involuntary dribbling of urine when standing or moving around.

PULSATILLA: for frequent, urgent need to pass water, slight dribbling, or incontinence with any movement such as coughing, laughing or sneezing.

NATUROPATHY

Stick to a varied wholefood diet, with plenty of fluids during the day to keep urine moving through the bladder, but reduce coffee, tea or alcohol which can all irritate. Zinc is of special benefit to the prostate. Pumpkin seeds are a good food source and a supplement (up to 20 mg) may be needed daily for a while if symptoms of enlarged prostate develop.

Hydrotherapy treatment is a valuable aid; use alternating hot and cold water for the low abdomen (3 minutes hot and maximum 1 minute cold), either using a shower or splashes in the bath. The ideal method is using Sitz baths, as in hydrotherapy spa clinics.

THRUSH

Thrush is the common name for a fungal infection of the mucous membranes by the yeast *Candida albicans*. It can affect the mouth, and this is sometimes seen in tiny babies, or around the anus or on the penis, but most commonly it is a vaginal infection. A number of things can trigger off an attack of thrush; one of the major causes is often a course of antibiotics, which seriously destroy our helpful, defensive bacteria.

AROMATHERAPY

One of the most significant natural anti-fungal agents is essential oil of Tea Tree. This is available in pessary (insertable) form in some countries, but the oil can be used in the bath or in more concentrated form in a hand-basin of water; use 6 drops in warm water and bathe the vaginal area with it. Although Tea Tree oil is much more soothing than most anti-fungal drugs, do use it well diluted at first in case of any irritation. Other useful oils to use in this way are Lavender and Myrrh, and they could be blended with Tea Tree to help speed up healing.

HERBALISM

Herbalists will probably give much of the advice discussed under Naturopathy below, and are equally likely to recommend the above oils for local use; other herbs that have healing, soothing and anti-fungal effects include Marigold (*Calendula officinalis*) and Cone Flower (*Echinacea angustifolia* or *E. purpurea*). These are best used in tincture form (see page 14); dilute at the rate of 5 ml (1 tsp) to 600 ml

LAVENDER (*Lavandula angustifolia*)

OTHER POSSIBLE CAUSES OF THRUSH

Quite often a vicious circle can be set up by an infection: cystitis – treated by antibiotics – leading to thrush. Other factors can be the contraceptive pill, frequent digestive infections, a diet high in sugars, or generally being over-stressed and run-down.

Conventional treatment involves the use of anti-fungal creams, or pessaries; both of these treatments may be irritating to the membranes, and self-help measures can often be the best route to avoid repetition of the infection.

(1 pt/2½ cups) of warm water, and use as a local wash. For oral thrush in babies apply a little with a cotton bud (swab), and in adults use 5 ml (1 tsp) of the tincture in a little water as a mouthwash. A powerful internal anti-fungal remedy is garlic, and if thrush recurs frequently, taking either fresh garlic or garlic capsules daily can help to combat general yeast infection. It can also be used locally, although it may irritate the vaginal membranes if they are very inflamed – peel a clove of garlic, dip it in olive oil (you may want to tie a piece of cotton thread around it, so you don't lose it inside!), insert in the vagina and leave overnight.

HOMEOPATHY

Treatment will focus on internal remedies, backed up by local self-help measures (see next page). Practitioners may even prescribe homeopathic doses of *Candida* itself, but some other possible remedies are:
MERC SOL: for reddish patches, especially if oral thrush when there may be blisters on the mucous membranes, with thick, slimy discharge and some mould-like odour.

NAT MUR: for white spots, less of a discharge but more painful irritation; in oral thrush

CONE FLOWER (*Echinacea angustifolia*)

MARIGOLD
(*Calendula officinalis*)

there may be painful blisters on the lips or tongue. Drier and more inflamed symptoms make this more suitable as a remedy than Merc sol. SULPHUR: for an itching and burning sensation, and a thick, white discharge with some odour. In oral thrush, Sulphur may be indicated when there is a foul taste and odour, lots of white blisters or yeast coating in the mouth, and dry, rough lips.

NATUROPATHY

Fungal infections thrive in warm, damp environments, so it is important to keep the vaginal area cool and dry, and let it "breathe" more freely

Pure Olive oil, as used in salads, has a natural anti-fungal effect.

– only use cotton underwear, and avoid tights or tight jeans. Do not use bubble baths or strong vaginal deodorants as they can disturb your normal defences. Apart from the oils or herbs to use locally, you may find it helpful to wash with salt water – use about a handful of salt in a hand-basin of warm water. If you are in an active sexual relationship, it is important for both of you to look at these suggestions, as you may re-infect each other without joint treatments. Live, natural (plain) yoghurt can also be used locally, on a sanitary towel (napkin) or tampon; this helps to encourage the defensive bacteria to multiply. If a recent course of antibiotics seem to be the cause, then eating live yoghurt will aid the defensive flora in the gut too.

Since yeasts will flourish on sugars, reduce all concentrated sugar and refined carbohydrates in the diet, and also severely restrict alcohol. Eat plenty of vegetables and whole grains,

and use a fair amount of olive oil for any salad dressings, as this has a natural anti-fungal effect (it may be applied sparingly locally too, especially if the area is dry and inflamed). As a supplement, *Lactobacillus acidophilus* has a significant effect on suppressing yeast invasion and encouraging the gut flora; it is the bacteria which converts milk into yoghurt, but occurs in much higher concentrations in the capsules or powder that are quite widely available. If diarrhoea develops, then stop taking it immediately.

A diet high in fresh vegetables, and low in refined sugars, helps to prevent recurrent thrush.

THE URINARY SYSTEM

O ur general health and vitality are often mirrored in the health of our urinary system. If we are chronically stressed or run-down, we are much more likely to be prone to recurrent cystitis or other urinary infections. Conversely, disorders of our kidneys have a weakening effect on our energy overall, and need to be treated by professional practitioners.

The urinary system is essential in maintaining the fluid balance within the body, and together with the heart and circulatory system it controls blood pressure. Equally importantly the kidneys keep our electrolytes, or fluid-soluble minerals, in balance and aid in removing toxins. Problems of urination can arise not only from infection or serious illness, but are affected by hormonal changes and in men the functioning of the prostate (see The Reproductive System, page 64), and by stress. Muscle tone is also important, especially as people get older and the bladder tends to shrink, or atrophy, and exercises can be helpful for maintaining control of bladder function.

ABOVE: Dandelion (Taraxacum officinale) is a highly effective diuretic. It is also rich in potassium, thereby counteracting any loss of potassium that occurs through urination.

CYSTITIS

Cystitis is an acute infection of the bladder, which may often recur and become a chronic condition. It is more common in girls and women than in boys or men, due to the much shorter length of the urethra in women; in many women it can be triggered off by irritation during sexual intercourse, and useful advice can include emptying the bladder before sex (if pre-meditated enough!) and certainly afterwards.

AROMATHERAPY

Essential oils have quite powerful antiseptic properties, and should be used at the earliest possible stage of cystitis. A useful way to use them is to add them to the bath, up to 10 drops in total added just before getting into the water. Some of the most suitable oils are Bergamot, Chamomile, Lemon (perhaps only use 5 drops if this oil is chosen), and Sandalwood. A warm compress (see page 15), with 3-5 drops of Chamomile or Lavender oils added, can be placed over the lower abdomen if there is a lot of discomfort.

HERBALISM

There are many herbs which have specific effects on the urinary tract, so if the cystitis persists or recurs, do seek professional treatment. In the first instance, drink plenty of fluid,

BEARBERRY *(Arctostaphylos uva-ursi)*

CYSTITIS SYMPTOMS

Symptoms of cystitis can include frequent urging to pass water, accompanied generally by a sharp pain – in women this is usually felt in the urethra, and there is usually inflammation (urethritis) here too, while men tend to experience pain in the penis. The urine may look cloudy or strongly coloured and may have a strong smell. Sometimes there is pain just before or just after urination, perhaps with a feeling of needing to pass water again as fresh urine trickles into the inflamed and irritated bladder.

especially water or infusions (see page 12) chosen from the following herbs. In mild cases simply drinking plenty of herb teas such as Chamomile *(Chamomilla recutita),* or Meadowsweet *(Filipendula ulmaria)* may reduce the inflammation sufficiently to solve the problem. These two herbs can of course also be taken as stronger infusions in acute attacks. Buchu *(Barosma betulina)* is a particularly useful herb, not only acting as a urinary antiseptic but soothing the inflamed

BUCHU *(Barosma betulina)*

membranes too, and helping to escape the cycle of cystitis-antibiotics-cystitis which can easily occur with conventional treatment. Bearberry *(Arctostaphylos uva-ursi)* is another strong antiseptic remedy, most helpful when the urine is acidic and sharply burning. To these herbs can be added Celery Seed *(Apium graveolens)*, which has a very alkaline effect on the urine, Agrimony *(Agrimonia eupatoria)* to tone and astringe the swollen tissues, and/or Marshmallow *(Althea officinalis)* (ideally the root, but the leaf is also good) for its pure soothing properties. It is generally recommended to take plenty of garlic internally to fight infection and to cleanse the tissues for some time after the attack has subsided.

HOMEOPATHY

Symptoms of discomfort when passing urine are a feature of the "remedy picture" (see Introduction to

MAKING BARLEY WATER

Home-made lemon barley water is a nutritious drink to take in place of tea and coffee when suffering from cystitis.

1 Cover 100 g (4 oz) of pearl barley in a little water and bring to the boil, strain and throw away this water. Pour 600 ml (1 pt/2½ cups) of boiling water over the barley (or ideally simmer the barley in 750 ml (1¼ pt/3⅔ cups) of water for 5 minutes, to extract the full benefit.)

2 Add the zest of a lemon and leave to cool. Strain and keep the liquid in the fridge. Drink often.

Homeopathy, page 10) for a large number of homeopathic medicines, so the professional practitioner has a wide choice. For self-treatment, choose initially from:

CANTHARIS: for the classical symptoms of cystitis, burning pains with passing water, which comes only slowly, and also a frequent urge to urinate.

PULSATILLA: for a great urge, and urgency to urinate, causing some pains and distress. Urine may easily dribble out, when coughing or laughing.

STAPHYSAGRIA: when the vulval area is sore or bruised – often given for "honeymoon cystitis".

NATUROPATHY

In the first place, as soon as you feel the twinges of cystitis coming on, drink plenty of water, or herb teas. Avoid alcohol, or strong tea and coffee, which can irritate the bladder lining further. Sometimes it can be helpful to add a pinch of bicarbonate of soda to water to make it alkaline. Avoid obviously acidic foods such as vinegar, unripe fruit or ones like gooseberries, plums, rhubarb or tomatoes.

Many people tend to suffer periodically with cystitis, and for recurrent problems, look at things such as not wearing tight jeans or trousers,

avoid vaginal deodorants and be careful to rinse underwear thoroughly (biological washing powders or detergents can leave irritant traces). If you have had antibiotics, it is very helpful to take plenty of live yoghurt afterwards to repopulate the defensive gut bacteria; a little can also be applied to the vaginal and urethral openings for local effect, especially if you are prone to cystitis.

This helps to alter the local acidity, which encourages the body's natural defences to multiply, and it is also quite cool and soothing to the irritated and inflamed surface.

FLUID RETENTION

Excess fluid in the tissues, or oedema, can happen in a variety of ways. Local, temporary swelling will occur with an injury, for instance a sprained ankle or a large bruise (see First Aid, page 104, for treatment). Fluid retention in the thighs and hips in women is often associated with a build-up of toxins, as in cellulite, and a general detoxifying programme of diet, exercise and massage will be most effective.

AROMATHERAPY

For problems such as fluid retention linked to cellulite, or temporary ankle swelling due to heat or long flights, massage the legs and thighs in an upwards sweeping movement, with a 1-2 per cent dilution of essential oils in a base oil (see page 17). Beneficial oils are Geranium, Grapefruit, Lemon and Rosemary; Juniper has an even stronger diuretic effect, stimulating the kidneys to excrete excess fluid, but do not use if there is any

FENNEL
(*Foeniculum vulgare*)

OTHER CAUSES OF FLUID RETENTION

Fluid retention is often aggravated during the pre-period phase (see also Pre-Menstrual Problems, page 71), especially in the breasts and abdomen. In hot weather most people find that they have some fluid retention, and ankles tend to swell during long plane flights – drink plenty of fluid (but *not* alcohol), and move about the plane as much as possible.

Severe leg and ankle oedema is often a sign of kidney and/or heart malfunction, and should be treated professionally, without delay, as should any unexplained or prolonged fluid retention.

kidney problem or in pregnancy. Another essential oil of value is Fennel, but this has a mild oestrogenic action too, so be careful not to use for long if oedema is hormone-related.

Pregnancy is a time when ankles might swell, but use essential oils sparingly (less than 1 per cent), if at all, and get professional advice if you are unsure. Do not use Fennel or Juniper, and only use Rosemary later on, from the fifth month of the pregnancy, if ankle oedema is a problem.

HERBALISM

In order to encourage the removal of fluid, the simplest approach is to use herb teas which have a diuretic effect. Do not use for more than a week at a time; long-term stimulation of the

---

THIGH AND LEG MASSAGE

1 To improve circulation in the legs, firstly oil the legs. Place hands on the thigh and stroke upwards to the buttock a few times, with light but steady sweeping movements, hand-over-hand.

2 Move hands down to the lower leg and stroke up to the back of the knee a few times. Repeat steps 1 and 2; always start this movement on the upper leg, and always stroke up towards the heart.

urinary system can be tiring and if the swelling has not subsided within a short period, qualified advice and treatment may be necessary.

One of the best herbal diuretics is Dandelion Leaf (*Taraxacum officinale*), indeed its common name in many languages translates as "Wet-the-bed"! When you pass urine, potassium is lost in the fluid, and with some prescribed diuretics this can lead to a potassium deficiency, which is itself a serious condition. Dandelions are so rich in potassium that this loss is counteracted. Make a tea and drink three cupfuls a day initially.

Other common and useful herbs are Chamomile (*Chamomilla recutita*), Fennel (*Foeniculum vulgare*) (but see Aromatherapy section earlier), Meadowsweet (*Filipendula ulmaria*) and Yarrow (*Achillea millefolium*), all of which are diuretic among their other properties.

For just increasing the amount of urine passed, without strain on the kidneys, the best herb is the creeping rhizome of Couch Grass (*Agropyron repens*). In the short term this can be taken as a decoction (see page 12).

HOMEOPATHY

Because of the complexity of the causes of fluid retention, and the fact that homeopathic remedies are aimed at the person's constitutional make-up as far as possible, it is much better to seek professional homeopathic treatment for any water retention. For purely first aid problems such as bruising causing some local swelling, see First Aid, page 104.

NATUROPATHY

Since fluid retention in the ankles and legs is often associated with circulatory problems like

Dandelion leaves can make a strongly diuretic tea.

Yarrow (*Achillea millefolium*)

varicose veins, all the general advice given under that section (see page 53) will be useful. Exercise is vital to improve the blood flow, and hence speed up the removal of fluid. Look at the diet, and in particular at salt intake; in most cases it will be very beneficial to reduce salt intake, since excessive amounts of sodium encourage fluid retention and also place an undue burden on the kidneys.

Massage is most helpful, especially gentle lymph drainage techniques – for self-massage, lightly and repeatedly stroke the affected areas in movements directed towards the heart. If the swelling is in the legs for instance, stroke the upper legs first in an upwards direction, before repeating the action to the lower legs, so that the fluid has somewhere to drain into from the ankles.

Try to have the legs raised, supported on something soft such as a cushion, to allow gravity to assist in draining fluid back towards the heart. In a similar way, swelling of the wrist can be eased by raising the arm or supporting it in a sling. Continued swelling, in any part of the body, requires medical attention.

URINARY INCONTINENCE

The inability to control the bladder and prevent dribbling of urine, or bed-wetting, is something that can affect people at both ends of life in particular. Children may get into problems with involuntary bed-wetting through something simple such as a chill or shock, or from a deeper upsetting worry, or just because they sleep too deeply (see Children's Ailments, page 112).

AROMATHERAPY

Alongside any self-help measures such as pelvic floor exercises, an excellent essential oil to use is Cypress, which is astringent, toning up the tissues and encouraging efficient excretion of fluid. Use it in the bath, about 6 drops, or make a compress with 2 drops in a small bowl of warm water and wring out a small towel in the liquid, placing it over the low abdomen. For daily use it may be easier to use a diluted oil, 2 per cent dilution (about 50 drops in 100 ml (3½ fl oz/½ cup) of base oil), and massage a little into the lower abdomen each day. Another oil that may help in this way is Pine, but use 1 per cent of this only. In either case do not use daily for more than 10 days at a time.

HERBALISM

Probably the foremost herb for this condition is Horsetail (*Equisetum arvense*), which is quite a strong diuretic, but more significantly it contains appreciable amounts of silica. This has an astringent and toning effect on the bladder tissues, encouraging it to empty efficiently and regain some of the lost muscle tone. Horsetail is perhaps best taken as the fresh juice, available in some countries, take 10 ml (2 tsp) twice a day; otherwise a decoction may be taken (see page 12). If emotional upset is a part of the problem, then also taking St John's Wort (*Hypericum perforatum*) may help a good deal – use the juice at the same rate or take an

HORSETAIL *(Equisetum arvense)*

infusion (see page 12) for a week or two (take care not to overdo this remedy if going out in strong sunlight, as it can increase sun sensitivity). For individualized treatment get professional help.

HOMEOPATHY

Several possibilities exist within homeopathy for treating this condition, some suggestions with a brief "snapshot" of the symptom picture for each remedy are:

ARGENT NIT: with incontinence at night in particular, although also possible in the day, brought on by nervousness, restlessness and anxiety. This remedy is useful for older people who may easily get anxious, perhaps over a move or travelling, and hence become incontinent; the urine may burn a little when passed.

BELLADONNA: with a constant urge to pass water when awake; there may be some involuntary dribbling when standing, and also during sleep.

PULSATILLA: this remedy is often appropriate for shy, sensitive people who are prone to crying. It is helpful if they experience bed-wetting at night, whether children or older people; there may be an easy tendency to dribble in the daytime too, with difficulty in retaining urine.

NATUROPATHY

One of the first things to look at is the muscle tone within the pelvic basin generally. Exercises such as alternately tightening and relaxing the buttocks can help to regain control of the bladder and urethra. Another exercise that may be useful is to try and stop in midstream while actually urinating, and hold for a couple of seconds before restarting to pass water. If done regularly, this can be a great aid in tightening and strengthening the muscles of the bladder.

Another approach is to employ hot and cold water applications to the lower abdomen and back. This can be via alternating hot/cold compresses, around 3-4 minutes hot and 1 minute cold, repeated once or twice. A simpler method is to have a fairly warm bath, followed by a short splash of cool water around the waist and bladder, or else when finishing a shower turn the temperature down to cool and use on this area for a minute. These methods will help to stimulate pelvic circulation, which in turn will encourage better muscular control.

THE MUSCULO-SKELETAL SYSTEM

Problems of the muscular and/or skeletal systems are for most of us simply a fact of life, ranging from simple aches and pains after unaccustomed exercise or effort, to the inevitable wear and tear on our bodies as we get older. In the great majority of cases these problems represent "everything that we don't die of", yet their impact on our health, vitality and mobility can be enormous, causing great problems. Back pain alone is the major cause of time lost from work in most industrialized countries, and the often crippling discomfort of chronic arthritis reduces the quality of life for sufferers by a considerable amount.

While it is true that wear and tear are a part of living, their effects *can* be lessened and much greater levels of comfort and mobility are possible. It is perhaps a sobering thought that much of our predisposition to problems with skeletal disorders in later life is established in the first few years of childhood; prevention, especially in terms of diet, is an important part of the equation therefore, and very hard to achieve when adult. Changes to lifestyle later on can make differences however, together with some of the suggestions under the sections that follow.

ABOVE: Massaging with aromatherapy oils is a wonderful and natural way to ease the body.

ARTHRITIS

Although specialists identify up to 200 divisions of arthritic conditions, it is useful to think of arthritis falling into two categories: osteoarthritis (OA) and rheumatoid arthritis (RA). Osteoarthritis is the natural wear and tear of the joints that occurs with ageing, as the cartilage surrounding the bones becomes thinner and the surface becomes rougher. This leads to friction and degeneration occurs as the joint gets deformed.

AROMATHERAPY

The two principles of many natural approaches to arthritis, namely detoxification and improving circulation around the joints, are the main aims of aromatherapy treatment. Essential oils which aid tissue cleansing include Cypress, Juniper and Lemon, and these can be used as bath oils (see page 8) regularly. Juniper also has an anti-inflammatory and mildly analgesic effect; similar properties are found in Chamomile, Lavender and Rosemary oils. These may all be used either in the bath or diluted in a base oil and gently massaged into the affected areas. If this is painful or difficult to do, they may be used in a hot compress (see page 15); try combining any two of these oils for greater effect, varying them to avoid overuse of any one oil. To stimulate the circulation, use oils such as Black Pepper, Ginger, Marjoram and Rosemary in any of the above ways. As you can see, some oils have overlapping effects and can help with relieving arthritic discomfort in many ways.

HERBALISM

The herbal pharmacopoeia are full of herbs that can be of benefit in treating arthritis; as mentioned above, it is useful to think of treatments in terms of detoxifying and stimulating the circulation, thus removing the need for local inflammation, as much as any simply pain-relieving action. For self-help treatment, apart from the dietary advice discussed below, an initial cleansing programme can be adopted. In order to remove acidic toxins, make a tea from Celery Seed (*Apium graveolens*), which has an alkaline effect on the whole system. Use just 5 ml (1 tsp) of the seed, perhaps lightly crushing the seeds with the back of a spoon before making the tea.

Another herb which increases elimination, via the urine, is Parsley (*Petroselinum crispum*); add 5 ml (1 tsp) of the chopped fresh herb to the above tea for maximum effect. Two cups of this tea daily for a week or two can have considerable benefits.

To improve the circulation you need

A warm compress on the affected area can help relax muscles.

OTHER CAUSES OF ARTHRITIS

Other factors include previous injuries and occupations – high amounts of some sports, or physical jobs such as farming can lead to greater wear on certain joints. Since it is sometimes associated with an excess of acid waste matter in the body accumulating around the joints, diet is important too.

RHEUMATOID ARTHRITIS

Rheumatoid arthritis is a different problem altogether. It is an inflammatory process that seems to be what is called an auto-immune disorder, meaning the body's defences for some unknown reason start to attack its own cells. In RA, not only are the synovial membranes lining the joints inflamed and thickened, but the bone underneath is steadily destroyed, leading to painful and often badly deformed joints. People are quite likely to feel ill in themselves as a result of this disorder, and professional treatment is essential to try to deal with the underlying condition.

look no further than Ginger (*Zingiber officinalis*); chop up a small piece and make a tea from it, or add to the mixture above. For a more direct anti-inflammatory action, a couple of suggestions are Meadowsweet

(*Filipendula ulmaria*) and Feverfew (*Chrysanthemum parthenium*). An infusion (see page 12) of Meadowsweet may be taken twice daily, while Feverfew may be taken in tablet form. The fresh leaves of Feverfew can also be chewed and eaten instead; just three leaves a day is a medicinal dose, but occasionally they can give mouth ulcers.

HOMEOPATHY

As a first treatment of arthritis, try one of these remedies:

BRYONIA: this is applicable for hot joints, when the pains are worse with warmth or with movements, and seem to be eased by the use of cold applications or compresses (see page 15).

PULSATILLA: if the pains and inflammation seem to move rapidly from one joint to another, with a quick change in symptoms. A pulsatilla-type of person usually feels much better in the fresh air, and this remedy seems to suit women better.

RHUS TOX: this is often the first remedy to be thought of in many rheumatic conditions; symptoms are better with warmth and after some movement, while the person is likely to feel stiff and painful after some time of resting. Cold, damp weather also makes the symptoms worse.

NATUROPATHY

Attention to the diet is an important part of treatment, and ideally this should be adapted individually by a practitioner. In most instances, it is essential to eat plenty of fresh vegetables, raw or cooked, and also fresh fruit – although citrus fruits are often to be avoided by sufferers. Other foods to reduce include red meats, cheeses, sugary foods and excessive coffee or tea. An approach that

Place 5 ml (1 tsp) of lightly crushed celery seeds in a teapot. Pour on boiling water and leave for 5 minutes to infuse. Sprinkle 5 ml (1 tsp) chopped fresh parsley on top of the tea, strain and drink a cupful.

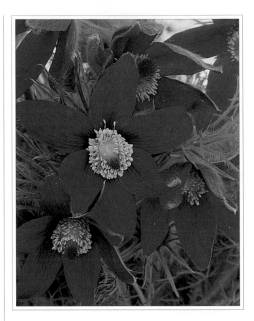

PASQUE FLOWER (*Pulsatilla vulgaris*)

has found some popularity is the Hay diet, named after its originator Dr Hay. The diet essentially involves avoiding combinations of proteins and carbohydrates at any one meal; this is beyond the scope of this section, but has been written about in other books.

To relieve stiffness, especially in winter in cooler, less sunny climates, there is a lot of value in taking cod liver oil capsules, one or two a day. The occasional use of a bath containing Epsom salts is also excellent to ease stiffness and discomfort; dissolve 60 ml (4 tbsp) of the salts in a hot bath and soak for 15 minutes. In an acute inflammatory stage of arthritis, with very hot joints, try using an ice-pack or cold compress. Often in chronic conditions, with cold, stiff joints, a warm compress is better (see page 15).

CRAMP

Acute and very painful contractions of muscles produce the feelings of cramp. It is probably most common in the calves, but can occur in any large muscles, for instance in the thighs, back, neck or abdomen. It can occur suddenly, often without warning and can be frightening for children the first time it occurs.

AROMATHERAPY

In order to improve the local circulation and so bring in more blood and oxygen to the muscles, massaging the area is often very beneficial. Firm effleurage, or stroking movements, are particular helpful, always done in a direction towards the heart. To aid this action, diluted essential oils like Juniper, Lavender, Marjoram, Rosemary or even Black Pepper should be used. These are all rubefacient, meaning they dilate the local blood vessels and encourage increased blood flow. The muscles become warmed and relaxed. For frequent leg cramps for instance, regular massage of the legs and thighs with one or more of these oils can help a good deal.

HERBALISM

One of the most effective treatments for cramp is the aptly named Cramp Bark (European

To ease stiff, aching arm muscles, oil the arm and then massage deeply down the length of the arm with the thumbs.

CAUSES OF CRAMP

A major factor is inadequate circulation to the muscles, especially if cramp comes on with exercise or effort (see also Poor Circulation, page 51); with athletes or people doing hard physical work there may also be a problem of salt deficiency from excessive sweating.

Repetitive movements, such as typing, can provoke cramping and lead on to inflammation – repetitive strain injury is a potential consequence of overuse of a set of muscles in this way. Night cramps are probably due to a combination of reduced circulation, tiredness and stress, and the whole person needs to be treated.

Cranberry Bush) (*Viburnum opulus*), better known to gardeners as the guelder rose. The bark is made into a tincture (see page 14) that is almost a specific remedy for muscle spasms, both internally in instances of, say, period pains or abdominal cramps, and used locally for leg cramps. Either make a warm compress using the tincture diluted about 1:4 with hot water, or incorporate it into a cream (see page 16) and massage into the affected areas. Internally, take 5 ml (1 tsp) once or twice daily, ideally in a little hot water. It is very effective, but unpleasant! For reduced circulation leading to cramping sensations, you may also find it helpful

to drink Ginger (*Zingiber officinalis*) tea, especially in the evening for helping night cramps.

HOMEOPATHY

Some possible remedies are:
COLCHICUM: for cramps usually in the soles of the feet.
CUPRUM MET: for severe cramps, often starting in the toes or fingers and spreading up the limb; symptoms are aggravated by cold winds, and often come on in the evening.
GELSEMIUM: for writer's cramp, especially if associated with mental exhaustion or tension.
NUX VOMICA: this is most often used for digestive problems due to over-eating, but can be helpful for night cramps.

NATUROPATHY

When a cramp occurs, the first self-help action needs to be to stretch the affected muscle; for example if the calf muscle has gone into spasm, it can be relieved by pushing down with the heel to elongate the muscle again, even though this initially feels very painful! If taking hard physical exercise in very hot weather, there may be a case for ensuring you have more salt in the diet, although this should be temporary and not overdone.

Using alternate hot and cold compresses on the affected areas is another way to improve local circulation in cases of repeated cramps. For long-term problems look at one of the many relaxation techniques around.

FIBROSITIS

This is inflammation of the muscle fibres, often a chronic condition which can lead to the formation of hard nodules within the muscle. Fibrositis particularly affects the large muscles of the back, neck and shoulders, and sometimes into the buttocks. It may occur as a result of an injury, but is equally likely to arise from chronic stress and tension or poor posture. It needs to be differentiated from arthritis or other causes of pain.

AROMATHERAPY

Massage of the affected area is one of the most effective forms of treatment, and professional massage may well be needed to get deep into the tight muscles. At home, stroking and kneading the muscles with an oil containing essential oils of Eucalyptus, Lavender, Marjoram, Pine or Rosemary will help to warm and relax the affected fibres, stimulating the local circulation.

HERBALISM

Any anti-inflammatory herbs that might be taken internally can often be used in conjunction with local agents, for instance the oils suggested above. Furthermore, since stress is often a factor, look at herbs for easing tension generally (see Stress, pages 28-9). A couple of herbs that may be appropriate to take are Meadowsweet (*Filipendula ulmaria*) as an infusion, or Willow Bark (*Salix alba*) taken as a decoction (see page 12), unless tablets are available. Both these plants contain substances that are related chemically to aspirin; indeed this was first synthesized from extracts of Willow, and was named after an older Latin name for Meadowsweet, *Spiraea*. They are, however, much safer for the stomach, notably Meadowsweet, but seek advice before using if you are allergic to aspirin.

MEADOWSWEET
(*Filipendula ulmaria*)

HOMEOPATHY

In the first place try Rhus tox if the pains are aggravated when first starting to move after resting, but gradually ease with continued steady movement. For other suggestions see Rheumatism, pages 88-9.

NATUROPATHY

Massage, stretching exercises and attention to posture will all help greatly, as will proper rest and relaxation. See a Naturopathy therapist for the best advice which will suit your own health and lifestyle.

MASSAGE FOR FIBROSITIS

1 To ease stiff muscles in the shoulder, oil the back, using a base oil and essential oils as recommended. Place fingers just inside the shoulder blade, supporting with the other hand. Keep a relaxed but firm pressure.

2 Move fingers steadily around the shoulder blade, pressing in firmly but within comfort limits. Repeat several times. Ease the pressure if too uncomfortable. Try this massage daily for a week.

GOUT

This condition occurs when there is an excess of uric acid in the body, and the kidneys cannot get rid of it effectively. The acid crystallizes into tiny sharp deposits like miniature needles; these collect in joints, often in the toes or feet but sometimes elsewhere such as the earlobes, causing intense pain and inflammation. The first signs of an attack may in fact be a feverish feeling, before the joint swells.

AROMATHERAPY

In an acute attack it is definitely not appropriate to massage the affected area – there is too much inflammation. Instead, use oils in cool or cold compresses to reduce the discomfort. For a detoxifying effect, try Cypress, Fennel, Juniper, Lemon or Pine oils. These may also be used in the bath. As the swelling and inflammation reduce, perhaps switch to oils such as Lavender or Rosemary for inducing local warmth and flushing toxins out of the joints.

HERBALISM

The classic herb is undoubtedly Celery Seed (*Apium graveolens*); this may be taken in tablet form or by making a tea from 5 ml (1 tsp) of the seeds, lightly crushed with the back of a spoon, in 300 ml (½ pt/1¼ cups) of boiling water. Take 2 to 3 cupfuls a day for acute attacks of gout, to encourage strongly the excretion of uric acid. More directly anti-inflammatory herbs

CELERY SEED (*Apium graveolens*)

SELF-HELP FOR GOUT

Uric acid may accumulate within the kidneys themselves, leading to kidney stones, which may have to be surgically removed. Generally speaking, all the advice for Arthritis (see pages 83-4), will be applicable to gout.

An acute attack of gout is extremely painful and may require medical treatment. Try reducing food to a minimum but make sure to drink plenty of water, which will encourage removal of uric acid from the body.

such as Meadowsweet (*Filipendula ulmaria*), Willow Bark (*Salix alba*) or Devil's Claw (*Harpagophytum procumbens*) may be taken alongside the Celery Seed.

The first two are described under Fibrositis (see page 86) while Devil's Claw is widely available in tablets or capsules, which are probably the easiest method in which to take it, up to 3 g per day. A general cleansing herb which is excellent to use regularly for chronic gout is Nettle (*Urtica dioca*) – simply drink it as a tea, 1 or 2 cups a day for a month or so.

HOMEOPATHY

A couple of remedies that often give some relief are:
ARNICA: for repeated attacks of gout, especially affecting the big toe, with

DEVIL'S CLAW
(*Harpagophytum procumbens*)

hot, painful and very tender joints.
RHUS TOX: a versatile remedy for most rheumatic or arthritic problems; suitable for hard, painful swelling of the joints – these can be mistaken in mild attacks for a bunion.

NATUROPATHY

Use cold compresses (see page 15) to reduce the swelling, switching to hot/cold applications in the longer term to encourage better circulation around the joint. Increase vegetable intake, especially raw or juiced, for a more alkaline intake, and cut out cheese, red wine (in the short term all alcohol), red meats, coffee and strong tea. When the swelling and inflammation has subsided, increase exercise to maintain joint mobility.

Drink plenty of mineral or spring water to encourage kidney action. Pain can be eased with some of the herbs discussed above.

RHEUMATISM

This is a general term which covers any inflammatory process in the muscles or joints; here its meaning will be limited to muscular rheumatism as Arthritis has already been covered (see pages 83-4). Much of the advice for Fibrositis (see page 86) is also relevant here as this is sometimes simply placed under the heading of rheumatism.

AROMATHERAPY

To aid the cleansing of the tissues, essential oils are probably best used in the bath (see page 8); appropriate oils are Cypress, Juniper, Pine and Rosemary, while Lavender may be added for greater muscle relaxation. Lavender and Rosemary are in addition quite analgesic in effect, giving some welcome relief from the pains and stiffness. If not too uncomfortable, massaging in a choice from these two, or else Juniper or Marjoram, diluted to 2 per cent in a base vegetable oil, speeds up the removal of toxins and

DANDELION
(Taraxacum officinale)

RHEUMATISM

As a rule, the emphasis of natural treatments is placed even more on detoxifying the system than is the case with joint problems, removing waste matter that congests and irritates the muscles to allow greater freedom of movement. A combination of dietary changes, exercise within limits of comfort, and other natural methods outlined in this section can dramatically improve rheumatic disorders over time.

improves blood supply to the affected muscles, and can be done regularly.

HERBALISM

Elimination of irritant waste materials can be encouraged very effectively by herbal remedies. Try Dandelion *(Taraxacum officinale)* as a first choice for home use; the leaf is more diuretic, increasing output from the kidneys, while the root is a gentle liver tonic and mild laxative. For maximum benefit, make the leaf as an infusion and the root as a decoction (see page 12), and take each for a week. They can be combined with a herb such as Nettle *(Urtica dioica)*, which is not only rich in various minerals but acts as a "blood cleanser", helping to provide the means for tissue repair and renewal. If pain is a significant factor, a remedy like

GINGER *(Zingiber officinalis)*

Meadowsweet *(Filipendula ulmaria)* can be very useful. These last two herbs can be used as infusions for a couple of weeks; for persistent discomfort get professional treatment.

If the circulation is definitely restricted, and the aching and stiffness are made worse by damp, cold weather, add a small amount of fresh Ginger *(Zingiber officinalis)* to any infusion. Ginger root is a strong circulatory stimulant and has a large part to play in treating many rheumatic/arthritic disorders.

HOMEOPATHY

Here are a few potentially helpful remedies; also compare with the suggestions for other conditions in this section which may be appropriate.
ACTAEA RAC: particularly good for painful, stiff muscles in the back and neck; also good for aching muscles after exercise or for neuralgic pains.
ARNICA: for general aching of limbs, with a feeling of being bruised (see also First Aid section, page 102).

Compresses can stimulate circulation and reduce inflammation.

BRYONIA: for stiffness and swelling, for instance of the hands and arms; if the joints feel uncomfortable and "crack" with movement, this remedy may well be very useful too.

RHUS TOX: for the typical stiffness pattern of rheumatic disorders, aggravated after resting and improving after some movements. The remedy for lumbago, with low back pains on rising or after long periods of sitting.

RUTA GRAV: for pains felt in the tendons and muscles, and joints such as wrists, knees and ankles. May also be helpful in relieving sciatic pains (see page 25).

ARNICA (*Arnica montana*)

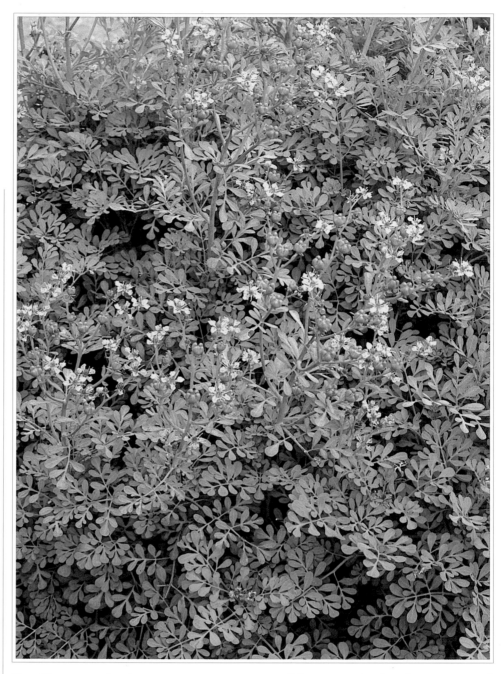

RUE (*Ruta graveolens*)

NATUROPATHY

Often a good soak in a hot bath (perhaps with a handful of Epsom salts) cases the stiffness and aching of muscular rheumatism, but too frequent a use of hot applications may produce too much congestion, so try alternating hot/cold compresses, if you can, in order to stimulate blood flow. A brisk rub with a thick, coarse towel will certainly aid this process. It is important to keep active as far as possible, so exercise is to be encouraged within individual limits of ability. Diet should be aimed at reducing acid waste matter, with plenty of vegetables and fresh fruit (with the probable exception of oranges) and very little refined carbohydrates or sugary foods. A supplement may be useful: take a multi-vitamin and mineral tablet once a day, or else initially just take a Vitamin B supplement. In winter, especially in cooler climates, taking a fish oil supplement such as cod liver oil capsules may ease stiffness.

THE SKIN

The natural approach to skin problems starts by taking the view that most disorders of the skin reflect inner imbalance, and that the whole person needs to be treated for truly effective results. This is especially so in conditions such as eczema or psoriasis, which can be highly complex disorders requiring professional treatment on an individual basis. Chronic or persistent problems should be referred to a practitioner. Given the potential negative effects of orthodox treatments such as steroid cream for eczema, there is much to be gained by looking at natural therapies.

The traditional treatment of many skin problems involves considerable attention being paid to the cleansing of the whole body. Both Western and Eastern (for example, Chinese or Indian) systems of herbal medicine have developed successful strategies for treating the skin. The role of other factors such as hormone balance, stress and lowered vitality also needs to be considered; for self-help other sections of this book may therefore be very useful.

As with all the conditions discussed in this book, do not overdo any of the self-help treatments suggested; if any skin problems get worse or continue for more than a short time, then stop the treatment and/or get professional help. Do not mix therapies; this is particularly true of homeopathy since the pattern of individual symptoms will be affected by other treatments, making the choice of homeopathic remedy more difficult. Small is beautiful in all the therapies – if a dose of something is helpful, do not think that doubling the dose will have double the benefit; quite often it is the opposite!

ABOVE: Herbal creams and ointments can bring relief to problem skin sufferers.

ABSCESS

An abscess is a localized inflamed swelling, containing pus. Abscesses can develop externally on the skin, but also internally in the mouth or on other mucous membranes – these should be referred for qualified medical treatment. Treatments locally on the skin will generally involve hot compresses or poultices to draw out the toxic waste matter; recurrent abscesses often indicate a weakened immune system. See also Boils, page 95.

AROMATHERAPY

Apply a hot compress (see page 15) to the area, by adding 5-6 drops of essential oil to a bowl of water as hot as you can bear, and soaking a piece of absorbent material in it. Suitable materials include lint, a clean handkerchief, or a face flannel. Fold over a couple of times for a thicker pad, and place on the abscess, covering with a bandage or piece of cling film (plastic-wrap) to hold in position. Renew when cooling to body temperature, and keep on for at least 30 minutes.

Appropriate essential oils for this process are Bergamot, Chamomile, Lavender and Tea Tree, either separately or in a combination such as Bergamot for its antiseptic properties, together with Lavender (also antiseptic) for a greater anti-inflammatory effect. (Remember that the number of drops suggested is the *total* amount used, not the number for each herb.)

HERBALISM

Make a hot poultice (see page 15) from a herb such as Marshmallow (*Althea officinalis*) for external treatment of the area. Either pour boiling water on to some fresh leaves, or mix the powdered root with hot water to make a paste. It may be helpful to use a little oil on the skin first to stop the poultice sticking, then place the herb on the abscess and cover with a clean gauze or strips of cotton, holding in position as above. Such a poultice can be kept on for several hours, but

Apply a hot poultice on to the affected area, applying a little base oil to the skin first so that the poultice does not stick.

may need replacing every couple of hours. Another excellent herb to help draw out pus is Slippery Elm (*Ulmus fulva)*; use the powdered inner bark as for the Marshmallow root above.

For mouth abscesses, it may be appropriate simply to place a hot compress, made with an infusion of Chamomile (*Chamomilla recutita*), on the cheek over the area until a doctor or dentist can be seen. Internal treatment, as described under Boils (see page 95), will be most helpful in cleansing the system as a whole and boosting immunity.

HOMEOPATHY

Hot compresses are likely to be suggested by practitioners here too, perhaps using tinctures of Hypericum or Calendula. Pour 15 ml (1 tbsp) of hot water on to 2 drops of either remedy, and soak a piece of

gauze in it. Place on the area and cover, renewing when cooling down.

Internally, take a few doses of either Hepar sulph if the abscess is hot, throbs with pain and is very tender to the touch, or else Silica if the abscess, although equally painful, feels cold to the touch, and the discharge is slow to clear up. These two remedies are very good for suppurating (oozing) skin conditions generally, given their different symptom pictures.

NATUROPATHY

If nothing else is available, use just hot water to make a compress, or put a hot water bottle over the affected area. You can use cabbage leaves from the garden with excellent results; take a few of the outer leaves, cut out the central rib and coarsely chop the leaves, pour on boiling water and make a poultice as outlined above. This is very soothing and helps to draw out infection. You may obtain Kaolin from a pharmacist to make a poultice, spread on a dressing and use over the area. When an abscess bursts, cover with a sterile dry dressing. For repeated problems a programme of dietary reform will be most helpful; for further information, see Boils, page 95.

MARSHMALLOW (*Althea officinalis*)

ACNE

This is a very common skin condition during puberty, although it may continue into later life for some people. Increasing levels of hormones during adolescence lead to greater activity of the skin's sebaceous glands, and if this becomes too great, excessive amounts of sebum, our natural oily skin lubricant, are produced. This in turn can cause the glands and hair follicles to become blocked and infected.

AROMATHERAPY

Many essential oils are not only antiseptic but also promote healing or generation of new healthy skin cells. Some of the best are Bergamot, Geranium, Lavender and Lemon; these may need to be used in varying combinations depending on the state of the skin and the person as a whole. Bergamot, for instance, is an effective antidepressant, and this emotional quality may be helpful at times as acne can understandably make the sufferer feel low (adolescence is a time of fluctuating self-esteem at the best of times), and as an astringent, antiseptic oil it is excellent for greasy, infected skin. Do not, however, overuse this oil as it increases the skin's sensitivity to the sun; moderate amounts of sunlight are generally good for drying and healing the skin too.

These oils may be used in a light carrier vegetable oil such as Grapeseed, which has a

WITCH
HAZEL
(*Hamamelis
virginiana*)

SELF-HELP FOR ACNE
The most common reaction of most people is to squeeze the spots; this almost always serves to spread the infection into surrounding tissues, and if done repeatedly can damage the local skin areas, producing scarring. Any programme of treatment therefore needs to include a lot of self-help to be successful. The natural therapies offer the most successful and safest ways to improve the condition and rebalance of the skin.

The best approach is to combine local, external cleansing with internal treatment; all therapies are likely to emphasize the importance of diet in treating acne.

Where acne persists for years after adolescence, there may well be a hormonal imbalance that needs to be addressed, and again there are appropriate natural remedies that may be used – seek professional treatment if needed.

slight astringency of its own, or Coconut, or else mixed into gentle cleansing creams for regular use on the affected areas. Another base might be a toning lotion such as triple-distilled Rosewater, Orange Blossom water or perhaps distilled Witch Hazel for extra astringency. Use 1-2 per cent of essential oils in any of these base carriers. If there is much

evidence of scarring after the condition has improved, use the essential oils in a carrier which includes 10 per cent Wheatgerm oil to promote skin elasticity and healing.

HERBALISM

Initial treatment should be firmly geared towards cleansing of the skin and of the whole system. Locally, any of the essential oils described above may be used, or else cleanse the skin with an infusion of herbs (see page 12) such as Elderflower (*Sambucus nigra*), Lavender (*Lavandula vera*) or Marigold (*Calendula officinalis*); adding 5 ml (1 tsp) of distilled Witch Hazel (*Hamamelis virginiana*) to 300 ml (½ pt/1¼ cups) of the infusion will gently increase the astringency if needed.

The main use of herbal remedies though will be internally: choose a mixture of the following herbs: BURDOCK (*Arctium lappa*): a powerful tissue cleanser, encouraging the removal of waste matter from the skin via the blood supply, and equally helping the transport of nutrients to the skin. The root is more powerful, and a decoction should be used (see page 12), the leaf is made into an infusion.

Start by taking small amounts of this herb (about 45 ml (3 tbsp), 3 times a day) as it can initially stir things up and the skin seems to get worse. CONE FLOWER (*Echinacea angustifolia* or *E. purpurea*): the best all-purpose immune stimulant, aiding resistance

MARIGOLD *(Calendula officinalis)*

and speeding up our reactions to infection. Used together with the above herbs, this creates a strong detoxification process.

DANDELION *(Taraxacum officinale)*: the root in particular is helpful in improving the detoxifying action of the liver, and also as a gentle laxative, taking pressure away from the skin as an organ of elimination.

RED CLOVER *(Trifolium pratense)*: another excellent blood and tissue cleanser, the infusion can also be used externally to carefully bathe inflamed spots and is gentle

enough to use on children in this way.
REMEMBER: if using more than one herb in an infusion or a decoction, the amount of each herb included is reduced to maintain the given overall maximum amounts.

HOMEOPATHY
In the short term try one of these remedies (also refer to the remedy suggestions for Abscesses and Boils, pages 91 and 95).

CALC SULPH: for spots that never come to a real head, but get tender and inflamed and then seem to subside after a while (suitable for "blind boils").
HEPAR SULPH: for lots of pus-filled spots, which feel hot and tender to the touch, and generally unhealthy-looking skin.
SILICA: for slow-healing of the skin, spots that develop pus which is slow to clear; this remedy is particularly good for helping the healing of scarring.

NATUROPATHY
The first basic principle of the naturopathic approach (as with all the other natural therapies) is to overhaul the diet, as far as is

possible given teenage fads! A reduction of sugary, fatty foods is essential, shifting the balance towards fresh fruit and vegetables, whole grains and lean forms of protein. It is often desirable to reduce dairy products for a while, especially milk or strong cheeses. Taking plenty of fluids regularly is important, *not* fizzy drinks or tea and coffee, but water or fruit juices. Alcohol should also be reduced.

Stimulating the circulation, either by self-massage or using hydrotherapy – for instance, by briskly rubbing the trunk and limbs with a loofah dipped in cool water – is a helpful aid to cleansing of the skin. Allow the skin to breathe by wearing cool clothes, and pay strict attention to hygiene. Sunshine is usually helpful, although be careful not to stay in the sun too long, and take adequate sun-protection measures.

Supplementation of the diet can speed up the cleansing/ healing processes initially; important vitamins are A (around 2,500 iu daily), B complex and C (up to 300 mg daily), while one of the most useful minerals is zinc (up to 15 mg daily). Evening Primrose oil has been found to be of benefit in some cases; take up to 1,500 mg daily.

RED CLOVER *(Trifolium pratense)*

ACNE AND THE ADOLESCENT
Acne can be a major blight on adolescence, causing much emotional upset and even relationship difficulties, so it is important that familes and all concerned do not exaggerate the condition. Concern and practical help are better then either dismissing the problem or worst still, making negative comments. Gentle, but regular, cleansing of the skin, attention to hygiene and diet will all help keep acne to a minimum, so encouragement of these activities is useful, even if met with opposition!

ATHLETE'S FOOT

This fungal skin condition can be produced by a number of different microscopic fungal growths, causing inflammation and itching. Despite its name, it is neither confined to the feet nor only restricted to athletes!

AROMATHERAPY

The most suitable anti-fungal essential oils to use are Lavender, Myrrh and Tea Tree, all of which not only tackle the infection directly but are also soothing and healing. Initially they may be best applied dissolved in a little neat alcohol, at 2-3 per cent dilution, or even used sparingly on their own on the moist, infected skin; when the skin is drier, they might then be incorporated into a cream base, up to 3 per cent dilution (see page 16).

Another useful base is Olive oil, which in itself seems to have some anti-fungal activity (see also Thrush, pages 74-5). Oil of Calendula, or the Old English Marigold, has very helpful healing properties and may be used as a base too. It may be helpful in the beginning to use a footbath, with 10 drops of one of the essential oils mentioned, but it is essential that the feet are dried thoroughly afterwards, and kept aired as often as possible.

MARIGOLD (*Calendula officinalis*)

SELF-HELP MEASURES

The commonest sites are where the skin gets moist and hot, such as between the toes or in the groin, and on the scalp where it may take the form of ringworm.

The most important self-help measures involve keeping the affected area cool and dry, and paying scrupulous attention to hygiene as the fungus can accumulate under the nails causing infection between the fingers or simply spreading by contact.

HERBALISM

External applications of tinctures of either Marigold (*Calendula officinalis*) or Myrrh (*Commiphora molmol*) are powerfully anti-fungal; leave the application to dry out on the skin. If the skin is very moist, these two herbs may be applied in powder form if available, either neat or by mixing with unperfumed talcum powder.

Widespread or recurrent infection may also require internal remedies to bolster the immune system – take Garlic (*Allium sativum*) regularly, either in food or perhaps as a capsule; a short course of Cone Flower (*Echinacea angustifolia* or *E. purpurea*), as an infusion, tincture (see pages 12 and 14 respectively) or in tablets (around 1,500 mg per day) may help.

CONE FLOWER (*Echinacea angustifolia*)

HOMEOPATHY

Homeopaths may well also recommend Calendula as a local treatment, the tincture at first and then perhaps the oil or an ointment. Internal remedies will depend on the nature of the condition – for instance, if the area is moist and suppurating, a choice may be made from Hepar sulph, Merc sol, Silica or Sulphur, among others, so it is most advisable to seek a qualified practitioner.

NATUROPATHY

The first action to take is to ensure that the affected area keeps as dry and well-ventilated as possible, as the fungi responsible love hot, damp conditions. Use cotton socks and underwear, changing the garments daily. Ideally avoid wearing trainers and use leather shoes. Wash feet and other affected areas at least once a day, drying very thoroughly by patting dry rather than rubbing and chafing the skin. Use talcum powder to help keep the feet dry. Wash underwear in very hot water; the fungi may survive a low temperature wash cycle. Do not share towels or flannels as the infection may be passed on through physical contact. Footbaths can have 10-20 ml (2-4 tsp) of cider vinegar added, for a stronger anti-fungal effect.

BOILS

A boil is an acute inflamed and infected area on the skin, often in a blocked hair follicle. If a number of boils occur together, they may produce a large inflamed lump with several pus-filled "heads", and are termed a carbuncle (the medical term for a boil is a furuncle; if they are recurring, you are suffering from furunculosis). A stye is effectively a boil occurring in the base of an eyelash.

SLIPPERY ELM *(Ulmus fulva)*

AROMATHERAPY

In order to keep the tissues surrounding the boil clean and free from bacterial infection, it is very useful to wash the area 2 to 4 times a day with a 2 per cent dilution of essential oil of Lavender in cooled, boiled water, using sterile cotton wool (cotton pad) if possible. For drawing out the boil, a hot compress (see page 15) with oils such as Bergamot, Chamomile, Lavender or Tea Tree will be useful. These are variously antiseptic, anti-inflammatory and speed up healing; they may additionally be used in the bath as more general detoxifying remedies. The oil of choice would probably be Lavender; this is the most versatile oil to have for home use.

CAUSES OF BOILS

Boils tend to occur when people are run-down, either by stress or through poor diet and hygiene, but can be more frequent in some other illnesses, such as diabetes when the higher blood sugar levels provide food for bacteria (see also treatment suggestions for Abscess and Acne, pages 91 and 92-3). Generally, treatments are geared initially towards bringing the boil to a head and allowing it to burst and discharge the pus. It is important that all external applications are as clean as possible – for example, use sterile dressings for applying any poultices. In the medium to longer term, the natural therapies are ideally suited to cleansing the system as a whole, building up immunity to further outbreaks and restoring health and vitality.

Deeper causes of lowered vitality, such as prolonged stress, will need attention too, and oils may be used in the bath or in massage to help restore normal functioning. For additional help with stress, see pages 28-9.

BURDOCK *(Arctium lappa)*

LAVENDER *(Lavandula angustifolia)*

HERBALISM

Treatment from a herbal practitioner will focus internally as well as on any local applications, and this is also a good approach for self-help – if boils recur or resist home treatments, seek professional advice. Many herbs are soothing and anti-inflammatory when used as a poultice (see page 15); two excellent ones are Slippery Elm *(Ulmus fulva)* and Marshmallow *(Althea officinalis)*.

Slippery Elm has been called the "herbalists' knife" for its ability to bring a boil to bursting point; simply thicken the powder with a little boiling water and apply as a paste, as hot as you can bear. Powdered Marshmallow root can also be used, or else the fresh leaves can be softened with boiling water and applied as a hot poultice. When the boil has burst, wash the area with cooled Lavender *(Lavandula vera)* tea or else keep using Slippery Elm as a cool poultice to speed up healing. If no other herbs are available, use fresh Garlic *(Allium sativum)* on the inflamed area, gently rubbing a cut clove over the skin.

Internally, Garlic may also be helpful, as a powerful antibiotic and immune-booster. Blood-cleansing herbal remedies include Burdock *(Arctium lappa)*, Yellow Dock *(Rumex crispus)* and/or Dandelion Root *(Taraxacum officinale)*, all most effectively taken as decoctions (see page 12), and Cleavers *(Galium aparine)* or Red Clover *(Trifolium pratense)* made as infusions (see page 12). It may be valuable to take Cone Flower *(Echinacea angustifolia* or *E. purpurea)* tablets or drops for a couple of weeks afterwards to help restore natural immune function.

HOMEOPATHY

Remedies to choose from are:
BELLADONNA: for very reddened skin probably in the earlier stages of developing a boil when it is throbbing and feels burningly hot to the touch.
HEPAR SULPH: for a hot, pus-filled boil which is coming to a head; this remedy will help it to mature and burst.
SILICA: this remedy is appropriate when the boil, although painful, feels if anything cold to the touch. This remedy

MARSHMALLOW *(Althea officinalis)*

and the previous one, with their differing symptom patterns, can be thought of as the "homeopath's knife", helping the boil to discharge.

NATUROPATHY

The diet definitely needs to be overhauled in the short term at least, to clear waste matter out of the system and provide essential nutrients for the immune defences to do their job properly and to aid tissue healing. If possible, try to have a strict diet for a week, cutting out all sugar, refined carbohydrates, tea,

GARLIC *(Allium sativum)*

coffee, alcohol, cheese and fried foods; eat plenty of fresh vegetables, raw or cooked fresh fruit, whole grains and a little lean protein.

Fluids should mostly be water, especially spring water, or else fruit juices (diluted in hot weather) or herbal teas. Alcohol should be avoided if at all possible.

There may be a case for taking extra nutrients in the form of a supplement: if the diet has been poor for a while, take a high quality multi-vitamin and mineral supplement, or else try taking zinc, up to 25 mg daily for a week and then 15 mg daily for another month.

Locally, bathing the boil in hot water may bring it to a head, or use a hot poultice (see page 15) made from the outer leaves of a cabbage, roughly chopped.

If boils recur, or continue, then seek professional help.

Fresh green salad leaves can greatly assist in clearing out the system.

COLD SORES

These are caused by the virus herpes simplex, another strain of which produces genital herpes (although it may be the same virus behaving differently). This virus is able to lie dormant in our tissues almost indefinitely until conditions trigger off an attack; it is probable that nearly everybody has acquired this virus at an early age from another person, so the key factor is what allows the virus to multiply and erupt.

AROMATHERAPY

Some essential oils are excellent for local use, and at the earliest stage possible of an outbreak are probably the most effective treatment for cold sores. Particularly good are Bergamot, Eucalyptus, Lavender, Lemon and Tea Tree. These may be applied neat, using just 1 drop on a cotton bud (swab), but may be better if diluted in a little alcohol; for home use a spirit such as vodka will do very well: add 5 drops of essential oil to 5 ml (1 tsp) of alcohol and dab on frequently. Neat Lavender oil may be dabbed on a little later to speed up healing.

HERBALISM

Local applications of herbs are most effective when they are used in tincture form (see page 14), dabbed on to the cold sores frequently to dry and heal the area. Some of the best are Lavender (*Lavandula vera*), Marigold (*Calendula officinalis*), Myrrh (*Commiphora molmol*), Wild Indigo (*Baptisia tinctoria*) and Witch Hazel (*Hamamelis virginiana*).

Where the appearance of cold sores indicates overall exhaustion, the herb St John's Wort (*Hypericum perforatum*) is an excellent choice; the tincture can be used locally as above, and may be taken internally as a calming restorative for the nervous system, 20 drops 3 times a day. *CAUTION*: this herb increases sensitivity to sunlight, so avoid prolonged exposure to strong, bright sunshine while taking internally.

ATTACK TRIGGERS

One of the most common predisposing factors is the ordinary cold, hence the name, but any respiratory infection can trigger an attack, as can being generally run-down. Extremes of temperature, or exposure to strong sunshine are other possible causes.

When an attack does occur, small blisters come out on the lips or at the corner of the mouth. These form a crust and remain moist underneath for up to 10 days or so before drying out. They are highly infectious during all the moist, weeping stages.

HOMEOPATHY

For a first-time eruption, try one of the following remedies, for up to 5 days at 30c potency (see Introduction, page 10, for explanation of potencies). If cold sores persist or recur, see a homeopath.

NAT MUR: for cold sores associated with a swelling of the lip, possibly even causing a deep crack, the sores forming several blisters.

RHUS TOX: for when the corners of the mouth get sore and there is a burning sensation; the eruptions may also spread out on to the chin, and the remedy "picture" often includes a red tip to the tongue as part of the overall symptoms.

NATUROPATHY

A simple yet highly effective home remedy is to apply freshly squeezed lemon juice to the cold sore, at the first signs of the problem (since the zest contains the essential oil, there is an obvious connection with Aromatherapy treatment). For a drying effect, you may find good quality eau-de-Cologne dabbed on and left to dry can be useful. It is often helpful to take a short course of a Vitamin B complex supplement, backed up by zinc (10-15 mg daily), and Vitamin C (500 mg daily). This is especially true when cold sores are recurring frequently, since these nutrients help to boost the immune system generally, as well as enhancing our ability to cope with chronic stress.

ST JOHN'S WORT
(*Hypericum perforatum*)

ECZEMA

This is a complex skin condition, and in most instances will need professional treatment. The natural therapies have an extremely good record in treating people with eczema, and given the problems associated with the long-term, regular use of steroid creams, there is a lot to be said for looking at other options.

AROMATHERAPY

The most important thing to remember when trying to help ease eczema is to be as flexible as possible. You may well need to vary the oils, and change the way you use them, since the nature of the condition can be due to so many factors, and the skin can get better for a while with one oil and then may need something different as the symptoms change.

Some of the most useful oils to use on the skin are Chamomile, Geranium, Lavender, Lemon Balm (often listed as Melissa, the first part of its Latin name) and perhaps Rose. They should be used in at most a 1 per cent dilution initially, and can be incorporated in a light aqueous cream, or perhaps use a thicker cream, ointment or pure vegetable oil base if the skin is extremely dry or weakened (see page 16 for how to make creams and ointments). Try these oils one at a time at first, to see whether the skin reacts to any of them.

CHAMOMILE
(*Chamomilla recutita*)

LEMON BALM
(*Melissa officinalis*)

Another method for a larger area of eczema is to use the oils in a cool compress: start with just 5 drops to 500 ml (16 fl oz/2 cups) water.

HERBALISM

This is an area where herbal medicine can be highly effective, and nearly always involves internal treatment as well as any local applications. Apart from some of the oils mentioned above, creams or ointments made with Comfrey (*Symphytum officinale*) or Marigold (*Calendula officinalis*) can help to reduce inflammation and speed up healing. For the intense itching that often accompanies eczema one of the best herbs is Chickweed (*Stellaria media*); use the fresh herb to make a cream or ointment, or simply make an infusion and when cooled apply as a compress.

If the skin is weeping, then infusions of Heartsease (*Viola tricolor*), Red Clover (*Trifolium pratense*) or even Nettle (*Urtica dioica*) used in a similar way will help to dry the area. Applying Evening Primrose (*Oenothera biennis*) oil, either neat or in a cream base, can

CAUSES OF ECZEMA

Essentially, eczema is an allergic inflammation and irritation of the skin. There may be a fairly straightforward external cause – for instance, a reaction to nickel which is often found in cheaper jewellery, watch straps, zips (zippers), clips and so on. Cosmetics, perfumes and hair colourings are another source of potential allergens, and fur, feathers, mould spores or dust make up another major group of irritants. Occasionally people react badly to various plants, especially in bright sunlight, and keen gardeners need to be aware of possible dangers if they have sensitive skin.

For many eczema sufferers, however, any external irritants are secondary to inner factors. In what is termed atopic eczema, there is often a family history of eczema, asthma or hay fever (all similarly over-reactive disorders), and problem areas such as emotional upsets, stress and food intolerance play a bigger part in the individual's eczema pattern. Unravelling the particular combination of factors for each person is often a detective story, which is where seeking treatment from a qualified natural therapist can be so valuable, with their focus on the whole person.

EVENING PRIMROSE
(*Oenothera biennis*)

be very soothing and
healing.

The traditional herbal approach
to eczema focuses on cleansing the
tissues, and this can yield very good
results. Herbs with blood-cleansing
or "alternative" properties include
Red Clover and Nettle, as
infusions, and Burdock (*Arctium
lappa*) or Yellow Dock (*Rumex
crispus*) as decoctions (see page 12).
Two other herbs that are of value
in removing toxins are Cleavers
(*Galium aparine*) for improving
elimination via the kidneys, and
Dandelion Root (*Taraxacum
officinale*) to tone the liver and
gently open the bowels. The
former should be used as an
infusion and the latter as a decoction.
Mixtures may be made from the above
herbs. Do not use for more than 3
weeks and if the skin gets worse, reduce
the dosage by half.

HOMEOPATHY

Since eczema can initially flare up
with treatment, take just one dose
of a 30c potency (see page 10) per
week, selecting from the following
remedies (if there is no improvement
within a month, consult a qualified
practitioner):

GRAPHITES: for a moist, weeping skin
which forms scabs that easily break off.
The discharge is sticky, and the exposed

surface of the skin may also bleed.
This condition may be anywhere,
but typical areas are behind the ears
or on the face.

RHUS TOX: for a dry, very intensely
itching eczema, such as might occur
on the hands and wrists. Often little
blisters form in the patches of
redness.

SULPHUR: for hot, dry and burningly
irritating skin. There is acute itching,
but scratching makes it very sore.
Heat of any kind (for instance, hot
baths or lying in bed) makes the
irritation much worse.

NATUROPATHY

Given the importance of
stress in aggravating many
kinds of eczema, looking at
relaxation techniques may be
valuable (see also Stress, pages 28-9).
With regard to diet, many foods can be
potential problems, most notably dairy
foods. Where eczema has been
around from infancy, it is
often very beneficial to try
eliminating cow's milk,
cheese and other dairy products
from the diet for up to
three weeks. Reducing
sugar, spicy foods,
coffee, tea and alcohol,
and keeping food additives
to a minimum are other potentially
useful approaches. Taking a
supplement of Vitamin B complex

HEARTSEASE (*Viola tricolor*)

DIETARY ADVICE
Specific dietary advice will
obviously require professional
consultation, as there may be
particular foods which provoke or
aggravate an individual's eczema. If
the suggestions in the Naturopathy
section do not radically improve the
skin with 6-8 weeks, get
professional advice.

can help, and sometimes Vitamin A (up
to 5,000 iu for a month) is needed.
Evening Primrose oil can be taken
internally as well as
used locally; to boost
the essential fatty acids
within the body, take up
to 1,500 mg daily.

PSORIASIS

This is a skin disease where the skin cells start to grow too rapidly; the immature cells over-produce but fail to mature into proper keratin. The new cells grow more rapidly than the old dead layers can be shed and so thick, reddened patches form which are covered with a silvery scale. They can appear in patches almost anywhere, often on the outer surfaces of the elbows or knees, and in severe cases can cover the whole body.

AROMATHERAPY

Essential oils which help to reduce inflammation may help locally (see Eczema, pages 98-9), but it may be just as helpful to concentrate on lowering the stress levels. Thus oils may be added to the bath: choose from Bergamot, Chamomile, Geranium, Jasmine, Lavender, Neroli or Rose for their relaxing and/or uplifting qualities. Change the oils around depending on the emotional state, and be prepared for limited success and slow improvements in the skin! Do not despair, psoriasis is notoriously difficult to treat, and sufferers carry the possibility of a recurrence even after the skin has cleared.

HERBALISM

Traditionally, psoriasis was linked to liver sluggishness as well as stress, and so herbal liver tonics and tissue cleansers form an initial part of treatment. Look at the herbs discussed under Eczema, particularly Yellow Dock (*Rumex crispus*) and Dandelion Root (*Taraxacum officinale*). These may be combined and made as a decoction (see page 12), to

NETTLE (*Urtica dioica*)

SELF-HELP TREATMENT

Psoriasis can run in families, and is a very complex condition with no simple treatment. It is frequently aggravated by stress and by being run-down, and seems to be an example of an auto-immune disorder, that is, when the body's immune system fails to recognize its own cells and starts to react against itself. In nearly every case exposure to sunlight is helpful, and often the condition will disappear on a summer holiday, when sun and relaxation are combined.

stimulate bile flow and clear toxins out of the whole system. Nettle (*Urtica dioica*) is also valuable as a cleanser; ideally take the juice (available in some countries) or else combine in an infusion (see page 12), with Cleavers (*Galium aparine*) for added effect. Topically, the thickened skin can be encouraged to slough off by rubbing with moistened fine oatmeal. Marigold (*Calendula officinalis*) can be used in a

RED CLOVER (*Trifolium pratense*)

cream or ointment to reduce the inflammation, or else Red Clover (*Trifolium pratense*) may be tried in similar fashion. If stress is an obvious factor, taking teas of gentle relaxants such as Chamomile (*Chamomilla recutita*), Lavender (*Lavandula vera*), Lemon Balm (*Melissa officinalis*) or Lime Blossom (*Tilia europaea*) over a period of time may help to restore balance.

HOMEOPATHY

Some short-term suggestions are:
ARSEN ALB: for roughened, scaly skin that may have a burning sensation, although often cold to the touch. The skin is exceptionally dry.
GRAPHITES: for when the skin dries out and cracks, producing a thick, sticky discharge. The cracked areas may also bleed, and the skin itches considerably.
SULPHUR: for hot, dry and itchy skin which is made worse by heat (although not necessarily the sun). Scratching gives very temporary relief, but then causes soreness and burning.

NATUROPATHY

Much of the dietary advice echoes that given under Eczema (see pages 98-9); there may be a case for looking at wheat as a source of food intolerance too; try eliminating

suspected foods on a rotation basis, a
couple of weeks or so off each food
group. For a short while Vitamin A may
be taken in quite high doses (up to
7,500 iu daily for 2-3 weeks), but this is
stored in the liver and can be toxic in
over-large amounts. A multi-vitamin
supplement may give a gentler but safer
effect over a long period of time.

Sunshine is most likely to benefit,
but do not get sunburnt! It is still
necessary to take sun-protection
measures when exposing skin to
sunlight for any prolonged period of
time (see pages 110-11). The Dead Sea
is famous as a treatment area for
psoriasis, using the mineral salts from

*Natural creams and oils can be gently
massaged into affected areas of skin.*

CLEAVERS *(Galium aparine)*

the sea together with sunbathing. These
salts are now available in many
countries, and can be added to the bath
or a wash-basin to bathe smaller areas
of skin. Evening Primrose oil may be of
help, both locally and internally (take
up to 1,500 mg daily). Relaxation
techniques or classes can be important
parts of self-help, learning how to cope
with stress and not internalize it.

Due to the complexity of factors
involved, psoriasis is not easily treated
with self-help, and professional
treatment may be the best course of
action. It can be associated with other
disorders, such as digestive problems,
and may lead on to a specific form of
arthritis, so read the suggestions
under these headings (see pages
61 and 83-4) to see how the
natural therapies can work on
the whole person, and to
suit your own condition.

Lime Blossom (Tilia europaea)
tea can help reduce stress levels.

IMPROVING THE CONDITION

One cannot really say that psoriasis
can be cured, but natural treatments
can greatly improve the condition
for long periods of time.
As psoriasis sufferers often have a
tendency towards tense, insular
personalities, the following Bach
Flower Remedies (see page 102) can
sometimes help: Agrimony, Crab
Apple, Water Violet or Willow.
Whatever treatment is used,
patience is required as visible
improvement can
take a while to
show through.

FIRST AID

There are a number of instances when natural remedies can be used for first-aid treatment, and you may find it useful to build up a natural first-aid kit, to go alongside items such as plasters, bandages and so on. The important feature to remember is that situations needing first-aid treatment are acute, so prompt help is essential, and also they should be limited in duration anyway, such as a bruise.

If symptoms get worse or persist, despite first aid, seek medical help. In this section some of the common problems that might arise are listed and possible forms of treatment identified.

A choice of items for a natural first-aid kit is up to each individual, but some excellent remedies are Comfrey ointment for bruises, sprains and strains; Lavender essential oil for burns, bruises, sprains and strains; Calendula cream (herbal or homeopathic) for cuts and grazes; homeopathic Arnica tablets at 6c or 30c potency for bruises and shock; and Rescue Remedy for all types of shock. The last is not technically part of mainstream herbalism, but is one of Dr Edward Bach's Flower Remedies. These are a series of gentle plant remedies which are intended to treat various emotional states, regardless of the physical disorder. For practical purposes, the Rescue Remedy is the finest treatment available for alleviating symptoms of shock.

Above: The distinctive smell of peppermint is highly effective when used as a smelling salt.

BITES AND STINGS

Bites and stings can occur from any number of insects, some being much more painful than others. In any situation where a bite or sting affects the mouth or even the throat, and also if there are signs of an allergic reaction, with distress and/or difficulty in breathing, get medical help immediately.

AROMATHERAPY

A drop of Lavender or Tea Tree oils may be applied to the area, ideally in a little iced water. This may be repeated every 10 minutes or so until the pain and irritation has subsided, or it can be made into a cold compress (see page 15) and left on for a couple of hours.

HERBALISM

A cold dressing made from an infusion (see page 12) of Chamomile (*Chamomilla recutita*), Elderflower (*Sambucus nigra*), Lavender (*Lavandula vera*) or Red Clover (*Trifolium pratense*) can be used over the area. Other herbal help can be to use fresh leaves of plants such as Lemon Balm (*Melissa officinalis*) or Plantain (*Plantago major* or *P. lanceolata*), or Yellow Dock (*Rumex crispus*) leaves – famous for treating nettle stings – directly on to the skin. Fresh onion may give quick relief from insect stings, placed over the area. For continued irritation, apply a cream (see page 16) made with Chickweed (*Stellaria media*) or perhaps Marigold (*Calendula officinalis*). For bites, Marigold, Myrrh (*Commiphora molmol*) or St John's Wort (*Hypericum perforatum*) tinctures (see page 14) can help – use a drop or two neat on the bite or dilute 5 ml (1 tsp) into 15 ml (1 tbsp) of water for a cold dressing.

Use either water or a herbal infusion, with ice added. Wring out a cloth and hold over the inflamed area.

REMOVING A STING

Some stings, for instance from bees, result in the sting being left behind in the skin, and this should be carefully removed first. This is probably best done by flicking the sting out with a sharp knife; tweezers may be used, but these can result in squeezing the poison sac of the sting and thereby sending more toxin into the puncture hole.

HOMEOPATHY

Two classic remedies are Ledum, the remedy of choice for puncture wounds generally, or else Apis mel when there is much redness and swelling around the sting. Use 30c potency (see page 10), and take a dose every 20 minutes until the symptoms are much relieved. If there is a rash around the sting, apply a cold dressing using 2 drops of Urtica urens tincture to 15 ml (1 tbsp) of water. If there are symptoms of shock, the remedy to choose is Arnica, 1 dose per hour for 4 hours if needed.

CHICKWEED (*Stellaria media*)

NATUROPATHY

If possible, apply ice to the area as soon as possible to reduce inflammation and swelling. If the sting is from a bee, there may be some value in using diluted bicarbonate of soda to clean the area; conversely, if it is a wasp sting, it may be helpful to use diluted lemon juice or vinegar for the same purpose. Bites should be thoroughly cleaned before any treatment.

BRUISES

Bruises can happen for several reasons; a knock, crushed finger or toe, sprain or other injury are the normal causes. However, if bruising is severe, frequent and without obvious cause, then it may indicate a lack of Vitamin K, or even be a sign of diabetes or kidney disease; get professional advice if dietary changes (see below) do not help.

AROMATHERAPY

Immediate use of oil of Lavender, in an ice-cold compress, can be the most effective treatment to avoid swelling and widespread bruising. If a bruise has developed, at a later stage when it is changing colour and resolving, use Rosemary essential oil diluted in a vegetable oil base to massage gently into the tissues to increase local circulation and speed up the healing process.

HERBALISM

Ice-cold compresses can be made with distilled Witch Hazel (*Hamamelis virginiana*); either dilute 15 ml (1 tbsp) in 300 ml (½ pt/1¼ cups) of cold water and apply on a dressing, or else be prepared beforehand and keep some ice-cubes made with the Witch Hazel in a separately

WITCH HAZEL
*(Hamamelis
virginiana)*

COMFREY *(Symphytum officinale)*

labelled bag in the freezer (this is a useful policy if you have children!). An infusion of Comfrey *(Symphytum officinale),* chilled with ice-cubes, can also be used for a cold compress. For aftercare, Comfrey oil or ointment (see page 16) is ideal, quickly healing the damaged tissues.

HOMEOPATHY

Probably the remedy of choice will be Arnica; this is excellent for any physical (or emotional) trauma and shock, and will help with bruising from a blow or injury. Take every 2 hours for up to 6 doses, then 3 times a day for 3 days, if needed. Keep an eye on symptoms; as they improve, reduce the frequency of dosage or stop taking the remedy altogether if much better. When the skin is unbroken, Arnica ointment may be applied to the bruised area; if there is damage to the skin, then Hypericum or Calendula ointments should be used instead. All the above ointments are available in most health shops. Other remedies for internal use could be Ruta grav or Rhus tox when the muscles, tendons or bones have been injured, for example in a sprain.

NATUROPATHY

Ice-cold compresses (see page 15) or packs should be applied as soon as possible – a bag of frozen peas makes a good temporary pack. If the bruise is severe or widespread, then try to raise the affected area to reduce local blood supply, and hence swelling. Repeated or very easy bruising may indicate Vitamin K deficiency; eat plenty of green vegetables such as broccoli, cabbage, spinach and so on, and also try taking plenty of live yoghurt to stimulate the gut flora that make this vitamin. To encourage dispersal of bruises, eat fresh pineapple, or drink the juice; it contains enzymes which aid this process. If bruises linger, it may be additionally helpful to take Vitamin C (500 mg daily for a few days).

ARNICA
(Arnica montana)

BURNS

Severe burns require urgent medical assistance; do not delay in getting treatment, especially for children and babies. The immediate treatment should be to apply cold water for up to 10 minutes if necessary, to reduce the heat. If the burn is from a chemical, remove any clothing that might have been affected. However, if there is burnt clothing stuck in the burn, then generally do not remove as this might do more damage.

AROMATHERAPY

Essential oil of Lavender is almost a specific treatment for burns; it is anti-inflammatory and analgesic, and promotes healing of the tissues. If applied quickly it can prevent scarring in many instances (I speak from personal experience). For a larger area put on to sterile gauze or smooth lint; otherwise drop on neat.

HERBALISM

In herbal practice Lavender (*Lavandula vera*) oil will most likely be used, as described above; another option for minor burns is Tea Tree (*Melaleuca alternifolia*) oil, a couple of drops applied to prevent blistering. If available, fresh Aloe vera gel is an excellent first-aid treatment for burns and scalds. Break open a leaf and spread the thick gel directly on to the

LAVENDER (*Lavandula vera*)

burn – again, this can produce completely scar-free healing if done as soon as possible. Other possibilities are infusions of Chamomile (*Chamomilla recutita*) or Marigold (*Calendula officinalis*), applied on a smooth dressing. Marigold cream (see page 16) may be used after some time has elapsed to ease continuing inflammation and soreness.

HOMEOPATHY

Probably the most-used homeopathic remedy for the first-aid treatment of burns is Arnica, followed by Cantharis; this helps to remove the burning pains that accompany blistering of the skin. For very minor burns Urtica urens may be suitable; probably only a couple of doses will be needed in this case. Urtica is also available as an ointment and is very effective for soothing superficial burns. Alternatively, after cooling of the skin it may be appropriate to use a commercial cream on a small burn.

CAUTION
Burns larger than the palm of your hand should be seen by a doctor immediately, regardless of any self-help treatment that has been advised here. All burns are painful and should be touched as little as possible.

MARIGOLD (*Calendula officinalis*)

REMEMBER, do not use greasy ointments, butter or other fats on new burns as all this does is simply fry the skin. Always cool the area thoroughly as the first treatment.

NATUROPATHY

Once the skin has been cooled, a valuable home remedy is honey; this is both antiseptic and promotes healing. When healing has started, a Vitamin E cream can aid restoration of tissue elasticity and reduce scarring. Do not give hot drinks to someone who has a burn; frequent small sips of cool water can help to replace lost fluids in more serious cases.

CHAMOMILE (*Chamomilla recutita*)

CUTS AND GRAZES

The first priority is to clean the area gently but thoroughly to remove any dirt. If the wound is deep, needing stitches, cover with a dry dressing and get medical help. It may be a sensible precaution to consider a tetanus jab (shot) if the cut has been from a dirty object or an animal, especially if there is a puncture wound.

AROMATHERAPY

The two oils of choice are probably Lavender and Tea Tree. These may be used neat on small cuts and scratches; they will sting temporarily but this soon passes. They can be added to a bowl of water for bathing (see page 8) and cleaning the affected area initially, or a couple of drops may be placed on a plaster or other clean dressing and applied over the site of the injury. Both these oils fight any infection as well as stimulating healing, and are generally very safe to use neat in this way.

To soothe and cool the wound, apply a cold compress to the area.

COMFREY *(Symphytum officinale)*

HERBALISM

Wash the area with distilled Witch Hazel *(Hamamelis virginiana)*, or apply it diluted (15 ml (1 tbsp) to 300 ml (½ pt/1¼ cups) of water) on a dressing. Tinctures (see page 14) of Marigold *(Calendula officinalis)* or Myrrh *(Commiphora molmol)*, similarly diluted, are alternatives for use on a dressing, or use an infusion (see page 12) of Yarrow *(Achillea mille-folium)*. Marigold cream is an ideal soothing healer applied to minor cuts and grazes. Comfrey *(Symphytum officinale)* ointment is a powerful tissue healer, so much so that it should only be used on clean cuts as it can seal dirt inside the wound. Fresh gel from Aloe vera is both soothing and healing, and should be applied 2 or 3 times a day, until fully healed.

HOMEOPATHY

Externally, a compress with either Hypericum or Calendula tinctures, 2 drops in 15 ml (1 tbsp) of water, may be used. This can be followed up by an

Add 2-3 drops of Lavender oil to a cold compress as a powerful antiseptic.

ointment from either of these (or any commercial cream made from both). Internally, take up to 4 doses of either Hypericum, especially if the injury has affected the fingers or toes and damaged local nerves, or Arnica for the shock of the injury, at 4-hourly intervals. For anything more serious get professional treatment.

NATUROPATHY

Clean your own hands thoroughly before cleaning the cut or graze, and apply a little honey or a Vitamin E cream on minor injuries. Keep the area covered if possible to avoid infection, and watch out for any swelling or inflammation.

YARROW *(Achillea millefolium)*

FAINTING

Feeling faint, or actually blacking-out, is due to a temporary lack of blood to the brain, and an isolated incident can be due to a number of immediate causes, such as excess heat or cold, fear, emotional upset, sight of blood, needles or something else that the person considers unpleasant.

AROMATHERAPY

For someone feeling faint, use one of the following oils like smelling salts, holding the bottle under the nose or else putting a couple of drops on a tissue and getting the person to breathe the aroma. Peppermint is particularly good, also Lavender, Neroli, Petitgrain and Rosemary. A drop gently massaged into the temples can be useful – a good commercial product for this use is Tiger Balm, which contains menthol and eucalyptol.

HERBALISM

Generally, any strong-smelling substance tends to stimulate the brain and relieve feelings of faintness. If available, tinctures (see page 14) of Lavender (*Lavandula vera*) or Peppermint (*Mentha piperita*) are pleasant and effective when used as smelling salts. One of the best remedies, especially when shock or upset has caused the faint feeling, is Rescue Remedy. If the person is conscious, put 4 drops under the tongue; if not, then moisten the lips with a couple of drops, and give 4 drops under the tongue when he or she comes round; repeat in half an hour if still feeling woozy.

HOMEOPATHY

Apart from the usual first-aid approach of making the person comfortable, if there is an obvious cause for the fainting, then a single dose of one of the following remedies may be called for.
ACONITE: for the effects of fright.
ARNICA: for faintness due to an accident, injury or shock.
IGNATIA: for over-excitement, or even feelings of hysteria.

POSTURAL HYPERTENSION
One of the commonest causes of fainting is postural hypotension (that is, a sudden change in position, such as standing up quickly), which lowers the blood pressure to the brain. Repeated fainting attacks call for expert investigation into the causes, which may range from low blood pressure or anaemia to changes in blood sugar levels. When someone has fainted, do not try to lift them up; falling down brings the head level with the heart and helps to bring blood to the brain more easily.

NUX VOMICA: for faint feelings associated with seeing blood, or from strong smells, or after a rich meal.
PULSATILLA: for the effects of being in a hot, stuffy atmosphere.

Finally, if the person has fainted, and on coming round feels chilly but desires fresh air, try a dose of Carbo veg – sometimes called the corpse reviver!

NATUROPATHY

Use basic first aid, such as ensuring there is enough fresh air if possible, helping the blood flow by sitting the person down and placing their head down between the knees, or else assisting them to lie down with their legs slightly raised. When recovering, give a few sips of water or better still warm peppermint tea.

FEELING FAINT

1 Put a couple of drops of essential oil on to a tissue.

2 Hold the tissue under the nose and lean the head slightly forward.

NOSEBLEED

This is most often due to a blow on the nose, rupturing some of the tiny blood vessels, and can be quite common in children. Occasionally a nosebleed is sparked off by very hot, humid weather, or by excitement, and if they occur frequently, professional treatment should be sought.

AROMATHERAPY

Soak a pad of cotton wool in cold, or even iced water with a couple of drops of Lemon oil added, and place firmly across the bridge of the nose. A more effective method is to place a small piece of this as a plug in the affected nostril. The essential oil helps to speed up clotting. Sometimes placing a cold compress on the back of the neck can be helpful in reducing the local blood flow too.

Make an infusion of Yarrow (Achillea millefolium) *(see page 12). When cool, soak a piece of cotton wool or soft cloth in the infusion and place on the soft part of the nose. Hold firmly in place.*

HERBALISM

The herb of choice is Yarrow *(Achillea millefolium);* even its Latin name is derived from its supposed use by Achilles in stemming bleeding from his heel. Make an infusion (see page 12) and cool with ice-cubes, soak a pad in it and use as described under Aromatherapy above. The tincture (see page 14) can also be used, 15 ml (1 tbsp) in 300 ml (½ pt/1¼ cups) of cold water, as can distilled Witch Hazel *(Hamamelis virginiana).*

Traditionally, a leaf would be placed in the nostril to act as a plug, the finely divided leaflets acting as a mesh for the blood platelets to produce a clot; however, removing this leaf often starts the nosebleed off again, so it is not particularly recommended.

HOMEOPATHY

Some useful remedies are:
FERRUM PHOS: for the results of a minor injury, or else from a head cold; a good remedy for childhood knocks.
HAMAMELIS: for profuse bleeding, with a feeling of pressure in the nose and sinus areas which is relieved by the blood loss to some extent.
PHOSPHORUS: for a heavy nosebleed associated with blowing the nose violently or sneezing, especially if occurring in the evening.

NATUROPATHY

In the first instance, get the person to sit down and lean forward slightly, pinching the soft part of the nose firmly between forefinger and thumb for several minutes. An ice-cube, or better still a pad of cotton wool soaked in iced water, can be held in place over this area too, to astringe the swollen blood vessels further.

CAUTION

In rare instances, conditions such as high blood pressure may be the reason behind the nosebleeds. Any unexplained or very heavy bleeds need immediate medical attention.

SPRAINS AND STRAINS

A sprain is an injury affecting a joint, with the tendons that attach muscles to the bones being overstretched and often torn. A strain is an injury to the muscles themselves, usually due to excessive or inappropriate exercise, lifting heavy weights and so on. The first treatment is a cold application (see Naturopathy entry below); massage of the area is not helpful at this stage, but can be used if the after effects linger on.

AROMATHERAPY

The most useful essential oil is Lavender; use 5 drops to 15 ml (1 tbsp) of iced water for a compress. Chamomile oil may be used in the same way; where there is a sprain, try to keep the affected joint as still as possible initially to reduce internal bleeding and to allow healing to start as quickly as possible, ideally with the limb raised.

HERBALISM

Make an infusion of Comfrey leaves (*Symphytum officinale*) and apply as a cold compress (see page 15), or use diluted tinctures (see page 14) of Comfrey or Marigold (*Calendula*

When treating a strain, the colder the water for the compress, the more effective it will be for the strain.

officinalis), 15 ml (1 tbsp) to 300 ml (½ pt/1¼ cups) of cold water. When the swelling has subsided, gently rub in Comfrey ointment to speed up healing of the damaged fibres. If muscles ache through over-exercise, this ointment is a good home treatment with massage of the surrounding area twice a day.

HOMEOPATHY

Choose from these remedies:
ARNICA: for the results of a fall or accident, with soreness and also a feeling of shock.
RHUS TOX: for muscular strains, from lifting heavy weights for instance, with pain, stiffness and swelling.
RUTA GRAV: for torn ligaments or tendons, especially in sprains of the ankles or wrists, with a feeling of bruising in the bones.

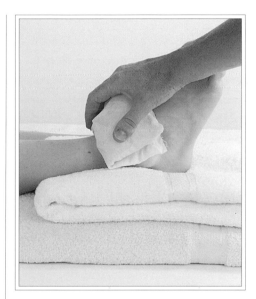

Raise the leg and support the ankle on something soft. Place an ice pack (a bag of frozen peas is a quick substitute) over the area and hold firmly in place.

NATUROPATHY

The immediate treatment is to apply the ICE approach : ice, compression and elevation. For example, a pack of frozen peas, held firmly around a sprained ankle, with the leg raised and supported, will help a good deal in reducing internal bleeding and joint swelling.

After the symptoms have subsided, there may be a case for using alternate hot and cold compresses (3 minutes hot followed by 1 minute cold, repeated for about 15 minutes) to improve local circulation to the relevant muscles, and later treatment may include massage to relieve muscular aches. Diluted oil of Lavender (about 2 per cent in a base oil) is helpful here.

SUNBURN

In most respects sunburn should be treated as for Burns (see page 105). The first thing to do is to avoid further exposure to the sun until symptoms have been cleared. Severe sunburn can produce bad blistering, dehydration and sunstroke, and occasionally people have an allergic reaction to the sun's ultraviolet rays.

AROMATHERAPY

For mild, widespread sunburn use Chamomile oil, either in a bath, or add 5 drops to a small bowl of water and carefully dab on to unbroken skin. With children, essential oils for the bath should ideally be pre-diluted in 5 ml (1 tsp) of Sweet Almond or similar oil. If the sunburn is more severe, use Lavender oil in similar ways, or apply neat on to any blistered areas.

As aftercare for the dry, leathery-looking skin, use essential oils of Chamomile, Lavender, Rose or Sandalwood diluted at 2 per cent in a base oil such as Sweet Almond and gently massaged in twice daily. Very dry skin may benefit from the use of

ELDERFLOWER *(Sambucus nigra)*

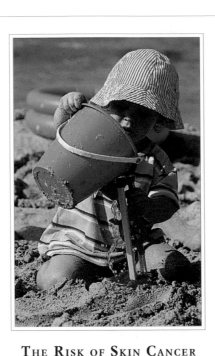

THE RISK OF SKIN CANCER

An increasingly frequent sequel to excessive exposure to the sun is skin cancer, and reductions in the Earth's ozone layer make this likely to become dramatically more common in future years, even in countries some distance away from the Equator.

In any case, the sun has an ageing effect on the skin, so enjoy it but use good suntan creams and after-sun moisturizing creams, and keep out of the midday sun if possible.

REMEMBER: sunbeds do not protect against sunburn so you still need to take it carefully when out in hot sunshine, and use the appropriate sun protection factor (SPF) lotion.

FRENCH LAVENDER *(Lavandula stoechas)*

Wheatgerm oil at 10 per cent of the base oil for extra nourishment.

HERBALISM

Firstly cool the skin as for Burns (see page 105), or by applying a chilled infusion (see page 12) of either Chamomile *(Chamomilla recutita),* Elderflower *(Sambucus nigra)* or Lavender *(Lavandula vera)* flowers. Marigold *(Calendula officinalis)* cream may be used afterwards, or else apply the blood-red oil of St John's Wort *(Hypericum perforatum),* which

Although expensive, Rose oil is wonderful for treating dry skin.

will take away much of the burning
pain very quickly – it has been used to
good effect on radiation burns. Pure
Aloe vera juice is another highly
soothing, cooling and healing herb.

HOMEOPATHY

Apply Cantharis, for when there is
an intense burning sensation,
before or after blisters have formed,

and Urtica urens, for sunburn with an
intense and persistent stinging
sensation. For milder burns, then apply
Hypericum and/or Calendula cream.

NATUROPATHY

After cooling the affected areas,
apply Vitamin E cream, as well as
taking Vitamin E internally (up to 500
iu daily) to improve healing and stop

*Young children should always have plenty
of sun-protection lotion on.*

scarring. Widespread sunburn may heal
more quickly if additional Vitamin C is
taken (up to 1,000 mg daily for a few
days). Sunburn is likely to mean
dehydration, so take plenty of fluids
(spring water and fruit juices, but not
alcohol) in the short term.

CHILDREN'S AILMENTS

In general, children and adults are treated in the same way by the natural therapies, each person's health being considered individually and treatment given accordingly, and the same approach applies to self-help measures. There is of course the matter of dosage of remedies, and these should be reduced or adapted as explained below. There are a number of illnesses that tend to occur in childhood, such as chickenpox, German measles and measles, and children are also more prone to colds, coughs, ear infections and the like. As well as any specific treatment for such conditions, it is worth bearing in mind some general considerations.

Children usually react quickly to any illness, showing acute symptoms that can then often subside equally quickly (much to the amazement/relief/annoyance of parents!). Due to their high levels of energy and faster metabolism, children often show signs of illness through a high temperature, and this should be looked at as part of the ailment, not as the whole problem (see Fever, pages 48-9). Because of this, it is easier for children to become dehydrated, and an essential part of treatment is to give plenty of fluids – with vomiting and/or diarrhoea in infants this can be literally life-saving. Conversely, if a child is unwell, he or she can go off food for a while, and provided fluid intake is adequate, this is not normally a major problem in the short term.

> REMEMBER: Keep all medicines and essential oils out of the reach of children.

Here are some comments about each of the therapies in relation to treating children, and some of the most useful remedies.

*ABOVE: Self-help treatment may not always be appropriate for children.
If in any doubt, seek medical advice.*

AROMATHERAPY

All the various methods of using essential oils discussed through the book – baths, inhalations, massage oils, compresses and creams – can be used for children as well as adults, with a few safety provisos.

❧ Do not use any oil undiluted on a child, except for Lavender oil on small burns or bruises.

❧ Dilute essential oils in a base oil before adding them to a bath for a child; they tend to enjoy splashing around in the bath more than adults and could get the oils in their eyes otherwise. Reduce dosage too, to a maximum of 4 drops per bath. For young infants, perhaps simply make a tea, of Lavender flowers for example, and add that to the bath.

❧ In massage, use lower dilutions of essential oils: a maximum of 1 per cent for ages 12-16; ½ per cent for ages 8-12; and ¼ per cent for ages 4-8. Under 4-year-olds will need just a drop or two in 100 ml (4 fl oz/½ cup) of base oil.

❧ Never leave a young child alone with bottles of essential oils, and always supervise their use.

❧ Use steam inhalations only briefly, and not at all if breathing is affected. Sometimes it is better to put a drop or two into a wash-basin of steaming water and sit with the young child next to it, rather than bending over a bowl.

Although aromatherapy oils may appear harmless, they are very strong and should always be kept out of the reach of children.

EUCALYPTUS (*Eucalyptus globulus*)

❧ A good way to help to fight infection, suitable for all ages, is to use a few drops in a plant spray, typically 600 ml (1 pt/ 2½ cups) capacity, fill with water, shake and spray the room at regular intervals. Use oils such as Lavender, Eucalyptus and Tea Tree.

Probably the two most suitable essential oils for use in childhood ailments are Chamomile and Lavender. They are both soothing, relaxing and anti-inflammatory, and help to calm the child as well as help to fight the illness. For instance, in a condition such as chickenpox, 2 drops of Lavender oil in 5 ml (1 tsp) of water can be dabbed on to the emerging spots to soothe the irritation and heal them at a much faster rate; Chamomile cream is very versatile, soothing many inflamed skin disorders. Additionally, the aroma of these oils helps to calm the child and give them a more restful sleep.

For colds and such like you may consider Benzoin, Frankincense and perhaps tiny amounts of Eucalyptus or Peppermint (also see other ailments).

PEPPERMINT (*Mentha piperita*)

HERBALISM

Since children have a higher metabolic rate, and good underlying energy in most cases, herbs which stimulate the circulation are generally to be avoided. Herbal teas are one of the most suitable forms of treatment. With stronger preparations such as infusions and decoctions (see page 12), it is sensible to work on the principle of reaching an adult dose at age 16; hence, a child of 8 will be given half the dose, and at 4 only quarter the adult dose. This can be achieved either by reducing the amount of herb used in the prepara-

Actually preparing your own infusions can become part of the healing process.

tion per given amount of water, or by reducing the amount of the preparation given to the child.

Some of the most suitable remedies to give as teas to children are:

CATMINT *(Nepeta cataria):* for nasal congestion and catarrh, repeated colds or blocked ears; of special benefit if there is a tendency to get feverish and restless with a respiratory infection or cararrh. Both this and Peppermint *(Mentha piperita)* have a slight underlying bitterness, which indicates their usefulness too in picking up the appetite after a feverish illness.

CHAMOMILE *(Chamomilla recutita):* for most digestive upsets, from stomach pains to indigestion, the effects of overeating, flatulence and diarrhoea. As a mild relaxant, it is a valuable remedy for calming children who get irritable and cross when they are ill, or who find it difficult to get to sleep. Do not make a tea of Chamomile too strong, in the hope of knocking the child out at night, as it can have the opposite effect at an overdose level and make them more stimulated, or irritable!

ELDERFLOWER *(Sambucus nigra):* this is the best temperature regulator in feverish illnesses; give a hot tea when the child's temperature is too high and it will induce sweating, so cooling the system. It is very helpful in feverish colds and flu, and will help to relieve catarrh as well.

LEMON BALM *(Melissa officinalis):* this is a wonderful herb for gently aiding relaxation, at the same time acting as a digestive and nervous tonic. It is very helpful in convalescence,

Picking herbs can be fun for children too.

and makes a refreshing cold drink in summer; make a tea, ideally from the fresh leaves, and after infusing for a few minutes strain and keep in the refrigerator. It will keep for 2-3 days, and a slice or two of lemon can be added for extra flavour and additional benefit.

LIME BLOSSOM *(Tilia europaea):* for tension headaches, mild digestive upsets and colds/flu with aching in the limbs. A tea of Lime Blossom at night can induce a calm and restful sleep.

PEPPERMINT *(Mentha pip-erita):* this is one of the best remedies for trapped wind, nausea and indigestion from rich or heavy foods. Another area where Peppermint is excellent is in the early stages of a cold, with fluctuating temperatures and nasal congestion.

Many of these teas may be blended together (although Chamomile and Peppermint seem to be better kept apart) for extra benefit, and can be used, suitably diluted, for infants – sometimes it is best to add 5 ml (1 tsp) to a bottle of their normal juice or water.

A posy of fresh, sweet-smelling herbs was called a tussie-mussie or nosegay in Elizabethan times and was used to ward off foul odours and potential germs.

HOMEOPATHY

Since children react in general very quickly to treatment, any homeopathic remedies can usually be given in fewer doses than might be the case with an adult. If the symptoms are less acute, or in any case for young children, try the 6c potency (see page 10) first; in more acute circumstances give the 30c potency. As soon as the symptoms are less pronounced reduce the frequency of the medication, or stop it altogether. If in any doubt about the right potency, get professional advice. Homeopathy is a wonderful system of treatment for children, with no problems of taste to overcome, and the range of remedies is very wide.

Here are some typical remedies for childhood ailments:

ACONITE: give at the earliest onset of symptoms, very good for ailments brought on by catching a chill, getting wet and so on. The child may be upset, with a hot, dry skin and a thirst for cold water, and restless at night.

ARGENT NIT: for agitation and anxiety, perhaps when anticipating some event; the child is fidgety and restless. This remedy is strongly indicated if the child has a craving for sticky, sweet foods or ice-cream, but gets an upset stomach, nausea or even vomiting after eating.

ARNICA: this is the remedy for shock, given after any minor bump or fall. It can be excellent to give before, and after, a visit to the dentist, to reduce tissue damage or bruising, and to help the healing process.

ARSEN ALB: for the child who gets fractious after any exertion, easily gets a stomach upset or mild food poisoning, and wants to be carried. Usually, the picture for indicat-

ACONITE
(*Aconitum napellus*)

CHAMOMILE (*Chamomilla recutita*)

PASQUE FLOWER
(*Pulsatilla vulgaris*)

ing this remedy is one where the child is peevish, wants to go from one person to another, and gets very thirsty, taking frequent, although small, sips of fluid.

BELLADONNA: for sudden onset of symptoms, associated with great redness of the skin and face. All symptoms tend to be violently acute, there may be over-excitability or a bad headache. This is a good remedy to give a child who has had too much sun.

CHAMOMILLA: for whining, cross and irritable children who can only be calmed with constant soothing and attention. In granule form, often at a very low potency such as 3c (that is, diluted at one part in 1,000), this makes a highly useful remedy for infants who are teething.

PULSATILLA: for mild-natured children, who are easily moved to tears, yet can be obstinate. They often fear the dark, and generally liked to be fussed over and cuddled. If the child's temperament is suited to Pulsatilla, then this remedy should be given no matter what the physical ailment.

SULPHUR: for the child who demands things quickly, and sulks if they do not come immediately. Babies get hot easily, kick off the bedclothes, demand feeding often. This is a remedy that is often used in skin conditions, such as eczema or psoriasis, and suits children with rough, scaly and itchy skin.

CAUTION
Some of the plants used in homeopathy are poisonous, for example Aconite (*Aconitum napellus*) and Belladonna (*Atropa belladonna*). Do not try to use them as herbs!

NATUROPATHY

Probably the most significant time for having a healthy diet is in the first seven years of our lives, when we are most actively developing our body, and our whole system. This is unfortunately not the easiest time to get healthy food into children. The need for energy-giving foods is high, and the metabolic rate burns calories up very fast, so snacks of fruit, fresh or dried, can be given ad lib. Intake of vegetables by children is mostly too low; encouragement and a varied diet can help, and in winter, soups and stews can be a way of disguising vegetables.

Although children love to eat sticky, chocolatey things, make sure their diet contains plenty of fresh fruit.

In acute, febrile illnesses such as chickenpox or influenza it is often helpful to allow a virtual fast for up to 48 hours (preferably check with your doctor first), but give plenty of fluids, especially fresh fruit juices. This stimulates a higher white blood cell count, improving the child's resistance to infection. Do not feed heavy stodgy foods in these illnesses; the appetite will nearly always come back with a vengeance after the acute stage has passed.

As for supplements, a multivitamin and mineral tablet can be useful, especially in winter. If the child is prone to colds, then Vitamin C is most important; dietary intake can be topped up with a supplement of 100 mg (1-3 times a day, depending on age and need). As girls move into puberty and menstruation starts, a multi-supplement containing a little iron can be a useful boost to the system.

The use of water applications, footbaths and so on, as described throughout the book, can be used quite effectively on children. For reducing fevers, sponge the face and/or upper body with water that is tepid, not cold, and allow to dry off naturally for a cooling effect. For dehydration, try a home-made rehydration preparation: dissolve 5 ml (1 tsp) of salt and 15 ml (1 tbsp) of sugar in 600 ml (1 pt/2½ cups) of freshly boiled water, leave to cool and keep in the refrigerator in a screw-topped bottle. Give 5 ml (1 tsp), up to 5 times a day if needed.

On the following pages are some suggestions for a few of the ailments that occur in childhood. Using the above information about the use of the natural therapies for children, and the other sections of the book, should help you treat most other common complaints. If in doubt get professional advice or treatment.

When a child is running a temperature, cool compresses can help calm and soothe the child and reduce body heat.

A well-balanced, sensible diet is the best start in life you can give to your child. Healthy eating habits, begun now, will reap rewards in later adult life.

CHICKENPOX

This is a highly infectious disease, not just restricted to childhood in fact, which is due to the same virus, herpes zoster, that gives adults shingles. It can be transmitted from an adult suffering from shingles, and in turn a child with chickenpox can give an adult shingles. The first signs may simply be a raised temperature and general feeling of malaise, and then a day later the spots appear, quickly developing into blisters containing a clear fluid. This is the most infectious stage, as the fluid contains the virus; after a few days the blisters dry up and form scabs which slowly drop off.

AROMATHERAPY

There are a few essential oils that are excellent for treating chickenpox, speeding up the drying and healing process and soothing the irritation. One of the best is Tea Tree oil. This can be made into a lotion to dab on to the spots – add 10 drops to 100 ml (4 fl oz/½ cup) water, or better still Rosewater, and shake. Since oils do not mix with water, you will need to shake before use each time. Add the oil to 50 ml (2 fl oz/¼ cup) distilled Witch Hazel for extra astringency and mix with 50 ml (2 fl oz/

LIME BLOSSOM *(Tilia europaea)*

Chamomile tea is a soothing drink for children.

¼ cup) of Rosewater. To soothe the itching skin, add 5 drops of Chamomile oil as well, or else use 10 drops of Lavender oil with the Tea Tree to give the best healing results (use fewer drops for young children, see the Aromatherapy section, page 13 and 113). Other essential oils that are effective anti-viral agents are Bergamot and Eucalyptus: use 5 drops of each as above.

HERBALISM

If the child is a bit feverish, give teas of Chamomile *(Chamomilla recutita)*, Yarrow *(Achillea millefolium)* or Lime Blossom *(Tilia europaea)* – or all 3 mixed – in 5 ml (1 tsp) doses (15 ml (1 tbsp) for over 3-year-olds) every 2 or 3 hours. Give plenty of fluids generally, and sponge with tepid water if the temperature is too high. To soothe itching on the skin, apply a little Aloe vera gel, which will also promote healing of the blisters.

COLIC

Colic in babies and infants is usually a sign of trapped wind (gas), but it is a problem that seems to affect bottle-fed babies more than breast-fed ones; this is partly due to the richness of cows' milk, and sometimes may indicate an intolerance to it. Colic, for this reason, can be noticed even in babies who are breast-fed, and may be due to the mother drinking a lot of cows' milk herself. If colicky symptoms are frequent then get advice.

Colicky symptoms can cause anxiety and sleeplessness in both the parents and the child.

HERBALISM

Where babies are breast-feeding, and having problems with wind and colicky pains, it may be easier to give herb teas to the mother which will then work through into the milk. Some of the most effective herbs are Dill *(Anethum graveolens)*, Fennel *(Foeniculum vulgare)* and Aniseed *(Pimpinella anisum)*; a tea may be made by lightly crushing 5 ml (1 tsp) of the seeds and pouring about 300 ml (½ pt/1¼ cups) of boiling water over them. Leave to stand for a few minutes and strain. The mother should drink a couple of cups a day. For slightly older infants, make a tea in the same way and give in 5 ml (1 tsp) doses (10 ml (2 tsp) for children over 3 years) every couple of hours until the symptoms have gone. Another useful herb is Chamomile *(Chamomilla recutita)*, given in the same way.

Peppermint *(Mentha piperita)* is another traditional herbal remedy for colic, taken as a tea; this tends to counteract a number of other

DILL *(Anethum graveolens)*

homeopathic remedies, so do not mix therapies (homeopathy generally should be used on its own anyway, although there is a tradition in some countries of using combined herbal/homeopathic tablets in over-the-counter medicines). Peppermint *(Mentha piperita)* is better for slightly older children, say over 3-years-old; peppermint oil capsules are available, which dissolve lower down in the gut and so have a stronger effect on colon spasm; these should be kept for children over 8-years or so, and only used for a short time (up to 2 weeks maximum) before getting professional advice.

HOMEOPATHY

Chamomile is also a favourite homeopathic remedy for colic, given in 3c potency initially (see Homeopathy advice page 115) for infants. For children who have got colic after over-eating, or eating food that is too rich, give a dose of Nux vomica (6c potency probably will be appropriate).

FENNEL *(Foeniculum vulgare)*

HYPERACTIVITY

This is a difficult problem to identify, since the boundary between normal energetic behaviour and abnormal activity is a subjective one. There are a number of factors that may contribute towards hyperactivity, such as psychological disturbances or social pressures, and it may be the result of a brain disorder. In general, therefore, this problem needs careful assessment and qualified help.

NATUROPATHY

One factor that had been overlooked in conventional medicine for some time is that of food intolerance. Studies have indicated that food additives in particular, especially some colourings and preservatives, can trigger off hyperactivity as well as other reactions; many of these additives have been steadily removed from foods as consumers have successfully protested at their use. If your child has a high proportion of foods containing colourings etc. then it may well be worth exploring a diet without such additives to see if this makes a difference. Changes in behaviour may take 3-4 weeks to be noticeable, although strong reactions to additives can be eased within a day or so.

Children naturally seem to have boundless energy and it can be difficult to spot the first signs of hyperactivity.

MEASLES

This is one of the more serious of childhood ailments, since there are possible secondary infections that can occur. These include middle-ear infections, bronchitis or even pneumonia. These complications are often more of a problem than measles itself, so preferably get professional advice. Initial symptoms are often those of a cold and cough, although a disliking of bright lights and sunlight is quite common at the outset. A clear diagnosis of measles can be made from the appearance of small white spots on the inside of the cheeks; 2-3 days later the rash appears, spreading from the face down the body to the legs. The red spots often join together to give a blotchy appearance, and the child normally has a fever, nasty cough and feels unwell. As the rash fades, it can leave a brownish stain that disappears by itself shortly afterwards, but can linger. The child starts to feel better as the rash spreads and then fades.

AROMATHERAPY

Since the immune system is temporarily lowered (hence the possibility of secondary infections) self-help measures to enhance this can be very helpful. Constant evaporation of essential oils like Tea Tree and Eucalyptus in the child's sick room can be important; use a burner or else add 20 drops of each oil to a 600 ml (1 pt/2½ cups) plant spray full of water. Shake and spray frequently into the air.

HERBALISM

For the fever, herb teas of Elderflower (*Sambucus nigra*), Chamomile (*Chamomilla recutita*) and Lime Blossom (*Tilia europaea*) will help to induce sweating and cool the temperature; the last two herbs are additionally calming, helping to reduce the upset and aid sleep.

HOMEOPATHY

Suitable homeopathic remedies are:
BELLADONNA: for a bright red rash, sore/hot throat and overall heat, not helped by cold air or cold drinks.
EUPHRASIA: for the beginning of the ailment, with runny nose and eyes, and reaction to bright light and strong sunlight .
PULSATILLA: for itching and burning spots, causing the child to cry a lot; a dry throat and troublesome cough.

DEADLY NIGHTSHADE
(*Atropa belladonna*)

NATUROPATHY

Garlic capsules, and/or Echinacea tablets may be given as immune-stimulants. Vitamin C is valuable: give 100 mg per day for 4-8-year-olds, 300 mg per day for 8-12-year-olds, and 500-800 mg per day for over 12-year-olds, for the first week of symptoms. Half this dose may then be given until all symptoms have gone.

MUMPS

An acute viral infection, producing the typical swollen parotid (salivary) glands on either side of the jaw. It can affect one side only, in which case the other side can, although only rarely, be affected if exposed to the virus later in life. The most worrying complication for adults is a secondary swelling and inflammation of one or both testicles (*orchitis*), but this only rarely causes any long-term problems. Alongside the swelling of the parotid gland(s) there is usually a fever, symptoms settling down in a week or so.

If there is difficulty in eating, give liquids or nourishing foods. Fluid is important because of the fever too, but avoid citrus juices which may increase saliva flow and add to the pains. A cold compress can be used to reduce the swelling; a drop of Lavender oil may be used in this, or perhaps use iced Lavender tea. Vitamin C may be given to boost the immune system, and herb teas taken to control the fever and act as general tonics (see Measles for suggestions).

Homeopathic remedies to look at include Belladonna where the face is red and burning hot, and Pulsatilla for a high temperature but a feeling of chill.

NAPPY (DIAPER) RASH

An irritation of the skin around the baby's bottom when urine and/or loose bowel movements have been left in contact with the skin for too long. Small, red pimples develop, these can break open and blister, and thrush can be a complication. Try to keep the area as dry as possible, use a little talcum powder with powdered Marigold *(Calendula officinalis)* for added anti-inflammatory effect. Calendula may also be used as a cream, or Comfrey *(Symphytum officinale)* ointment may suit better. Infusions (see page 12) of Marigold or

MARIGOLD *(Calendula officinalis)*

Chamomile *(Chamomilla recutita)* may be dabbed on to the sore area and allowed to dry. Aloe vera gel can be both soothing and healing, as can a Vitamin E cream. Where the baby is breast-feeding, it is helpful for the mother to avoid strongly spiced foods, citrus juices, coffee or alcohol to reduce the irritation of the baby's urine.

SLEEPLESSNESS

Sleeplessness in children is normally due to the same reasons as in adults, i.e. over-stimulation or anxiety. There may also be pains, such as from teething, that can stop a child getting off to sleep. In the first instance, use herbal teas to act as gentle relaxants; Lime Blossom *(Tilia europaea)*, Chamomile *(Chamomilla recutita)* and Hyssop *(Hyssopus officinalis)* are good choices. Give 5 ml (1 tsp) to under 3-year-olds, a 10 ml (2 tsp) for 3-to 8-year-olds and 15 ml (1 tbsp) to over-8s, shortly before bed, with a little honey if needed. A tissue with a drop of Lavender oil on it can be tucked under the pillow to have a steady calming effect too. Look at Insomnia, for other suggestions (see page 23).

TEETHING

The pain from teething can make children very fretful, with disturbed sleep. Probably the classic remedy is Chamomile *(Chamomilla recutita)*, which can be used in aromatherapy, herbal or homeopathic ways. Use one drop of Chamomile oil in 5 ml (1 tsp) of a carrier oil, and gently massage into one or both cheeks – if possible get essential oil from the Roman Chamomile *(Chamaemelum nobile)*, but the German Chamomile *(Chamomilla recutita)* is almost as good. The latter is the one used in teabags etc. and a teaspoon or two of a tea from this can help to relieve the pain and calm the infant. It can also be used in a warm compress, held over the affected cheek. Homeopathically, Chamomille will be prescribed for the typical pattern of one red cheek, one pale one, with restlessness, irritability and wanting to be carried.

TRAVEL SICKNESS

Children are more prone to travel sickness generally, and this can be accentuated if the blood sugar level drops too low, so keep a sweet handy when travelling. The best remedy is ginger *(Zingiber officinalis)*, and chewing a small piece of crystallized ginger can be the simplest way to relieve the symptoms. Peppermint *(Mentha piperita)* tea, sipped frequently, may also help; add a little ginger to it for extra benefit.

Homeopathic remedies that may be suitable include:
PETROLEUM: for when there is waterbrash and belching.
COCCULUS: when the smell of food makes the nausea worse.

IMPORTANT NOTICE

All the treatments suggested in this book are deemed safe and have been used by professional practitioners for many years. However, any treatment could cause an adverse reaction in an individual, and if this happens to you, stop the treatment immediately and seek professional advice. Do not try self-diagnosis or self-help treatment on any prolonged or serious problem without seeking medical advice or talking to a professional practitioner. Do not begin a course of self-help treatment when undergoing a prescribed course of medical treatment without seeking medical advice first.

Detailed below are some important reminders regarding the application of aromatherapy, herbalism and homeopathy treatments at home.

AROMATHERAPY

Essential oils should never be taken internally except under strict professional supervision. Do not increase the dosages suggested in this book. Essential oils are very powerful and doubling the number of drops is much more likely to do you harm than good.

Many essential oils should not be taken during pregnancy. Only use the doses recommended in the section on Reproduction and avoid the list of essential oils listed on page 64. All the dosages recommended in this book assume a dropper that gives 20 drops to 1 ml.

HERBALISM

As with aromatherapy oils, it is important to limit yourself to the dosages suggested herein – exceeding the dosages may cause more harm than good.

If pregnant, or likely to become pregnant, only use the herbs recommended in the section on Reproduction, and seek professional advice if in any doubt. Specific herbs to be aware of are:

SAGE: Avoid therapeutic doses if pregnant, or likely to become so. Sage should also be avoided by epileptics as sage contains thujone, which may trigger fits.

COLTSFOOT: Although there is no medical evidence of Coltsfoot causing liver damage in humans, some rats who have been exposed to large amounts of the herb have had liver damage. It should be taken internally only for a short period of time and preferably under professional guidance.

RESTRICTED HERBS IN AUSTRALIA AND NEW ZEALAND: The sale, supply and use of Borage, Coltsfoot and Comfrey is restricted in New Zealand and in some states of Australia.

HOMEOPATHY

Do not mix herbal or aromatherapy remedies with homeopathy – you will only confuse the treatment. It is also important to take the correct dosage as stipulated in this book. Potencies over 30c should always be checked by a professional before taking.

NATURAL THERAPIES

In a world of ever-increasing technology and machine-controlled medical interventions, people are beginning to feel the need for a human, individual touch; for a more natural approach to health that seeks to enhance life rather than dissect illness into more and more obscure diseases. Fortunately, there are a number of natural therapies which have just such a positive, holistic approach, and have also stood the test of time, to emerge as the most rational way to sustain our health into the twenty-first century. In the second section of this book the natural therapies are explored in five broad categories: Health from Plants covers herbal medicine, aromatherapy, the Bach Flower Remedies and Homeopathy; Naturopathy explores diet and exercise; Stress Management explains self-hypnotism and meditation as well as pyschotherapy, autogenics and healing; Bodywork offers detailed step-by-step routines in massage and reflexology, and the final category, Eastern approaches, covers shiatsu, makko ho, yoga and moxibustion with exercises that will introduce you to the benefits and theories of each discipline.

We have become accustomed to thinking of medicine as a crisis treatment for when we are sick, but one of the strengths of these therapies is their value in countering the effects of stress and helping to actually prevent illness. By reducing the impact of worries and stresses, many natural systems of treatment work to restore our vital energy and inner harmony. Eastern cultures have retained a strong tradition of therapies aimed at balancing energy, and in recent years these have gained increasing attention in the West. Our own traditional forms of treatment, such as herbalism and massage, have also undergone a resurgence in popularity, and there are the beginnings of major research projects to confirm their value. Natural therapies not only have a long history, they have a bright future.

HEALTH FROM PLANTS

The most basic and the most pervasive source of medicines throughout the world ever since time began has been the plant kingdom. From our earliest origins we can trace the use of plants for health; even today most people rely on herbal medicines for most of their primary health care.

In ancient cultures, diet and medicine were inextricably linked – let your food be your medicine, and your medicine be your food – and the importance of diet to health is discussed in another section, but plants provide an additional healthy element to our food. Herbs not only enhance the flavour of what we eat, but often contain useful trace elements and also help with the digestion of many foods. Herbal teas are low-caffeine drinks that carry many health benefits too.

Professional herbal medicine may use plants with quite profound effects on our systems, while other therapies such as homoeopathy utilize the energetic qualities of plants, among other substances. In aromatherapy, the essential oils of plants are used to affect our emotional states, as well as for quite powerful anti-infective properties. As well as these therapies, requiring treatment from qualified practitioners, the plant world also offers many home remedies, and equally importantly plants can be used in many ways to maintain good health. This section shows some of these ways, and when to seek help.

ABOVE: A selection of herbs and dried flowers used in teas and tisanes.

OPPOSITE: A garden overflowing with plants used for centuries for their health-giving and medicinal qualities.

HERBAL MEDICINE

HISTORY AND ORIGINS

The history of herbal medicine is really the history of humankind, for every culture throughout time has relied upon herbs for its medicines. Some cultures – for instance, in India and China – have maintained a strong, unbroken tradition of herbalism for several centuries, while in Europe and North America its popularity has soared and plunged periodically as Western medicine achieved greater prominence. Today, however, interest in herbal medicine has increased once more, with an appreciation of its safer, holistic approach.

Probably the first system of herbal medicine, apart from the almost instinctive use of plants for healing that existed from the dawn of history and is still practised by remote tribes, was developed in India well over 4,000 years ago.

From India, the use of plants probably travelled with

RIGHT: Ma-Kou (a Chinese goddess) carrying her medicinal herbs.

migrating people into China; traditional Chinese medicine has developed a strong philosophical viewpoint on health and disease, with treatments ranging from herbal medicines to acupuncture, moxibustion and massage techniques.

Knowledge also travelled westwards, into the Middle East, and one of the significant influences on present-day European herbalism was the ancient Egyptian tradition. Papyri dating back some 3,500 years indicate that the Egyptians used several hundred plants for food and medicine. These two uses were inextricably linked for centuries, as one Greek writer put it: "Let your food be your medicine, and your medicine be your food."

As the ancient Greeks expanded their empire, so their knowledge and use of herbs was spread throughout the realm, and other plants were added to their *materia medica*. When the Romans superseded the Greeks, their army doctors carried herbs and herbal medicine all over the known world. A large number of Mediterranean herbs were thus spread through Europe and into Britain. During these two great civilizations, several major works were written on natural history and medicine which were to be fundamental to medical thought for centuries.

After the decline of the Roman Empire, much of its literature went eastwards to Byzantium and the Arabic cultures. Traditional medicine here has retained a good deal of this ancient philosophy, and some of it came back to Europe with the Moorish invasions.

After the printing press was invented, all the old Greek

BELOW: Although drying herbs alters their colour and flavour some, such as rosemary and thyme, keep many of their properties.

RIGHT: A traditional monastic layout is recreated in this twentieth-century garden, well stocked with a wide variety of herbs. Medieval monks kept physic gardens, growing herbs to make medicines for themselves and the local people, while the villagers would generally use simple plant treatments for all manner of ailments.

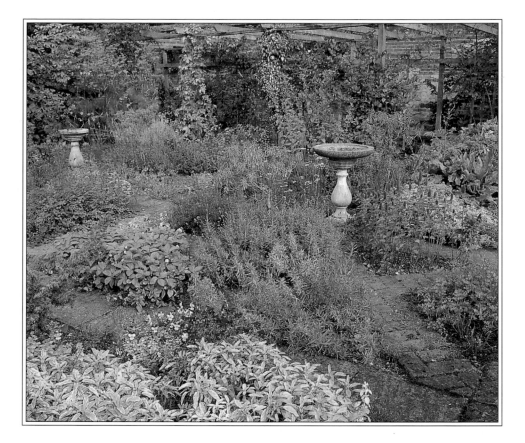

and Roman texts could be reproduced for a much wider readership. This coincided with the rapid expansion of towns and cities, and for the next three hundred years or so, knowledge and interest in herbs, in all areas of life, was greatly increased. By the sixteenth century, books about herbs were being published in the contemporary languages rather than Latin, and herbalism was an integral part of life. Books by authors such as Matthiolus, Turner, Gerard and Culpeper became bestsellers with practical advice on the uses of herbs; indeed Culpeper has never been out of print to this day, for over three hundred years.

Meanwhile, herbal medicines had been taken over by the settlers to America and used much as in Europe. It is possible to trace the spread of herbs along the eastern seaboard of the United States of America from early plantings by these settlers. Some of the more inquisitive migrants tried to learn from the Native Americans, since they were, before the importation of different diseases by the colonists, a healthy race.

The Native American system of health relied upon the use of herbs, simple yet nourishing food, fresh air and exercise. They also successfully used heat and water applications such as sweat lodges – teepees heated by a fire – with their physical and spiritual benefits.

The last ten to twenty years have seen another great resurgence in interest in natural medicine, and herbalism is both highly popular and increasingly respected as a safe and effective system of general medicine.

While today's professional practitioner of herbal medicine may see a wide range of people, often suffering from serious and chronic ill-health, the emphasis is always on the individual, looking at the whole picture of a person's health and not just any specific symptoms; this holistic approach is one good reason for its renewed popularity. Herbalism is also equally concerned with prevention or maintaining good health outside times of illness, and it is this aspect which attracts many people to use herbs in their daily lives.

LEFT: Native Americans used sweat lodges – teepees with a fire inside – as part of their natural medicine treatments.

HERBS IN FOOD

A number of widely used herbs have appreciable amounts of vitamins, minerals and trace elements, and can be thought of almost as nutritional supplements. Many others have excellent digestive qualities, helping the body cope with oily, fatty or gas-producing foods. For these reasons, as well as the extra pleasure given by their flavour, one of the earliest and best uses of herbs to help maintain health is in one's food.

LEAFY HERBS

BASIL, BAY, CORIANDER LEAVES, MARJORAM, MINT, OREGANO, PARSLEY, ROSEMARY, SAGE, SORREL, THYME.

These plants are essential ingredients in many culinary traditions, for their flavour and digestive properties. Most of these leafy herbs aid digestion, stimulating the production of enzymes that help break down fatty foods and aid absorption.

Mint sauce for example, traditionally used with lamb, helps to make this fatty meat easier to digest. Rosemary is often used with similar dishes for the same reason, stimulating the liver to work more effectively. Soups and stews are made much more tasty by the use of bay, marjoram or thyme; their aroma gets the digestive juices flowing before you have started the meal.

BASIL *(Ocimum basilicum)*

Most of these herbs contain important trace elements, and

BELOW: Sage, mint, rosemary and chives; herbs used in fresh and dried form for cooking and in salads.

ABOVE: Leaves such as rosemary and parsley are essential in many culinary traditions for their flavour and as aids to digestion.

if the diet is restricted or lacking in nourishment then these nutrients can be very important in maintaining health. The herbs then become foods in themselves, and may be used in larger amounts such as in a sauce.

Parsley for instance is rich in iron and other minerals, while sorrel is a useful source of Vitamin C. Neither should be used all the time, but may add to the nutritional value of a meal. Like many other herbs, sage is a mild antiseptic and has a wide medicinal application in liver disease and respiratory tract infections. The oil is used in both the pharmaceutical and culinary industries.

CORIANDER *(Coriandrum sativum)*

The best way to benefit from herbs is to grow them yourself so that you always have a fresh supply. All the herbs mentioned above are easy to grow. You can even grow herbs inside on a sunny windowsill. Concentrate on the more common ones first and expand your collection as you go.

AROMATIC SEEDS

ANISEED, CARAWAY, CARDAMOM, CORIANDER, CUMIN, DILL, FENNEL, STAR ANISE.

These aromatic seeds are all to some extent carminative, that is they help almost immediately to reduce the build-up of excessive wind in the digestive tract, and to release any trapped gas. They have traditionally been used with foods that are notorious in creating wind. This carminative

ANISEED (*Pimpinella anisum*)

BELOW: To make the most of the beautiful fragrances and flavours of aromatic seeds, grind them in a pestle and mortar as required.

CUMIN (*Cuminum cyminum*)

effect is contained within the essential oils in the seeds, and they have quite strong fragrances; usually only small amounts are needed to enhance the taste and flavour of a dish.

Caraway is a good example: used with foods such as cooked cabbage (a traditional association in Germany) or baked apples, it helps to prevent the bloating and discomfort that these can produce from trapped wind. Dill and fennel have been major ingredients in gripe water for babies for centuries, easing colicky pains. Coriander and cumin are important flavourings in curries and other Eastern dishes.

FRUITS AND BULBS

CHILLI PEPPERS, GARLIC, JUNIPER, PEPPERCORNS.

The general effects of these fruits is to speed up metabolism or to act as an antiseptic. Chilli peppers and peppercorns are both highly stimulating to the circulation; the effect of creating temporary heat in the stomach is to encourage gastric secretions, which in turn kill off potentially harmful bacteria in food. Traditionally this meant these herbs could be used in foods that might otherwise be toxic, the herbs providing protection as well as flavour.

RIGHT AND BELOW: The pungency of garlic and other fruits and bulbs such as chilli, juniper berries and peppercorns speeds up the metabolism and acts as an antiseptic.

RIGHT: Fresh green chilli.

The classic herb in this respect is garlic, which is not only warming, but helps lower cholesterol levels and fight infections. Juniper too is a powerful digestive antiseptic. Eating spicy, hot foods can make you perspire more, and this actually has a cooling effect which has long been appreciated by the inhabitants of hot countries.

Garlic and juniper have a traditional association with meats such as pheasant or hare, not just because their strong flavour calls for stronger-tasting herbs but because game can often be on the verge of going off. Any contamination is minimized by the antiseptic herbs.

ROOTS AND BARK
CINNAMON, GINGER, HORSERADISH.

These are all circulatory stimulants, creating an inner warmth and vigour that can be very useful in colder climates. By speeding up the metabolism, blood moves around the body better and keeps our energy levels higher. In the digestive system, the transient heat that is created helps both with digestion and in reducing trapped wind. Generally, the increased circulation helps the immune system to work better, and these herbs can be used in foods over the cold months of the year to increase the body's natural resistance to colds. Horseradish has a pungent

GINGER (*Zingiber officinale*)

ABOVE: The warmth and spiciness of ginger in all its forms is used in many herbal remedies.

flavour that lends itself to savoury dishes, the classic combination being with roast beef. It is a stimulant and a weak diuretic. Ginger is much more versatile, and will go well with savoury rice dishes and apple pies for instance. Cinnamon is also often used in both savoury and sweet dishes, its own sweetness perhaps making it more useful for puddings. It has a less hot effect than the other two, gently warming the whole system.

CINNAMON
(*Cinnamomum zeylanicum*)

HERB TEAS

One of the most widespread methods of using herbs to maintain good health and ward off illnesses is by drinking herb teas, or tisanes as they are known in France. For medicinal purposes, when treating an actual ailment, stronger preparations such as infusions or decoctions are prescribed, but in general it is possible to make a simple tisane at home.

Herb teas can be used as everyday hot drinks, to replace tea and coffee and hence reduce the caffeine intake in the diet. As each herb differs greatly in taste and flavour, it is very much an individual choice. A couple that have some of the taste qualities of ordinary tea are rooibosch and maté. The former has long been the daily drink for many people in South Africa, and is now grown in several countries; it makes a very enjoyable, low-caffeine tea. Similarly, maté is well-known in South American countries for its refreshing effect, with a smoky flavour reminiscent of Lapsang Souchong tea.

In general, it is sensible to vary herb teas, not only to enjoy a variety of flavours but to ensure that their medicinal properties are not overdone. Some can, however, be drunk over some considerable time, to maintain health and prevent ailments. In winter, especially in cooler climates, rose-hips might be a good choice. These contain considerable amounts of Vitamin C, which is an excellent way to sustain resistance to colds, flu and so on. Vitamin C can have something of a laxative effect, but the tannin content of rose-hips helps to balance this out. Many of the early naturopathic clinics in

ABOVE: Most warm herbal teas have a comforting effect and are very easy to prepare.

Switzerland, such as that run by Dr Bircher-Benner, the creator of muesli, insisted that their clients drank a few cups of rose-hip tea daily. Tea bags are easily available in many countries and are very convenient to use, although quality varies.

A SIMPLE TISANE

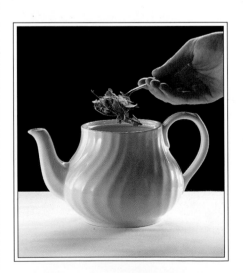

1 Warm a teapot and add one heaped teaspoonful of dried herb per person, or double for fresh herbs.

2 Pour on boiling water and allow to infuse for 2–3 minutes.

3 Strain and drink without milk or sugar (if you prefer a sweetener, use a little honey).

DANDELION TEA

Dandelions are a diuretic and can help to reduce water retention and bloated feelings. They can also help rheumatism. This tea acts as a mild laxative so should not be drunk in large quantities.

1 Remove any stems from the dandelion leaves. Tear them into strips and place in the bottom of a mug. Pour on enough boiling water to fill the mug and leave to stand for 5–10 minutes.

2 Strain, discard most of the dandelion leaves and drink. If you prefer a sweetener, add a small teaspoonful of honey.

A pleasant summer tea can be made from fresh lemon balm leaves: gather a few sprigs of the leaves, and make a tea, leaving it to stand for a few minutes. This herb reduces the impact of stress and anxiety on the system, especially where nervous indigestion is involved, and its balancing effects make it suitable for morning or evening drinking. The dried herb can be used too, but its flavour is inferior.

MINT (*Mentha x piperita*)

In hot weather, keep a jug of the tea in the refrigerator, perhaps with a slice or two of lemon for added flavour, and drink as you wish.

Peppermint and rosemary are both good pick-me-up teas, to prevent or overcome tiredness, and may be made from either fresh or dried leaves as a morning cup of tea – many blends of herbs in tea-bags are based upon the taste of peppermint. Peppermint tea is becoming more popular as a digestif drink to replace coffee after a heavy meal. Cinnamon and ginger make pleasantly warming drinks, separately or mixed together, for colder weather; just coarsely break a cinnamon stick into the teapot, while fresh ginger root may be sliced or grated. Chamomile flowers are one of the best digestive remedies, and the tea is often drunk in the evenings to aid restful sleep, or to soothe upset stomachs. Elderflowers make a thirst-quenching drink, with beneficial properties for warding off colds and catarrh, which is best made from dried flowerheads. All the above herbs can be used in combinations for extra flavour and medicinal effect.

Used regularly, herbal teas can make a significant contribution to a person's quality of health and wellbeing, not simply as replacements for stimulants such as tea or coffee, but for their general health-giving properties and specific medicinal benefits.

HERB TEA CHART

HERB	PROPERTY	BENEFIT
Chamomile	Relaxant, digestive, anti-inflammatory	Settles digestion, aids restful sleep
Cinnamon	Carminative, warming, diaphoretic	Improves digestion and good when cold/chilled
Elderflower	Expectorant, diaphoretic	Clears catarrh, reduces fevers by sweating
Lemon Balm	Relaxant, digestive, anti-depressant	Relieves nervous dyspepsia, good tonic
Lime Blossom	Relaxant, analgesic	Eases tension headaches or aching colds and flu
Peppermint	Antispasmodic and digestive	Reduces flatulence, is good for head colds too
Rosehip	Contains Vitamin C	Helps build resistance to colds and flu

HERB SUPPLEMENTS

All in all, therefore, herbs can play an essential role in maintaining one's health and vitality on a daily basis. They provide much more than extra flavouring to food, enjoyable though this may be, and their continued and universal popularity demonstrates how much people rely on them to keep well. Many herbs can be used as effective, powerful yet safe remedies for all kinds of ailments.

Herbs in other forms can also be used to maintain good health. Many people's experience of herbal medicines is in the form of tablets or capsules obtained from health stores or other outlets. Some of these extracts are more valuable in preventing ill-health than as medications; if you are actually ill, it may be better to consult a herbal practitioner since the principle of herbalism is based on individual treatment.

ABOVE: Ginseng, renowned in China as a powerful natural remedy for hundreds of years, is now used more and more in the West.

GARLIC

One of the most effective herbal remedies is garlic, which can help tremendously in building up resistance to respiratory infections, warding off colds, flu and so on. Garlic needs to be taken daily during the late autumn, winter and early spring months to sustain this resistance. Undoubtedly it is most effective when a fresh bulb is used, ideally raw, but as you can lose most of your friends if taking garlic this way every day, it may be more suitable to take one of the commercial garlic capsules that are

GARLIC TABLETS

easily found. These are less powerful, but should impart less odour to the breath – the reason for garlic's actions in resisting respiratory infections is that the (smelly) essential oil which gives it a powerful antiseptic property is 99 per cent excreted via the lungs.

ECHINACEA

Another herb with very useful properties is *Echinacea* (sometimes called purple coneflower). This stimulates the immune system, boosting general resistance to infection and illness. If vitality has been lowered, or if you simply wish to strengthen the immune response, *Echinacea* is available in either a liquid form or as tablets (sometimes it can be found combined with garlic), and a course may be taken for three or four weeks to raise immunity.

GINSENG TABLETS

GINSENG

Chronic stress is one major source of impaired immunity, and it may well be useful before or during a time of increased stress, or indeed before the winter arrives in colder climates, to take a three-week course of herbs to improve your ability to cope with physical, emotional and mental stresses. The classic herbs for this are the various ginsengs. These are most suitable for waning energy and are to be used with caution (if at all) where people respond to stress with increased anxiety or tension and raised blood pressure. Korean, or Asiatic ginseng *(Panax schinseng)*, gives the most uplift, while American ginseng *(P. quinquefolium)* has a more relaxing effect. Siberian ginseng *(Eleutherococcus senticosus)* is a completely different plant, with similar effects to Korean ginseng in enhancing stamina. These are all available as tablets, and the two *Panax* species can often be found as the actual dried root, which may be chewed in small pieces or made into a tea.

EVENING PRIMROSE

A plant that has become very popular in recent years is the evening primrose; the oil extracted from the seeds is a potent source of essential fatty acids, particularly a substance called gamma-linoleic acid. Some people do not produce enough of this compound, which in turn can lead to a shortage of more complex compounds that have beneficial effects in a number of ailments, such as arthritis, eczema and even multiple sclerosis. Evening primrose oil, however, is perhaps best known and most widely used for its use in helping ease premenstrual problems or the symptoms of the menopause. Obviously, the full treatment of hormonal disorders requires professional attention, but there may be a case for taking evening primrose oil capsules daily (500–1500mg) as a preventive treatment in the early stages of the menopause.

FEVERFEW

Another good self-help herb to use in order to help prevent the occurrence, or recurrence, of ailment symptoms is feverfew. This is another plant which has gained in popularity, this time for its usefulness in warding off migraines. It is not to be thought of as a remedy to take when you have a migraine – the reasons for which can often be a detective story and need individual treatment – but as a preventive measure. The herb is now widely available in tablet form, daily dosage about 125mg, and as the fresh leaves taste very bitter and can occasionally cause mouth ulcers, the tablets are a convenient way to use feverfew.

ALFALFA AND KELP

Some herbs are sufficiently rich in nutrients to be thought of as food supplements, although it may be more appropriate to use them in different ways. Sprouted alfalfa, for instance, contains high amounts of several vitamins and minerals; this is best taken as part of the diet, eaten in salads where it gives a crunchy bite to the dish. Nettles are very rich in iron, together with some Vitamin C, and can make an energy-giving tea for people who are bordering on being anaemic. Kelp contains several minerals, notably iodine which acts as a tonic for the thyroid gland, and can aid those who have a sluggish metabolism; this herb should *not* be used by anyone taking thyroxine for an under-active thyroid gland – if in doubt, seek professional advice. Many seaweeds are used in cooking, especially in Japanese cuisine, and this is one way to take them; kelp is also easily found in tablet form, and this is a useful way to take a daily course for, say, four weeks to boost the system.

ABOVE: Clockwise from top left: alfalfa sprouts, nettles, kelp tablets, alfalfa seeds and dried kelp.

KELP TABLETS

RIGHT: Evening primrose is widely used to alleviate the side-effects of menstruation.

AROMATHERAPY

HISTORY

One of the most primitive forms of medicine involved burning aromatic plants in order to "smoke" illness out of a patient. This process was frequently interlinked with various rituals and religious practices, and sometimes plants with mind-altering properties were burnt too, to create a mystical, other-worldly experience as part of the healing ritual. The use of incense in the ceremonies of diverse religions through the centuries has perpetuated this aspect; many of the gums and resins that are used in incense have powerful therapeutic properties – for example, as respiratory antiseptics – as well as inducing a meditative, reflective state of mind in the worshippers.

Aromatic plants and extracts have been highly regarded by all the greater ancient civilizations, stretching through the Middle East from Babylonia and Persia to India and China. The oldest medical texts from these countries, dating back at least 3,000 years, list many aromatic plants and their uses. Some of the most detailed descriptions are to be found in ancient Egyptian writings; fragrant plants were employed in all aspects of life, from perfume and cosmetics to medicine and in the rituals for embalming the dead. Some of the ointment jars excavated from Tutankhamen's tomb contained

BELOW: Aromatherapy oils are now widely available and can be mixed with pure vegetable oils for use in massage.

preservative resins such as frankincense which still had an odour after some 3,200 years.

The Egyptians were very aware of the value of fragrance in enhancing mood, and developed a reputation as masters of perfumery; Cleopatra may have owed something of her fabled attractiveness to Julius Caesar and Mark Antony from her use of vast amounts of rose petals to scent her living quarters. Interestingly, however, the Egyptians do not appear to have discovered the process of distilling the essential oils from plants, relying instead on infused oils and ointments. These were later widely used by the Greeks and Romans, both as medicine and as part of the daily ritual of public bathing, which the Romans in particular so enjoyed.

Many Greek physicians were employed by the Roman armies, and they carried the knowledge of aromatic, and other, plants across many countries. Galen, who rose to be the personal physician to the Emperor Marcus Aurelius, invented the original cold cream and was a great writer on all matters concerning health and medicines. His and other works formed the basis of medicine for many centuries, and with the decline of the Roman Empire much of this knowledge went eastwards into Byzantium. It was the Arabic countries that made the next great leap forwards in aromatherapy. By the ninth century, Baghdad was thriving partly due to being the centre of the rose industry, exporting rose water as far as India. The principle of distillation was first applied to roses and is generally credited to Abu Ali Ibn Sina, better known as Avicenna (980–1037), a philosopher and physician from Uzbekistan. Steam distillation enabled the pure essential oil to be extracted from many plants.

In the West, aromatic infused oils had continued to be used, and during the period of the Crusades, essential oils, or "perfumes of Arabia" as they were known, spread extensively throughout Europe. As the gums and resins of Asia were not easily available, native Mediterranean plants such as rosemary and lavender were used for making essential oils too. The French were particularly enthusiastic in adopting these oils, laying the foundations for today's perfumery industry as well as therapeutic uses.

Burning antiseptic herbs such as thyme and rosemary, to fumigate the air and ward off disease, was carried out in several French hospitals until well into the twentieth century. Indeed, it was a Frenchman, René Gattefosse, a chemist working in the perfumery industry, who coined the term aromatherapy some 50 years ago. He burned his hand badly in an accident in his laboratory. He used essential oil of lavender to cool the tissue and found it healed the burned flesh remarkably quickly, with no infection or scar. During both

ABOVE: Essential oils are highly concentrated; it can take 5,000 roses to produce just one teaspoonful of oil.

World Wars, essential oils were used to treat wounds and infections, and one of the pioneers of this work was Dr Jean Valnet, who published his findings in the late 1960s. Respected medical establishments in France are now looking at the medicinal aspects of essential oils.

It should not be forgotten, however, that the power of aromatic plants extends beyond antiseptic or anti-inflammatory properties. It is well established that scent can evoke memories, change people's moods and make them feel good. Aromatherapy has developed in the UK, the US and many other countries in the last 20 years into a holistic system that tries to heal and balance the whole person. The oils are often incorporated into massage, or used in baths, or simply evaporated into the air in a burner to improve physical and emotional well-being. These methods would all be familiar to the ancients, and show a continuing tradition of usage of aroma in therapy. There are also more aromatherapy practitioners than ever before offering complete treatments.

OILS AND PREVENTION

Many of the beauty and cosmetic products now on the market contain essential oils, their popularity stemming both from their wonderful fragrance and the widespread interest in using as many natural ingredients as possible. Aromatic essential oils can also be used in a number of ways to maintain good health and prevent ailments; it should always be remembered, however, that self-help is not a substitute for seeking professional treatment for an illness or condition. Furthermore, the pure essential oils themselves are highly concentrated and should be treated with respect. For instance, it may have taken 5,000 roses to produce a teaspoonful of essential oil of rose!

A useful guideline when using essential oils at home – for instance, in the bath – is the 1–2 rule. Use only one or two oils together at any time; use one or two drops in the bath; and do not use any particular oil on a daily basis for more than one or at most two weeks.

Some essential oils have a stimulating effect on the uterine muscles and should therefore not be used if you are pregnant, or suspect you might be. The possibly problematic oils to be avoided during your pregnancy include basil, clary sage, fennel, hyssop, juniper, pennyroyal, peppermint,

BASIL (*Ocimum basilicum*)

ABOVE: *Lavender is one of the most loved and well-known essential oils and has been distilled for centuries.*

sage and thyme. Equally, if you ever get any skin irritation or allergic reaction to any oil, then you should of course stop using it. Many of these herbs are used in cooking and are quite safe for pregnant women in this form.

ESSENTIAL THERAPIES

AROMATHERAPY OIL	PROPERTIES AND BENEFITS
Lavender	Antiseptic, anti-depressant, healing; relieves stress and insomnia, soothes insect bites.
Rose	Anti-depressant, aphrodisiac, tonic; helpful for menstrual disorders; aids sleep.
Bergamot	Antiseptic, astringent, stimulative; helps to combat oily skin but can sensitize it to UV light.
Sandalwood	Healing, antiseptic; can relieve fluid retention, cystitis and insomnia.
Patchouli	Healing, soothing; helps combat dandruff and dry skin patches.
Ylang Ylang	Antiseptic, aphrodisiac, tonic.
Myrrh	Healing, antiseptic, calming; eases viral and fungal infections such as thrush (if added to a bath).
Juniper	Diuretic, antiseptic, cleansing, calming; avoid in first five months of pregnancy, not to be used by those with kidney disease.
Neroli	Calming; soothes nerves and upset stomachs; a good remedy for dry skin.
Chamomile, Roman	The most soothing oil; relieves anxiety, stress, allergies, and Pre-menstrual syndrome (PMS).
Basil	Reviving, decongestive.
Rosemary	Antiseptic, stimulating, balancing, diuretic, uplifting; not to be used in the first five months of pregnancy, or by those with high blood pressure.
Frankincense	Decongestive, relaxing; aids sleep.

OILS IN THE AIR

A widely used method of employing essential oils in the home is to fragrance the rooms by means of a vaporizer, or oil burner. Vaporizers are widely available, and range from the simple utilitarian version to the highly decorative, hand-crafted piece. Although they come in many forms, they all work on the same principle. The reservoir, or receptacle, is filled with water, to which are added drops of essential oil. The reservoir is then heated, causing the water to evaporate and the warm oil to release its perfume.

CHOOSING AND USING A VAPORIZER

When choosing a vaporizer there are two important points to consider. First, there should be a suitable distance between the source of the heat and the reservoir for oil and water. This will reduce the risk of completely evaporating the water and therefore burning the oil. Second, the vaporizer should be easy to clean, ready for use with a different oil.

The simplest type of vaporizer makes use of a candle as the heat source; a more efficient, but more expensive, type is the electric vaporizer. Under certain circumstances these are preferable to the type heated by a candle – for example in the reception area of an office, in a hospital ward, or at home, when you want to disperse oils for a long period of time without the necessity of frequent supervision. Some electric vaporizers have a silent fan that disperses the evaporating oils; others employ a heated ceramic dish. Either would be suitable for a child's bedroom, or a room occupied by someone who is bedridden. Whenever you use a vaporizer of any kind, do make certain that you place the burner in a safe position, out of the reach of children and pets.

The number of drops of oil used in a burner depends on the size of the room: two to three drops for a small room, and as many as six to ten for a larger one. It is better to use fewer drops and refresh the burner more frequently, rather than use too many and saturate a room with scent. Remember too that your sensitivity to the scent will decrease, but this does not mean that the

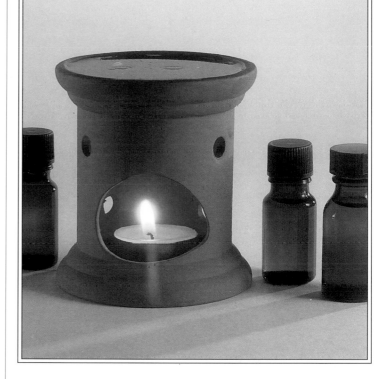

ABOVE: A terracotta vaporizer makes a lovely, warm, friendly glow as it burns and is as much a pleasure to look at as to smell.

aroma is not still present and probably still quite strong.

If you do not have a vaporizer, or you feel the need for an instant aromatherapy treatment, try applying just a few drops of oil to a handkerchief or paper towel and gently inhaling the perfume. Placing the handkerchief on your pillow at night should ease breathing if you have a blocked nose; some oils will help promote a good night's sleep. It is not wise to take essential oils as a medicine except on the advice of a practitioner, but some people do use essential oils in tea, adding two or three drops of a suitable oil to a pot of black tea for digestive problems, urinary problems or stress.

These are just some of the ways in which aromatherapy can be used as a preventive healthcare system in the home. In general, start with just a few oils, find out about their properties and uses, and go from there. One of the best things about aromatherapy is the pleasure to be derived from the aromas; keeping healthy can be enjoyable and fun.

LEFT: A porcelain vaporizer; do not leave these burning unattended.

OIL IN WATER

One of the most pleasant ways of using aromatic oils is to put one or two drops into a bath just before you get in; they form a thin film over the surface of the water, which coats and penetrates the skin while you lie in the heady aroma. If you have very dry skin, try adding a couple of drops of your chosen essential oil to a teaspoonful of pure vegetable oil, such as sweet almond, and pour this into the bath.

To help ward off the effects of the cold in winter, try using oils that have a warming effect on the circulation, such as black pepper, ginger, marjoram or rosemary. These are especially good in the morning, to stimulate the whole system. Respiratory infections can be another problem of colder months, and using essential oils through the winter months can help to build resistance to colds, coughs and so on. Oils to consider here are benzoin, eucalyptus, frankincense, lavender, pine, tea-tree and thyme, as well as the circulatory stimulants mentioned above.

After the winter, many people can feel rather sluggish and perhaps be overweight. This can be a good time to use refreshing essential oils that also help to aid digestion. Among others, choose from fennel, geranium, grapefruit, lemon, mandarin and orange – most of these are citrus oils, which have an uplifting, stimulating quality.

On the emotional level, several essences have quite remarkable effects in helping to keep our moods in balance. The best anti-depressant oil is undoubtedly bergamot, and

ABOVE: Essential oils have an ancient link with water and have been used since classical times as part of a bathing ritual.

this can be used to ward off low vitality at times of stress and depression. A note of caution though – bergamot increases sensitivity to the sun, so do not overuse before exposure to bright sunlight.

Other mood-elevators are neroli (or orange blossom), jasmine, melissa and rose. All of these particular oils are very expensive to produce, and this in itself gives a feeling of luxurious pampering when using them.

ABOVE: Add some pure vegetable oil and one to two drops of essential oil for a relaxing, steaming bath.

RIGHT: For a steam inhalation place ten drops of oil and a cup of hot water in a bowl. Inhale deeply through your nose.

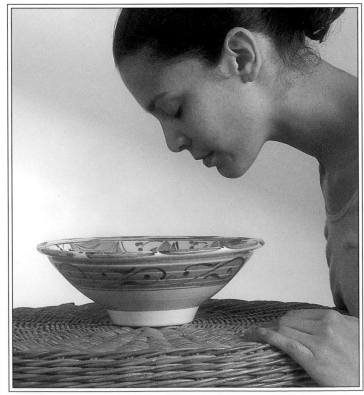

OILS IN MASSAGE

For direct use on the skin, essential oils must be diluted. Use a good, pure vegetable oil as the base, such as coconut, apricot kernel, jojoba (actually a liquid wax) or sweet almond. If your skin tends to be very dry, add about ten per cent of avocado or wheatgerm oil to the blend – avoid the latter if you are allergic to wheat. The essential oils are added at one or two per cent; assuming 20 drops to 1ml, this means using one or two drops per 5ml (1 tsp) of base oil.

All the above suggestions for bath oils apply equally to aromatherapy massage. Another area of use is in skincare itself. Some essential oils have a balancing, healing effect on the skin; frankincense, lavender, neroli, rose and sandalwood in particular can all be massaged into the skin regularly. It may be easier to mix them, at the same dilution, into your favourite skin cream; make up small amounts at a time, and vary them after a while.

SPORTS BLENDS

The oils listed below are grouped according to their usefulness before and after sporting activities.

BEFORE

❦ For stimulation: juniper, eucalyptus and rosemary.

❦ For supple, toned muscles: black pepper, ginger, rosemary, lavender, cypress, juniper, peppermint, grapefruit, orange.

❦ To aid a good strong respiratory system for aerobics: eucalyptus, peppermint, rosemary, geranium.

❦ To aid mental preparation before a competition: a blend of rosemary, lemon, lavender, chamomile.

❦ To promote good circulation: rose and palmarosa.

AFTER

❦ To soothe and prevent aching muscles: eucalyptus, ginger and peppermint.

❦ To eliminate stress following a competition: lemon, nutmeg, clary sage, orange.

LEFT: Massaging with essential oils is a good way to appreciate their benefits.

BELOW: Remember to bring the oil to room temperature before you use it, to help release its precious aroma.

DILUTING OIL FOR MASSAGE

1 Pour the equivalent of two teaspoonsfuls of pure vegetable oil into a bowl.

2 Very carefully add one or two drops of essential oil and mix together.

BACH FLOWER REMEDIES

The Bach flower remedies are named after their originator, a Dr Edward Bach. He was a medical doctor, immunologist and bacteriologist who developed a successful practice in Harley Street, London, at the beginning of the twentieth century. After several years of practice, he became convinced that much of the medicine of his day was counter-productive, depressing rather than enhancing our natural self-healing energies. For some time he was interested in homeopathy, but eventually felt that remedies should only come from nature – plants, sunlight and pure water. He gave up his lucrative practice, moved to Wales and spent the rest of his life developing a range of gentle plant-based remedies.

Dr Bach seems to have been something of a sensitive or medium, because after he had a severe illness, he found that he had an ability to assess the healing properties of various plants intuitively. Over the years he had come to the conclusion that behind all illness was an inner imbalance, an

ABOVE: The flowers for the remedies are distilled in pure spring water.

emotional or psychological state that affected the individual's health. He also felt that the vital properties of a plant were transmitted into the dew that would form in the early morning, and that this essence could be captured by floating the plant on pure spring water and leaving it for a while in the sunlight. These preparations are then preserved with a little brandy, creating in effect a diluted tincture, although not as extremely diluted as homeopathic remedies.

The flower remedies are prescribed therefore to treat negative emotional moods or states of mind, whatever the physical complaint. Their effects are thus rather difficult to evaluate – it is easier to note the disappearance of physical symptoms than a change in emotional make-up – but although sometimes subtle, the remedies can have profound effects on people's vitality and health.

Remedies may be prescribed singly or in combinations, but generally the fewer taken at one time the better. It therefore requires honesty and sensitivity when deciding what negative emotional aspect is dominant at that point. Self-prescribing is certainly possible, and Bach himself intended these remedies to be simple enough, and safe enough, for people to use on themselves. The remedies are sold in small bottles with dropper inserts, and from these stock remedies one takes four drops a dose. These may either be placed straight on to the tongue, or diluted further with a little spring water and then sipped frequently. The dose may be repeated four times a day. The high level of dilution means that the Bach remedies are usually safe for children.

Interestingly, Rescue Remedy, a compound of five of his original remedies, has become very popular as one of the finest treatments for shock, even with people who know nothing about the other remedies. Although research has failed to come up with an explanation for the effectiveness of Bach remedies, it is accepted that there is a physiological basis for its benefits, and its popularity is growing.

BELOW: An important part of developing Bach flower remedies is the application of sunlight and water to the plants.

HOMEOPATHY

Homeopathy dates back to the end of the eighteenth century, although it has much earlier antecedents. A German doctor, Samuel Hahnemann, gave up his medical practice in the 1780s in protest at the violent measures then practised, such as bloodletting and strong purging. He felt that such treatments often made patients weaker than their original illness, and for a time he turned to making a living as a translator of medical works. While working on a herbal by a Scottish writer called Cullen, he came across the assertion that cinchona bark (from which quinine was later derived) was a helpful treatment for malaria because it was a good astringent.

Since there were plenty of better astringents available, Hahnemann decided to test cinchona bark on himself to see its effects. After a few days, he started to get all the symptoms of malaria, although he did not have the disease. This led Hahnemann to the concept that symptoms were not a sign of disease but an indication of the body's attempts to fight illness; the cinchona strengthened this response. To test

ABOVE: The distinctive little white homeopathic pills prescribed to stimulate the body's immune responses.

this theory further, he tried out many more medicines on himself, friends and others, and eventually came to the principle of *similia similibus curantur* – "like will cure like"; that is, a remedy which induces certain reactions in a healthy person will be a valuable remedy for treating an illness in which these same symptoms are seen.

Hahnemann also found that symptoms often seemed to get worse initially when people were given a remedy. In order to overcome this, he diluted his remedies in a special way until they became almost undetectable, and yet the therapeutic effect seemed to get stronger. He reasoned that the healing effects must be carried out on a subtle, energetic level. He termed his system homoeopathy, literally meaning "like disease".

HOMEOPATHIC PRINCIPLES

❦ Homeopathic remedies act by stimulating our immune responses into greater action, to bring about a cure.

❦ The remedy itself does not bring about a cure, this comes from within us.

❦ The correct remedy for someone is the one that when given to a healthy person produces the same symptoms as the disease is producing in the ill person.

❦ To reduce or avoid aggravations of the symptoms, the remedy should be given in very small dosages.

❦ Dilution of the remedy, accompanied by a vigorous shaking, acts in such a way as to potentize its effects; the greater the dilution, the quicker and more effective the remedy.

Remedies are often diluted using the centessimal scale, that is one part of the original substance is diluted and succussed with 99 parts of a liquid, usually alcohol or water. This would make a 1c potency. One part of this is then diluted with 99 parts of liquid for a 2c potency, and so on.

Homeopathy has been widely used in some countries for a long time; in the last 20 years, its popularity has increased across the world and it has become much more accepted.

BELOW: Marigolds are an important ingredient in homeopathy.

NATUROPATHY

This section is intended to cover those areas of self-help and professional therapies that do not fit into the other categories of this book. More than that, however, they comprise those approaches that focus on our natural healing abilities and try simply to enhance them. Iridology has been included here since it aims to diagnose imbalances by "reading" our own natural body signs, and treatment is often along naturopathic lines.

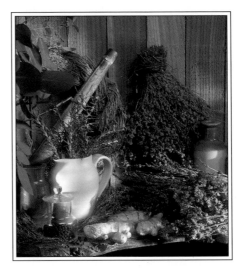

Naturopathy is itself a professional therapy, including diet, exercise, supplements and hydrotherapy within its field. Some traditions of naturopathic training also link with some of the hands-on professions such as osteopathy or chiropractic, and the practitioners of these latter disciplines may advocate other measures to help to restore full health. Hydrotherapy, or "water cure", has a strong tradition in Northern Europe, and is still carried out at centres in Germany, Austria, Switzerland and France. Increasingly it is also becoming more widespread in the US.

Both diet and exercise are vital elements in achieving and maintaining optimal health, and most of us can make adjustments in these areas. Some ideas for improvement are presented here; a key factor is to include exercises and dietary changes that you will enjoy, as a part of really appreciating life.

ABOVE: *A selection of natural herbs and plants.*

OPPOSITE: *A balanced diet gives us a secure foundation for good health and vitality.*

DIET AND EXERCISE

Probably the two most obvious and successful ways in which we can affect our health are through nutrition and exercise. Most of the natural therapies will include an assessment of and advice about these areas; indeed naturopathy focuses largely on them as a means of treating illness. A healthy diet and adequate exercise are essential for health, and although many books and magazines are devoted to encouraging us to work on these factors, they provide so much advice and differing theories and methods that it seems difficult to fulfil these aims.

A healthy diet involves eating foods that provide all the nourishment that our bodies need for growth, tissue repair, energy to carry out vital internal processes and to stay fit and active. In the last hundred years or so, the changes in eating habits in many countries have meant that large numbers of people have become overfed. Ironically, at the same time these dietary changes have left a lot of us undernourished, lacking in vitamins, minerals and trace elements that would help us to be in the peak of health.

Eating for health does not have to mean switching to a fussy, complicated diet, or adopting every new fad that comes

BELOW: Most people find it more stimulating to exercise in a group and there are many different classes to choose from.

ABOVE: A healthy diet is far from boring as long as you maintain variety and imagination in your food preparation.

along. In the first place, a healthy diet should be an enjoyable one. For conventional nutritionists, food intake is broken down into various essential ingredients, such as carbohydrates, protein, fats, vitamins and minerals; however, people generally do not think in this way but eat meals or snacks which are a mixture of various elements. What is useful is to have an understanding of which foods contain which of these ingredients, and then to look at the overall balance within the diet. Balance is probably the key word in nutrition, and it is the unbalanced nature of many Western diets that lowers vitality and may lead to ill-health. With a better understanding of the elements it is easier to create a healthy diet without too much thought and analysis.

CARBOHYDRATES

Carbohydrates are our main source of energy, and need really to form the major bulk of our diet. They are broken down in the body into glucose, and used immediately for energy or else converted into glycogen for short-term storage in the liver. An excess of carbohydrates over time will be changed and stored as fat. This is a particular danger with refined carbohydrates or sugars, which do not take much processing in the body and provide large amounts of instant energy. Since they have less starchy bulk, refined carbohydrates do not make you as full, and therefore it is easier to eat too much of them, leading to fat storage and obesity.

The main sources of unrefined carbohydrates, providing dietary fibre and trace elements, are flour and grains, beans, peas and lentils, and potatoes. With grains, this is especially true when they are unprocessed, like wholegrain bread, whole oat cereals, muesli, wholewheat pasta, brown rice and so on which supply long-term energy supplies. For more immediate energy, fresh fruit, dried fruit or vegetables such as carrots or beetroot are high in fructose, or fruit sugar. This is easily broken down by the body for energy use, and since fructose metabolism does not require insulin, it can be an essential energy resource for diabetics.

There is almost complete accord among official governmental nutrition advisers and natural dietary therapists, that carbohydrates should be the chief element in our diet. In practical terms that means eating plenty of fresh

BELOW: Eat plenty of bread, wholemeal or granary if possible.

ABOVE: Bread, rice and pasta are important for the carbohydrates which give us vital energy.

vegetables and fruit, grains of all kinds (unless there are specific reasons for avoiding a particular grain, such as with a wheat allergy), potatoes, beans and lentils. A recent piece of advice from official organizations, for instance, has been to consume five portions of fruit or vegetables a day.

FIBRE FACTS

Fibre is important to a healthy diet. Your body cannot digest it, so, in rather basic terms, it goes in and comes out, taking other waste with it. Fibrous foods include bread, rice, cereals, vegetables, fruit, and nuts. We should aim for about 30g (just over 1oz) of fibre a day. These are some examples of good fibre sources.

GOOD SOURCES	AVERAGE PORTION	GRAMS OF FIBRE
wholemeal pasta	75g/3oz (uncooked)	9
baked beans	125g/4oz	8
frozen peas	75g/3oz	8
bran flakes	50g/2oz	7
muesli	50g/2oz	4–5
raspberries	100g/3½oz	6
blackberries	100g/3½oz	6
banana	average fruit	3.5
baked jacket potato	150g/5oz	3.5
brown rice	50g/2oz	3
cabbage	100g/3½oz	3
red kidney beans	40g/1½oz	3
wholemeal bread	1 large slice	3
high-fibre white bread	1 large slice	2
stewed prunes	6 fruit	2

PROTEINS

Proteins are the essential body-builders, helping us to create muscles, bones, tendons, hair, skin and nails. They are also vital in most of our hormone and enzyme production. The first thing to say about protein is that in most developed countries people eat too much, so the problem is not so much increasing those foods that are high in protein but getting the balance right. An excess of high protein foods in the diet will be converted into glucose for energy use or else stored as fat.

Foods rich in protein include meat, fish, poultry, eggs, milk and other dairy products, nuts and seeds, beans and lentils, and grains (bread has a little under ten per cent protein). Human protein is made from a number of simple substances called amino-acids, and these need to be present in certain amounts or combinations in the protein in our diet for us to make use of them. Animal sources do contain the right amounts of these amino-acids, but also contain relatively high levels of fat. Plant sources of proteins often need to be combined in order to give adequate levels of amino-acids; this can be something as simple as beans on toast, or a spicy bean dish with rice, and generally means having a more varied, or even a more adventurous diet.

LEFT: Dairy products, such as milk, butter and cheese, supply us with not only protein but also fat.

ABOVE: Eggs are an important source of vitamins and protein but you should not eat more than two to three a week.

LEFT: One of the best sources of protein, fish is high in vitamins and minerals and is highly recommended by nutritionists.

BELOW: Eat unsalted nuts for their protein.

FATS

Fats are vital too, helping to form part of the cell structure and maintaining our inner organs and nerves. They also act to provide insulation and temperature regulation. It is, however, well-recognized that in the developed world much of our diet is too rich in fats, especially animal fats, and this is a major factor in heart disease, obesity and even some cancers, especially when we have such sedentary lives. Growing children, however, especially active ones, do need fats more than adults, and we should not reduce their intake so much.

Advice on fat-containing foods tends to be what to reduce rather than what to increase. Meat and dairy products can contain concentrated sources – a nice, juicy steak may have 30 per cent fat, for example. There are some differences between the effects of saturated fats (from animal products) and unsaturated fats such as are found in oily fish like salmon or plant oils like sunflower products. In general terms, move the emphasis towards the latter, using oils such as olive, sunflower, corn or safflower with salads or in cooking, but most people need to reduce all kinds of fats; they are the most concentrated sources of energy and anything over small amounts easily leads to obesity. There are plenty of reduced-fat items, particularly dairy products, which are now available and which can help in controlling fat intake.

ABOVE: *Oil made from the seeds of sunflowers is an unsaturated fat which should be used instead of animal fats in cooking. Avoid frying foods, however, and grill or steam instead.*

EASY WAYS TO CUT DOWN FAT AND SATURATED FAT

EAT LESS	INSTEAD
Butter and hard fats.	Spread butter more thinly, or replace it with a low fat spread or polyunsaturated margarine.
Fatty meats and high fat products such as pies and sausages.	Buy the leanest cuts of meat you can afford and choose low fat meats like skinless chicken or turkey. Look for reduced-fat sausages and meat products. Eat fish more often, especially oily fish.
Full-fat dairy products like cream, butter, hard margarine, milk and hard cheeses.	Choose skimmed or semi-skimmed milk and milk products and try low-fat yogurt, low-fat fromage frais and lower fat cheeses such as skimmed milk soft cheese, reduced-fat Cheddar, mozzarella or Brie.
Hard cooking fats such as lard or hard margarine.	Choose mono-unsaturated or polyunsaturated oils for cooking, such as olive, sunflower, corn or soya oil.
Rich salad dressings like mayonnaise or salad cream.	Make salad dressings with low-fat yogurt or fromage frais, or use a healthy oil such as olive oil.
Fried foods.	Grill, microwave, steam or bake when possible. Roast meats on a rack. Fill up on starchy foods like pasta, rice and couscous. Choose jacket or boiled potatoes, not chips.
Added fat in cooking.	Use heavy-based or non-stick pans so you can cook with little or no added fat.
High-fat snacks such as crisps, chocolate, cakes, pastries and biscuits.	Choose fresh or dried fruit, breadsticks or vegetable sticks. Make your own low-fat cakes and bakes.

VITAMINS AND MINERALS

Vitamins and minerals are needed for proper growth and development and body maintenance. They control the absorption of other nutrients and without them a series of complaints can develop, from headaches to sterility. There are 13 major vitamins which, apart from K and D, must be obtained from the food we eat. The fresher the food the higher its vitamin content. Food loses its vitamins through cooking, exposure to light or cold and storage, so buy small quantities of fresh food and eat it as soon as possible.

RIGHT: Supplements are an important source of vitamins but do not rely on them for all your requirements.

MINERAL AND VITAMIN VALUES

VITAMIN	SOURCES INCLUDE	BENEFITS
Vitamin A	Liver (especially fish livers), egg yolk, fortified margarine, oily fish, oranges, apricots, carrots, tomatoes, melons, dark green leafy vegetables.	Eyesight; skin; may protect against cancer.
Vitamin B1	Most foods – including wheatgerm and pulses, wholegrains, brewer's yeast, nuts, fortified breakfast cereals.	Helps break down carbohydrates; nervous system; repairs body tissues.
Vitamin B2	Brewer's yeast, liver, kidney, dairy produce, wheat bran, wheatgerm, eggs.	
Vitamin B3	Wheatgerm, wholegrain cereals, meat, fish.	Essential for tissue chemical reactions.
Vitamin B6	Avocados, liver, wholegrains, egg yolk, lean meat, bananas, fish, potatoes.	Nervous system; skin; red blood cells.
Vitamin B12	Liver, kidney, some fish (including shellfish), eggs, milk.	Healthy blood and nerves.
Vitamin C	Citrus fruits, potatoes, tomatoes, leafy greens.	Helps heal wounds, may fight colds, flu and infections; protects gums, keeps joints and ligaments in good working order.
Vitamin D	Fish liver oils, fatty fish, eggs, fortified margarine, also synthesized by ultraviolet light.	Calcium deposits in bones.
Vitamin E	Vegetable oils, some vegetables, wheatgerm.	Cell growth; antioxidant.
Vitamin K	Most vegetables – especially leafy green ones, liver.	Essential in production of some proteins.

MINERAL	SOURCES INCLUDE	ESSENTIAL FOR
Calcium	Cheese, milk, yogurt, eggs, bread, nuts, pulses, fish with soft bones such as whitebait and tinned sardines, leafy green vegetables.	Healthy bones, teeth and nails; muscle and nerve function; blood clotting; milk production in nursing mothers.
Iron	Liver, red meat, oily fish, wholegrain cereals, leafy green vegetables.	Makes haemoglobin, the pigment in red bloods cells that helps transport oxygen around the body.

HEALTHY EATING

So, what advice can be given on foods? Our needs do vary throughout life, so there is no single diet that can be suggested – thank goodness! Children and teenagers need more protein, and most other nutrients, due to their growth rates, and pregnant women have an extra need too. Hard physical work or other activity increases demand, while older and less active people may require fewer calories. What we all need is varied, healthy and enjoyable food.

Three key words are freshness, wholeness and variety. As far as possible make fresh foods the major part of your food intake – fresh fruit and vegetables, freshly cooked bread, pasta or other grains, and a little freshly prepared meat, poultry, fish or other protein-containing foods. Preparation of foods should aim to retain as much of the original goodness as possible, so grill or bake foods rather than frying them. Wholeness can be taken to indicate not just trying to use wholegrains but cutting back on processed foods as far as possible. Try to have fresh foods first, then frozen and only occasionally resort to packaged or canned food. Variety means exactly that; it is as unhealthy to eat just oranges all day as it is to eat nothing but hamburgers all day.

BELOW: Take advantage of the many kinds of fruit available around the year, and vary your intake as much as possible.

ABOVE: Steamed vegetables retain much of their vitamins as well as colour and flavour.

SOME IDEAS MIGHT INCLUDE:

❧ More fresh fruit and vegetables: they are high in vitamins and minerals and low in fats.

❧ Steadily increase fibre-rich foods, such as fruit, vegetables, wholegrains, beans and lentils.

❧ Eat fish, poultry and leaner cuts of meat, and avoid frying them as far as possible. Cut down on meat products such as pies, sausages and so on, which generally have high levels of fat.

❧ Eat fewer dairy products and use low-fat versions of, say, yogurt or milk.

❧ Keep pastries, cakes, biscuits and chocolates for special occasions.

❧ Drink plenty of water; many of us get dehydrated.

❧ Ease up on stimulants such as coffee and tea, and also alcohol.

❧ Try to use less salt – this also means reducing intake of processed foods, since they can often be high in salt.

❧ Enjoy food! There is a lot of pleasure to be gained from the taste and aroma of a varied diet.

7-DAY HEALTHY EATING PLAN

This healthy eating plan gives suggestions for a balanced way of combining foods. Try to choose low-fat, low-sugar foods aiming to include plenty of wholegrain high fibre foods and 5-6 portions of fruit and vegetables each day.

To the suggestions below add your own choice of fruit juices and water and limited wine, tea and coffee. Try drinking some of the many blends of herb teas which are now available and which are a delicious, healthy substitute for tea and coffee. For snacks and desserts choose fresh fruit, and low fat fromage frais or yogurt with occasional high fibre bran muffins or carrot cake for treats.

RIGHT: Make sure the fruit and vegetables you buy are fresh and flavoursome, and buy little and often to gain full vitamin benefit.

	BREAKFAST	**LUNCH**	**DINNER**
Monday	Fruit juice, porridge, fresh fruit.	Sardines or pilchards on toast.	Macaroni, cauliflower and broccoli cheese.
Tuesday	Grilled mushrooms or tomatoes on toast.	Homemade coleslaw with cottage cheese and rye crispbreads. Fresh fruit and oatbar or flapjack.	Salade Nicoise; lettuce, tomato, cucumber, new potatoes, tuna, olives, hard-boiled eggs, anchovies.
Wednesday	High energy drink, juice or milk, and banana, yogurt, honey and wheatgerm.	Onion soup with grilled cheese croutons. Fresh fruit and fruit cake.	Stir-fried vegetables and chicken or cashew nuts with rice or noodles.
Thursday	Muesli topped with low-fat live yogurt and chopped apple.	Wholemeal sandwich of cream cheese, avocado and salad. Fruit.	Pasta with tomato, bacon and mushroom sauce and parmesan cheese and mixed salad.
Friday	Fruit juice, cereal, toast and honey and fresh fruit	Hummous with crudites and wholemeal pitta bread or rye crackers.	Paella or risotto and green salad.
Saturday	Boiled, poached or scrambled egg on granary toast.	Jacket potato with baked beans and grated cheese, salad. Fresh fruit.	Grilled fish with fresh tomato sauce, steamed vegetables and new potatoes
Sunday	Fresh or soaked dried fruits with low-fat live yogurt. Wholemeal or granary toast.	Roast chicken joint with roast Mediterranean vegetables; whole garlic, peppers, courgette, aubergine etc, and potatoes or rice. Fruit and yogurt brulée.	Thick vegetable and lentil soup with wholemeal bread. Fresh fruit salad and cheese.

MOVE TO KEEP ALIVE

As far as exercise is concerned, the best phrase to sum up the importance of movement to your body and health is, "Use it or lose it". Inactivity, a sedentary lifestyle, means that our bodies steadily deteriorate and various health problems start to develop. Equally importantly, exercise helps to reduce the effects of stress and worry, and makes us feel better. The value of exercise is high at all times of life, for children growing up and developing strong bones and muscles, for adults to keep fit, active and healthy, and for older people to reduce problems like osteoporosis and simply to keep mobile and independent.

This is another area where official encouragement has occurred in recent years, with suggestions of a minimum of 20 minutes of brisk exercise three times a week as one example. Having activity goals can be very useful, but they should not act as a deterrent to getting started; any amount of exercise is better than none. It must be said, of course, that sudden, unaccustomed or inappropriate exercise can cause musculoskeletal problems, and people with certain conditions may need to seek medical advice before undertaking

Below: Exercise in the fresh air as much as you can with walks and cycle rides in the country.

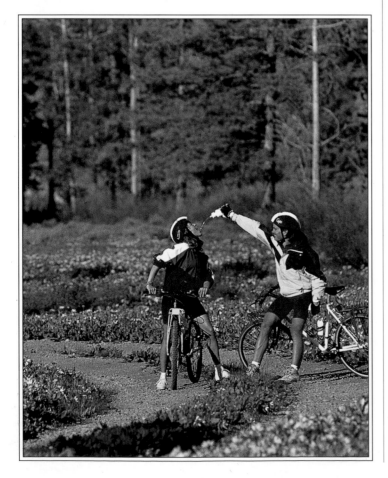

Right: Take small amounts of regular exercise.

exercise. Nevertheless, steadily increasing exercise is likely to benefit the great majority of us, improving the efficiency of our heart, lungs and muscles, improving our posture and making us feel fitter and look healthier.

The first advice is to take the kinds of exercise that you enjoy and that you can incorporate into your lifestyle. Walking up and down stairs rather than taking the lift can be a simple example of fitting more movement into your life. Weekend walks, gardening, cycling or dancing are some leisure activities that can also help you to get fitter.

If you have not done much exercise for some time, do try to warm up and loosen the body before doing anything more strenuous, and don't exercise straight after meals. If you are ill or very tired, then limit physical exertion too. To allow easier movement, try to wear loose, comfortable clothing when exercising, and use the correct shoes and clothing when playing a particular sport. A good idea may be to join a class; with exercise like aerobics, low-impact exercises or weight-training, a class is essential to make sure that you are doing the movements safely and correctly. Personal trainers can provide detailed exercise programmes for you, with advice on the training zone, or optimal heart-rate, that you should aim for. Serious exercisers have access nowadays to all kinds of scientific back-up on how to plan and carry out exercise, but for most people it is most important to get fun and enjoyment out of physical activity.

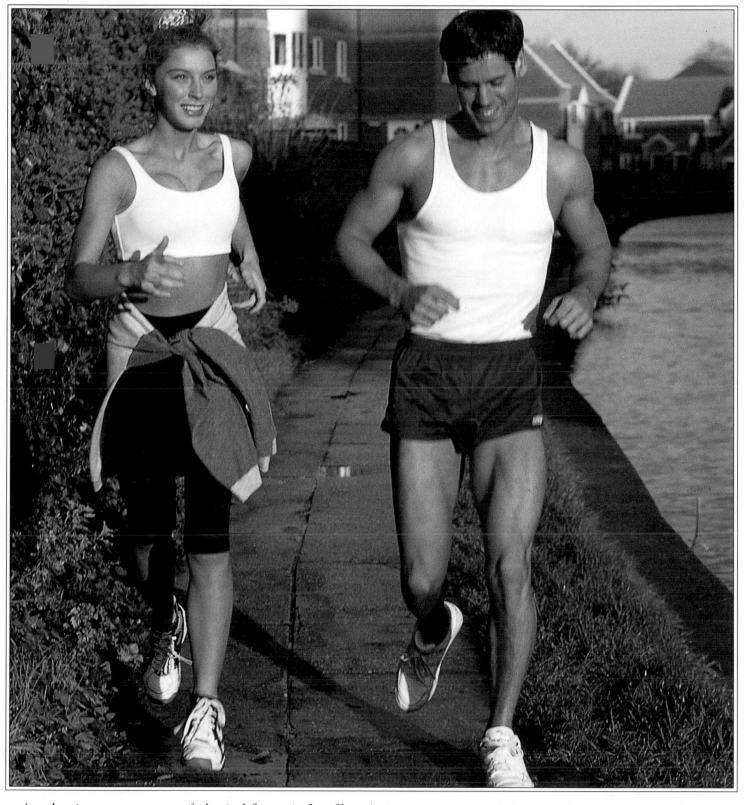

ABOVE: Exercising with friends adds encouragement and company.

Another important aspect of physical fitness is the effect it has on the way we feel about ourselves. Without becoming neurotic about your size and weight, try to take an interest in the state your body is in. An enjoyable and invigorating fitness regime, at a level you can sustain without undue stress, can enhance your mental and physical well-being. When you are unfit you tend to feel more lethargic and uninterested in the world and the people around you. A straight back, a spring in your walk and an alert, energetic expression will create a better impression than bad posture, slumped shoulders and uncoordinated movements. So improve your fitness and your self-esteem at the same time.

SHOULDER AND NECK EXERCISES

WARMING-UP EXERCISES

Some suggestions for warming-up exercises are given here. If you haven't done much exercise for a long time, or are recovering from a long illness, initially they may be enough on their own to get you more mobile. They will also be helpful to prepare you for something more strenuous. If you are exercising for the first time in a long while, pay attention to how your body responds. If you become out of breath or your heart races, stop, and ask your doctor's advice on suitable exercise. If you are more used to exercise, use this routine as a warm-up before moving on to something more strenuous. Try to breathe freely and comfortably when doing these and any other exercises, and remain aware of your body's responses to the movements.

1 To loosen the shoulders and ease neck tension, try slowly rolling your shoulders in a circle, lifting them right up as they move round, and then dropping them down again.

2 Stretch the neck muscles by dropping your head to the side, towards one shoulder and then the other, repeating three or four times.

3 Then slowly swing your head in an arc, from one side across your chest to the other side.

4 Repeat the swing three or four times, keeping control of the movement all the time.

ARM AND ABDOMEN EXERCISES

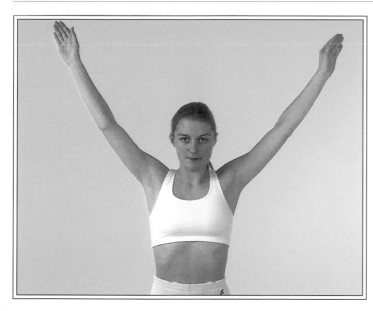

1 Swing your arms forwards in large circles, to begin to loosen the shoulder joints .

2 Then reverse the action and swing your arms backwards in large circles to open up the chest.

3 Facing forwards, twist your arms from one side to the other, letting them move loosely.

4 Continue the movement but begin to allow your head and trunk to move sideways with the arm swings.

5 Continue to twist right round, keeping your head in line with your arm movements.

6 Bend sideways from the waist, keeping your hips still and moving your hand down towards your knee.

7 Return to an upright position, then bend to the other side. Keep your feet firmly on the ground.

8 Extend this movement into a bigger stretch by raising one arm in the air and bending sideways.

9 Repeat the movement in the opposite direction.

BENDING AND SQUATTING

1 With legs about shoulder-width apart, bend forwards as far as you can, keeping your legs straight.

2 Steadily return to the upright. Repeat the action. If this is difficult, keep the legs slightly bent when bending forward, and gradually work on straightening the legs while you are leaning forward.

3 With hands on your head or hips, squat down, keep your back straight.

4 Come back to a standing position, returning to your tiptoes as you do so. Repeat the exercise serveral times.

5 Try jogging, running or jumping on the spot. If you suffer from any back problems, you may be better off with a rebounder or using a step to go up and down to reduce impact – get professional advice if you are unsure.

FLOOR EXERCISES

1 To tone and strengthen the abdominal muscles, try sitting on the floor, with knees bent and hands clasped around the knees. Lean back as far as comfortable, using your arms to support your weight, breathing out as you do so and holding for five seconds if possible.

2 Repeat at least five times. As your muscles improve, try placing your hands behind your neck, so that the abdominal muscles do more work.

3 Go on all fours on the floor, making sure your hands are directly below your shoulders, and your knees are in line with your hips. Keep your back and neck in a straight line.

4 Then stretch and arch your back upwards, dropping your head down, hold this position for a few seconds, then return to the first position. Repeat several times.

You may use these exercises before harder physical activity, and/or as a cooling-down period after strenuous exercise, or simply on their own if you have a very sedentary life. If you have any pain or discomfort, then you may need to get advice – the old slogan "no pain, no gain" has been sidelined by more positive attitudes to movement. If you find you prefer doing exercises with others, to music or even while singing along yourself, then do so and have fun.

HYDROTHERAPY

Hydrotherapy, or the use of water for healing purposes, has an ancient pedigree, and different applications of using water can be found in many classical civilizations. Both the ancient Greeks and Romans used hot- and cold-water baths extensively, and many of the modern spas throughout Europe owe their origins to Roman bathing centres. Similarly, the Native Americans were familiar with the use of sweat-lodges, for physical and spiritual cleansing, and were proficient in various hydrotherapeutic techniques.

In recent centuries, however, some of this knowledge and expertise was lost. The therapeutic uses of water were largely revived in Europe in the nineteenth century by a Bavarian Dominican monk, Sebastian Kneipp. He believed that people had considerable innate healing powers and that water applications were a medium for stimulating, or occasionally soothing, our recuperative efforts. His ideas have continued to be influential to this day, and in spas in Germany it is possible to experience one of 50 or so different water applications for a variety of ailments.

Typical treatments may include contrast bathing, using alternating baths of hot and cold water. These are usually what are termed sitz baths, a kind of hip bath that immerses the lower trunk, while the feet may be placed in foot-baths of contrasting temperature in order to stimulate the circulation. Other forms of treatment may include high-pressure hosing with cold water, hot or cold body wraps, friction rubs, or baths with various ingredients added for extra elimination – for example, mud baths, Epsom salts baths or thalassotherapy (seawater baths).

Cold body wraps are made by soaking a sheet in cold water and wrapping

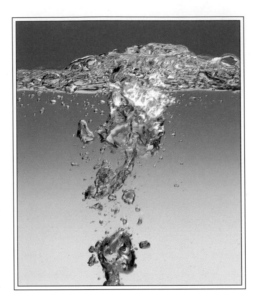

ABOVE: Fresh bubbling water is full of power and energy.

it around the body, then covering this with a dry sheet and blanket. The initial cold is quite quickly replaced by warmth. These wraps are used for a number of conditions such as chronic muscle strains and backache. The sitz baths are often recommended for conditions such as chronic constipation, congestion in the pelvic area, recurrent cystitis and period pains. The sprays have similar effects to the baths, depending on their temperature, but are generally more stimulating to the circulation. A milder effect is achieved by whirlpool baths, which are increasingly popular in homes, gyms and spas.

Some recent medical research has shown the benefits of cool baths for reducing high blood pressure and improving peripheral circulation, and the contrasting applications of hot and cold water compresses and such like have a strong effect on the immune system, so hydrotherapy has very definite physiological effects. As a note of caution, prolonged exposure to very hot water is not a good idea for pregnant women or anyone with hypertension or heart disease, so be careful with saunas, Turkish baths, whirlpools and so on. Regular shorter sessions are often more beneficial.

Home applications can be very simple; a sprained ankle or similar injury with swelling needs a cold application initially, such as an ice pack or cold compress. After a while, older injuries may respond to hot, then cold applications, while chronic areas of muscular stiffness often do better with just warm water treatments. Although largely neglected by orthodox medicine in the UK, European countries and indeed the US have been much more positive about hydrotherapy, and new research is confirming its potential.

BELOW: A soothing foot-bath will help everyday aches and stiffness.

IRIDOLOGY

Iridology is the study of health and illness by diagnosing changes to the iris, or coloured part of the eye. The eyes have always been considered of some importance as indicators of internal health, or ill-health, but iridology as a distinct system dates back to the nineteenth century, to a Hungarian doctor called Ignatz von Peczely. As a boy, von Peczely had cared for an owl that had broken a wing. As the wing mended, he noticed that a thin black line which he had observed in the bird's iris gradually faded to little marks around a small dot. As an adult and a physician, von Peczely became more and more convinced through observation of his patients that similar illnesses produced similar changes and patterns of markings in their irises.

He published his findings in 1881, and they caused much interest throughout European and later American medical circles. In the 1950s in the US, Dr Bernard Jensen produced a detailed chart of the iris, locating each organ in the body to a specific part of the iris. His mapping system is quite complex, with various rings or zones relating to different systems, such as digestive, circulatory, lymphatic, muscular, skeletal and so on. Overall, the left eye shows up problems on the left side of the body, and the right eye the right side, although many disturbances seem to produce changes in both irises.

The map that Jensen and others developed divides the iris

ABOVE: A healthy eye will be clear, with no signs of inflammation, soreness or discolouration.

into various sections, rather like a wheel divided by spokes. In each segment any markings within the iris are thought to be linked to different parts of the body, or else varying functions. Overlapping these divisions are the concentric rings mentioned above, which radiate from the centre of the eye outwards and are believed to show disturbances in the stomach, the glands and inner organs, the muscles and skeleton, and finally the skin and eliminative processes.

In the last 30 years or so, the knowledge of what an iris is able to show has increased, and a lot of work has been done on its complexity. There are some different schools of thought among iridologists and, in the main, although doctors find the general appearance of the eye – yellowing, dullness or unnatural brilliance, for example – an indication of ill health, conventional medicine dismisses completely the concept of specific, detailed links between parts of the body and markings in parts of the iris. Nevertheless, iridology has steadily grown in popularity among a number of therapists, who will use the technique as one of their diagnostic methods and as a non-invasive way of checking out internal functioning. An iridologist will diagnose rather than treat, and if any signs of degeneration, malignancy or disease are detected, patients are advised to see their GP.

Although many natural therapists are themselves sceptical of some of the claims of iridology, it is an area for fruitful research – our eyes are, after all, windows to the soul.

BELOW: Map of the eye showing which part relates to which part of the body.

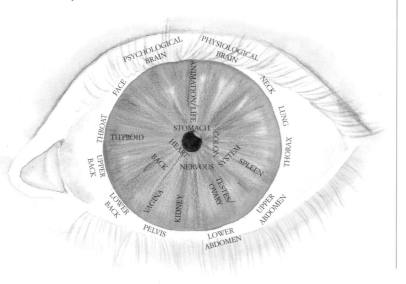

STRESS MANAGEMENT

It is probably fair to say that the greatest threat to our health today, at least in the developed countries, is having more stress than we are able to handle. The increasing pace of lifestyles, the complexity of many professions, not to mention changes and added strains in relationships due to greater mobility and thus distance from others, has placed considerable burdens on our stress-management systems.

Nearly all natural therapies place great importance on stress as a probable factor in ill-health, and yet people need a certain amount of stress in order to become motivated and develop; so what is the problem? Our internal stress-coping mechanisms originally developed to cope with potentially life-threatening situations, the so-called "fight or flight" adaptation. However, these biochemical changes are all too often brought into play by other factors nowadays, from meeting deadlines or work crises to receiving the latest bill. When the body is placed in an almost constant state of alert, the adrenal glands become tired eventually and people are depleted and panicky rather than stimulated and awake.

These problems have been recognized for a long time, and most natural therapies will offer some help with stress-related problems; in this section the focus is on some approaches which specialize in helping with stress-management directly.

ABOVE: Meditation is a well-known method for diffusing stress and tension.

OPPOSITE: Take time to relax and allow your body to rest during busy periods of life.

HYPNOTHERAPY

A person in hypnosis is not "asleep"; indeed they are often more aware of what is taking place than normal. Anybody (with a very few exceptions) can enter this deeply relaxed state, and indeed will, naturally.

It is believed that the state of hypnosis was used in ancient Egypt, South East Asia, and the Pacific island cultures. The hypnotic state is described in Greek and Roman writings too. The advent of Christianity appears to have marked the decline in its use, as it was then classed as witchcraft. It was, strangely enough, a Roman Catholic priest, Father Gassner, who in the late 1700s renewed public interest by using hypnotic inductions as a means of "casting out devils". Around the same time Anton Mesmer began to theorize about "animal magnetism", and the use of this phenomenon for medical purposes. He believed that Gassner was magnetizing his clients with the metal crucifix which he held. Mesmer attracted a lot of

ABOVE: Mesmerism: an operator and his patient from E. Sibly's A Key to Physic and the Occult Sciences, *London.*

attention in France, and was later investigated by the French government and denounced as a fraud. It was left to James Braid to investigate further in 1841, and he is responsible for renaming mesmerism as hypnosis, from the Greek word *hypnos* meaning sleep, later trying to rename it mono-idealism, as he recognized it was not sleep but a concentration of the mind upon one channel of communication. But the words hypnosis and hypnotism had caught on, and change was impossible. Many more people after Braid developed theories about hypnosis and used it in the medical world. Perhaps the best-known exponent is a surgeon called Esdaile, who performed many serious operations painlessly using only hypnosis as an anaesthetic; some three hundred of these are carefully recorded. This method might well have continued had it not been for the discovery of chloroform and ether as chemical alternatives. It is interesting to note that hypnosis as anaesthetic is returning to popularity, especially in the US.

What then is hypnosis? It is a state of deep relaxation, a state of heightened awareness, combined with a feeling of calm lethargy. It can be best described as similar to that state between sleep and wakefulness when you are aware of your surroundings but unwilling to move. Its characteristics are a heightened susceptibility to beneficial suggestion and a much improved memory with access to "forgotten" or repressed memories stored in the unconscious mind.

In itself, the hypnotic state is very pleasant, but nothing more than that. It is very similar to the mental states achieved during meditation and yoga. It is what the therapist and client do together within this state that makes it therapy.

LEFT: Mesmer's tub at his consulting room in Paris which he opened soon after his treatise in 1779. The tub was a vat of dilute sulphuric acid and patients sat round it holding hands or holding on to one of the iron bars which projected from it.

SELF-HYPNOTIC INDUCTION

Self-hypnosis may not be suitable for anyone suffering from mental illness, or taking medication for a nervous condition. It is also potentially dangerous to use self-hypnosis to mask pain as this could lead to a serious illness going undetected. Ask your doctor's advice before using self-hypnosis in the above situations or if you have any doubts as to its suitability for you. It is also advisable to have one or more sessions with a properly qualified hypnotist to establish suitability and to receive instruction on how to use self-hypnosis.

Hypnosis as a natural state can be created in a number of ways, by audio, tactile or visual means. People can be shocked into hypnosis or coaxed or even bored into it. Self-hypnosis can be attained in many different ways too, but many therapists believe that by using the patterns outlined below, anyone can achieve a state of self-hypnosis. Initially, when learning these patterns, it may be useful to read them, slowly, on to a cassette tape, and then, preferably with headphones, use the tape to guide you into self-hypnosis. You may be reassured that should anything happen that requires your immediate attention, you will sit up straight away and deal with it as you would normally do: you are in control at all times. Non-intrusive music in the background can be helpful, too. Once you have learned to gain the state of hypnosis, you will be able to do so anywhere at any time that is useful to you.

STRESS MANAGEMENT

There follow three methods of self-hypnotic induction that can be highly beneficial to break a stressful day, to take five minutes to clear the mind before that important meeting, or just to unwind at the end of the day, so as to be clear thinking and able to enjoy the evening at leisure without carrying the worries of work into other areas of your life.

1 PHYSICAL RELAXATION

1 Settle back and relax in a chair or on a couch, or lie on your bed and just gaze upward, as if you were looking up through your eyebrows. Fix your gaze on a spot, either real or imaginary, and count down slowly from five to one. As you count down, imagine your eyelids becoming heavy, your eyes becoming tired, so that when you get to one, you can allow your eyes to close. Now begin to relax deeply. Think of the top of your head, your scalp, and concentrate on all the muscles, skin and nerve-endings there, deliberately relax them all and let go of all the tension.

2 Tense your facial muscles, scrunch them all up, around the eyes, the forehead, around the mouth, scowling and grimacing for a count of five seconds, and then release and let go, and feel that beautiful relaxation in all those muscle groups.

Thinking down through the neck and shoulder muscles and on into the tops of your arms, allow those muscles to sag down and become tension-free. Thinking over the muscles of the upper arms, tense those muscles for a count of five and let them go, let them relax down into the elbows and on to the forearms, just letting all those areas relax and let go.

3 Clench your fists, really tight, for a count of five, and release any tension, leaving the hands and arms heavy, easy and relaxed. With each breath you breathe out say to yourself, in your mind, the word "calm". Let any tension in the chest area drain away, as you think down into the stomach muscles, letting them relax too. Let all the muscles of your back relax. Thinking into your waist, your hips, and thigh muscles, let tensions drain away as you think down towards your knees ... and on down into the shins and calves, allowing those muscles to relax, into the feet and toes, all muscles tension-free and feeling good.

2 THE STAIRS

Imagine a beautiful staircase stretching down in front of you made up of ten steps covered in a soft cream coloured carpet, perhaps lit with candles. Imagine you are standing on the tenth step up. Count backwards from 10 to 0, and as you count backwards, imagine each number as a step, and each step as a step down the staircase, into deeper and deeper levels of relaxation, so that by the time you get to 0, you can allow yourself to be as deeply relaxed as you can ever manage, while still aware of sounds around you.

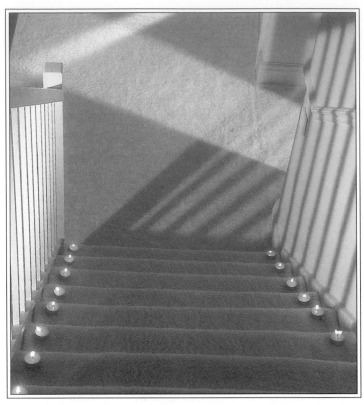

2. On step 6 you are becoming calmer ... and calmer ... even calmer still ... Halfway down the stairs and you are continuing to relax, continuing to let go and feeling good. On step 4 you are relaxing even more ... letting go ... and by step 3 – sinking deeper ... drifting further into this welcoming, relaxed state.

1 Imagine taking the first step down, relaxing and letting go. Take another step down, feeling beautifully at ease and at peace inside. On step 8 you are becoming more relaxed, and letting go even more ... on 7 you are drifting deeper ... and deeper ... and even deeper down still ...

3 On step 2, the last but one, you are enjoying those good feelings now, half-awake, half-asleep. By the time you reach step 1 you are nearly all the way down now, feeling beautifully relaxed. At the bottom of the staircase you are so beautifully relaxed, you can allow your mind to drift ...

3 THE HAVEN

Allow your mind to drift ... drift to a pleasant, peaceful place – a place that you know and where you can always feel able to relax completely. A safe, secure place where no one and nothing can bother you. It may be somewhere you have been on holiday, a beach or a place in the countryside. Or it may be a room you have had, one you do have or one you would like to have – an imaginary place. It's a place where you can always feel able to completely let go – a haven, a haven of tranquillity, unique and special to you.

In order to help you be in this place, notice first the lighting level. Is it bright, natural or dim, with any particular source of light – natural or manmade? Also notice the temperature level. Is it hot, warm or cool? Is there any particular source of heat? Be aware also of the colours that surround you. What are the shapes and textures and the familiar objects that make that place special?

Just be there, sitting, lying or reclining, enjoying the sounds, the smells and the atmosphere with no one wanting anything, needing anything, expecting or demanding anything from you. Now you can truly relax.

Now that you have reached that peaceful state of deep relaxation known as hypnosis, you can just relax and enjoy. You can bring yourself to full wakefulness at any time, by just slowly counting up from one to five, and allowing yourself to drift back to full physical and mental awareness, opening your eyes and getting on with the rest of your day, feeling restored and rested.

As with anything, the more you practise, the easier it will become, until you can shorten the patterns by just doing the following steps. You can achieve self-hypnosis in two to three minutes at most with these four steps.

1 Close your eyes.
2 Check that you are physically at ease.
3 Use the sound of the word "calm" with each breath you exhale.
4 Imagine yourself in your own "haven".

THE CALM TECHNIQUE

Once you have used the methods of self-hypnotic induction a few times, the mind has accepted the sound of the word "calm" as a signal for physical relaxation and mental calmness. This can then be used anywhere to control emotions and allow a return to clear thinking and just the right level of calm and relaxation for the situation. No one else will know you are doing it, but it puts you back in control. It is an ideal technique for a meeting that has become heated, and for immediately calming yourself before giving a presentation or having an interview.

BELOW: Your safe place might be a beautiful, sunlit woodland glade, with shafts of light illuminating the forest floor.

AFFIRMATIONS AND VISUALIZATION

Self-hypnosis can be usefully combined with affirmations, which have been brought into the forefront of psychotherapy in recent years. This deceptively simple device can be used by anyone and has proved remarkably effective.

It is recommended that you use this method while in self-hypnosis, having previously planned and memorized the affirmations involved. Thus you combine that ease of access to the unconscious mind and the effectiveness of repeated powerful positive phrases. You must say to yourself, out loud, a positive statement about yourself such as "I like my … (physical attribute);" "I am proud of my … (attitude or achievement);" "I love meeting people – they are fascinating;" or "I am quietly confident at meetings".

Notice the main points in these affirmations which can be used singly or together. They are in the present tense, and they are positively phrased and imply an emotional reward. You can create your own, and use them as often as you wish. The oldest and best-known affirmation is "every day in every way, I am getting better and better", written by Emile Coué at the end of the nineteenth century.

Yours is the most influential voice in your life, because you believe it. Used in this powerful combination, it can be truly effective in changing your expectations and reactions and in influencing outcomes.

In the same way that you can utilize your voice, so – and perhaps more powerfully – you can use your imagination. The imagination can stimulate emotions and can provide a direct communication with the unconscious part of the mind, and can also provide an impetus for registering new and more positive attitudes in the mind.

Visualization requires that you imagine yourself behaving, reacting and looking as you would wish to do in a given situation; for example a business meeting or a social gathering, and what that will mean for you. See your reactions, the reactions of those around you, and, most important, experience all the good feelings that will be there when this happens in reality. It is like playing a video of the event, on that screen on the inside of the forehead, the mind's eye, from the beginning of the situation through to the perfect outcome for you. Should any doubts or negative images creep into your "video", push them away and replace them with positive ones. Keep this realistic, and base it upon real information from your past.

Again the best time to do this is when relaxed mentally and physically – in self-hypnosis. Teach your mind to expect new, positive outcomes. This can be combined with affirmations and be doubly effective.

ABOVE: *Imagine yourself at a social function where you are chatting with people you have met for the first time, with confidence and charm.*

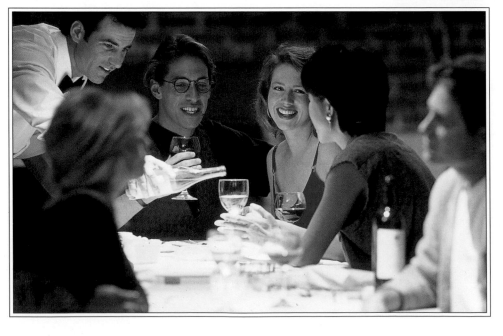

LEFT: *Imagine yourself at a social gathering, such as a dinner party, where you are relaxed, comfortable and happy. You know that others are enjoying your company just as you are enjoying theirs.*

THE SWISH TECHNIQUE

This technique is particularly useful to combat pre-interview or presentation jitters. It is a very effective method utilizing visualization and is derived from NLP (Neuro-Linguistic Programming), which is used throughout the world by therapists and patients alike. You can use this technique at any time when you feel relaxed. First thing in the morning, before getting out of bed, is a good time. Ideally, however, include this in your self-hypnosis programme and it will take just five minutes. Just work through it, with the instructions beside you, and then you will be able to do it on your own.

First, think of the event that is going to happen, an interview for example, about which you feel anxious. Focus in on that for a moment. You will probably find it much easier with your eyes closed.

Now create two pictures in your mind, filling the whole of the screen on the inside of your forehead, your mind's eye. The first picture is called "The Moment of Anxiety", and depicts the scene at the moment when you would expect to start feeling most anxious. Make the picture as detailed as you can: the room, the people, furnishings and so on – like a photograph you have taken yourself, so you are not in the picture, in full colour, detailed and brilliantly lit. When you are sure you have done that, put that picture to one side.

Next, form another picture; this one is called "The Moment of Achievement". This is a picture of you at the end of that occasion, looking really good, relaxed and happy, leaving the interview perhaps. Make this picture as detailed as you can: but most important of all – you, and the look on your face. The event has gone well and you feel really good. Make sure you have this in your mind as clearly as possible.

BELOW: The Moment of Anxiety.

ABOVE: The Moment of Achievement.

Now see both of these pictures in the following way. The first picture, "The Moment of Anxiety", in full colour and brilliantly lit filling the whole of your mind's eye except for one of the lower corners, where, like a snapshot tucked into the frame of a larger picture, there is a small, dull black-and-white picture, "The Moment of Achievement".

When you have them clear and steady, swish them over – the small becoming large and full colour, the large becoming small and black and white. Allow yourself a few moments to really enjoy the feelings displayed on your face.

Clear your mind by opening your eyes and looking around you. Then set the pictures up again as they were before, with the Moment of Anxiety large and full colour and the Moment of Achievement as a small black and white snapshot, then swish them over. Do that exercise three more times, making five times in all.

Use the SWISH technique once a day for about a week before the situation you have in mind. You will find that very soon it is impossible for you to hold the first picture in your mind's eye without the second one automatically taking over. When this happens, you know that you have reprogrammed your mind for success rather than failure. Then repeat the exercise for two more groups of five to make absolutely sure.

It is under your control now. You can use this exercise to help yourself to gain the right attitudes so that you can be successful in many different situations.

Under no circumstances should the patterns illustrated here be used on someone else, nor should any effort be made to delve into personal history or past lives without the aid of a professional therapist. It can lead to situations that can quickly get outside of your competence.

MEDITATION

The word "meditation" means different things to different people. In the Western philosophic and religious tradition it can simply mean turning an idea or concept over in one's mind. What it has generally come to mean today is some form of clearing or emptying of the mind. A word such as "contemplation" may have been used at other times to mean the process of coming to a central point, focusing and quietening the mind. These practices are often referred to simply as "sitting".

Very often the word "meditation" is associated, in many people's minds, with all sorts of bizarre practices involving wearing long robes and sitting on the floor with your legs tied in a knot for hours on end. In short, there is a lot of mystification surrounding the idea of meditation. By describing some basic principles and aims in this chapter, and intro-

BELOW: When you are meditating make sure you are in a quiet, peaceful place with no risk of interruption or distraction.

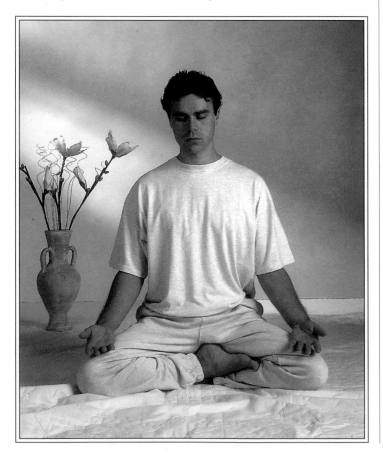

ducing some simple exercises which should benefit most people, some of that mystification should be dispelled.

There are hundreds of different schools of meditation, many associated with some form of religious practice, and many that are not. Some of these varied forms of meditation may include techniques such as complex visualizations or chanting words or sounds known as "mantras". Many of the world's great religions also make provision for retreat from the world in order to focus more closely on meditation for short or long periods. Practices of this kind have great value, but often form the basis for widely held and perhaps stereotyped ideas about what meditation involves. All of these techniques, and more, can also be practised without the necessity of being a follower of any particular religious tradition. (Incidentally, the exercises presented in this chapter are considered to be quite compatible with whatever religious belief, if any, an individual may already hold.)

Of course, you may choose to incorporate any, or all, of the above exercises into your practice, but none of them is strictly necessary in order to gain the benefits that meditation can bring to a modern, stressful lifestyle. Meditation is a truly holistic activity in that, ideally, the whole system of body, mind and spirit is involved and benefited.

BODY

The physical benefits of meditation are easily quantifiable and plenty of research documentation exists. These include relaxation, improvement of sleeping patterns, lowering high blood pressure, helping recovery from fatigue and a general beneficial effect on most stress-related disease. Posture can be helped, too, in that better posture leads to better meditation which in turn leads to better posture! The same can be said for relaxation. The mind cannot let go until the body relaxes, and vice versa.

Meditation is sometimes seen as a kind of vanishing upwards into rarefied heavenly atmospheres, rejecting all that is grossly physical. On the contrary, awareness of the body is an essential part of effective meditation. A kite can only fly if the string is firmly held on the ground. Many of the emotional stresses and upsets that people experience can be held as tensions in the body and therefore be fairly

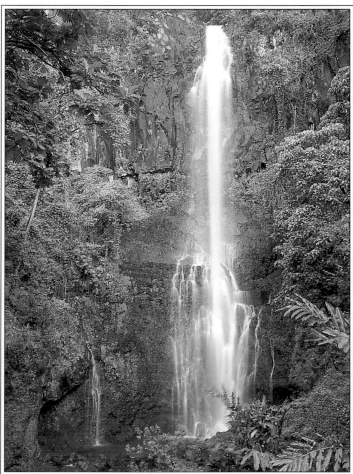

ABOVE AND RIGHT: A beautiful scene, such as mountains or a waterfall, can help evoke a feeling of wholeness, joy and peace. Use images such as this in your mind's eye when you are meditating. It may be a special place where you have been happy which holds personal significance for you, or it may be somewhere you have always dreamed of visiting which you have a strong mental picture of. Make the image in your mind as real as you can.

unconscious. Through the process of conscious relaxation of body and breathing that meditation entails, these stresses can be unlocked from their hiding places in the muscles and joints and simultaneously released. There was once a school of yogis in Tibet famous for their one principle or mantra: "Mind in the body, bum on the ground!" One can go a long way with a very simple awareness of body and breath.

Most traditions, both in the East and the West, agree that the body is bound together by a subtle form of energy (called *qi* in China, and a variety of names in other parts of the world) which manifests in forms known as the aura, acupuncture meridians or *chakras*. The increased sensitivity that develops from paying attention to natural bodily processes often results in a perception of this energy (perhaps as warmth, tingling, pressure, lightness or other such sensations). At this point the differentiation between mind and body begins to dissolve.

MIND

Meditation can improve the ability to concentrate, the ability to listen, both to others and yourself, and is a good way of monitoring the "internal weather". It is said that rates of depression and suicide are rising steadily in Western society and many commentators point to the breakdown of communities, people's divorce from the natural world and the poor living conditions of many. But if people cannot change their external conditions to any great degree, they can take responsibility for changing their attitudes and reactions – the way the mind interacts with the world. One of the safest and most effective ways to bring about this change is to meditate. People are able to be more self-sufficient and begin to let go of the addictions and dependencies they may have, such as drugs, food, television or sex, in which many seek refuge from reality. Paradoxically, meditation is not an escape from the real world; in fact it leads to a deeper engagement with, and awareness of, one's life in order to transform it.

The forms of meditation described in this chapter do not involve suppressing the thoughts or emotions with rigid self-control. What is required is more of a drawing together, paying ever closer attention, becoming absorbed in your object of meditation. If meditation is not a rejection of body, neither is it a rejection of mind – specifically of thoughts. Thinking is what the mind, or more accurately, the brain, is designed to do. This is its contribution to humankind's survival for the thousands of years we have been on this planet. In a way, trying to stop thinking would be like trying to stop breathing. What is even more important is to change one's attitude towards these thoughts, perhaps even the nature of them, not by rigid control but by developing what might be called a feeling of inner spaciousness that can include any thought or emotion. There is then less jostling for position, less anxiety and fewer demands for attention from one's thoughts.

Imagine a little girl, tugging at your sleeve persistently, determined to tell you something. You try to ignore her and perhaps even get angry, which then results in tears and uproar. If instead you turn round and give her your absolutely full attention, she may either suddenly become shy and run away, or whisper her few but terribly important words and then be satisfied to go and occupy herself elsewhere. Thoughts can behave in a very similar way. If your adult self is clear enough in its intention to meditate, the thoughts can continue with their play without causing disruption.

In a sense most people might be described as sleepwalking through life for all the engagement they have with it. The path of meditation offers a way of becoming more awake and alive to every aspect, inner and outer. The mind ceases to be a burden and distraction and instead becomes a tool for paying very good attention to the present moment. The practice known as "mindfulness" is simply carrying this present-centred attention into one's daily life and activities, whether walking, running or doing household chores. In this way meditation practice begins to become relevant to "real life" and not something separate and isolating.

RIGHT: *Adopt a position which you feel at ease and relaxed in when you are meditating. Wear clothing which is loose and comfortable and which does not restrict you in any way. There is no correct way to sit, it is up to the individual to find a posture which suits them.*

SPIRIT

The words "spirit" and "spirituality" can be very loaded for many of us with both negative and positive connotations. Those who may have suffered at the hands of dogmatic, judgemental or fundamentalist religion may feel understandably wary of this area and reject it altogether. However, spirituality may not necessarily have anything to do with any organized religion or philosophy. It need not even include the word "god". It might be useful to think of the word "spirit" in the context of phrases such as "in good spirits", "in the right spirit" or "a spirited horse".

Your spirituality is simply your relationship to whatever is most important or meaningful in your life – whatever nurtures you and fulfils your deepest needs. For some people this may be money, possessions or status, but going beyond these things, ask what it is they depend on and why you need them. You may not come up with any definitive answers, but it is the asking of the questions that is important. This inquiry may lead you to discover what is truly meaningful for you; perhaps loved ones, family, home, an appreciation of beauty, honesty, a desire to discover the true meaning of life.

WHEN AND WHERE?

How often should I practise? How should I sit? are questions often asked by those starting out on the path of meditation, once the basic exercises have been explored. For both these questions there are no "right" answers, no one "proper" way of meditating. Individuals explore for themselves, evolving an effective and appropriate practice.

As to frequency of practice, some schools suggest many hours a day, some advocate quality rather than quantity – a short, focused period of meditation of five or ten minutes. Regular practice is certainly helpful, preferably daily. Building a new habit into one's life may take time, but of course anything becomes easier with regular practice. Eventually, it may well feel indispensable. For some people self-discipline works well, although listening to the voice in your head which governs your discipline may be very interesting. Are you barking orders at yourself, judging yourself a lazy, useless slug if you cannot manage half an hour's meditation every day at 6.35 a.m. precisely? Or is the voice more of an invitation to participate in a restful exploration of your inner workings? Is there any sense of this five, ten or 20 minutes of your day being set aside gratefully as a gift to yourself? The greatest incentive known for doing anything is that it is enjoyable and makes one feel good. If meditation practice becomes as burdensome a necessity as, say, flossing your teeth or if it seems an indulgence that you do not have time for in your busy life, so full of important things to do, then you had better start examining your motives.

Sometimes being in a group or class to practise meditation can be very helpful. In a group one has the support of a roomful of people doing the same thing at the same time. A kind of synergy seems to exist in a group of people who are meditating together. Sometimes the reverse is true and solitude is what people need to get in touch with that single-pointed attention. Time, place and companions are all matters for individual choice and experimentation.

ABOVE: *Your body may take a while to adjust to the sitting position. Lie down and relax for a few minutes before you begin.*

What about ways of sitting? Generally, meditation seems to work best when the spine is straight, but relaxed and vertical. The reasons for this are several. First, sitting upright is a very good way of staying awake and alert while the eyes are closed and the attention drawn inwards. If the body is upright, the breath can begin to move in and out freely and without obstruction. Also the muscles of the torso and spine have a chance to unknot themselves of old tensions. This may not always be an entirely pain-free process. Until the body becomes used to sitting in a new more conscious way, it may fight to be allowed back to its habitual "comfortable" state. These conflicts will pass, perhaps aided by some exercises such as yoga, tai chi or chi gung.

Eventually, proper posture will prove to be the most genuinely comfortable way of sitting still for a period of time. Sitting upright sends a message to the unconscious that although your eyes are closed, you are not going to sleep, as you would when lying down. On a more subtle level the body's *qi* energy, or life force, is able to move more freely if the spine is straight. Energy cannot move through tense muscles, so as relaxed a way of sitting needs to be found.

There is not necessarily any inherent virtue in sitting on the floor to meditate. Some people are very comfortable doing so, but if this is difficult for you, sitting in a chair is perfectly acceptable. Given the basic requirement of an upright spine, the way of arranging the legs is a matter for personal preference and respecting the body's limits. If sitting cross-legged on the floor, you will probably find it helpful to have a firm cushion at least 5–7.5cm (2–3in) thick under your bottom. This lifts the spine so that it is easier to sit upright. You may choose to kneel, in which case a larger cushion or a meditation bench under your bottom would be advisable to prevent cutting off circulation to the legs. If you feel most comfortable sitting in a chair, choose one that is the right height for you, or use some books under your feet. A firm, straight-backed chair is better than an armchair and if you can sit up unsupported, all the better.

A major objective in this discussion of posture is to ensure the free flow of breath through an open posture. Why is the breath so important in meditation? On the physical level, if the body is taking in enough breath, the brain then has sufficient oxygen to function at its peak and thus remain alert and focused. Breathing in by allowing the lower abdomen to expand enables the lungs to expand to their full extent and also relaxes the muscles of the torso and the internal organs. Many people breathe in a very shallow way, using only their shoulders and the top part of the chest. This way of breathing can produce stress and anxiety as it provokes the "flight-or-fight" response, meaning that rather than being alert in a relaxed and open way, they are tense and watchful. Breathing deeply, with the muscles of the abdomen relaxed, enables you to let go of deep levels of stress and tension, continuing and deepening the process of relaxation that begins with an aligned posture.

ABOVE AND LEFT: Choose your posture, sitting on a chair or kneeling on the floor.

ABOVE: The traditional meditation position is sitting on the floor, with legs crossed.

FOCUSING

Your breath also provides an ever present and easily accessible focus for concentration. One is always breathing! Many schools of meditation teach focus on the breath in various ways. This may involve imagining that the breath originates in one particular point in the body. The points most usually focused on are the *hara* or *tan tien* – just below and behind the navel, or the heart – in the centre of the chest. The crown of the head, the base of the spine or the soles of the feet may all be included in the awareness. Focusing on the breath can also take the form of noticing the physical changes as the breath moves in and out, either at the nostrils or the abdomen. Meditation can be as simple as this, just breathing while sitting.

There are many ways of concentrating the mind in order to occupy that part of the mind that chatters incessantly, worrying and obsessing.

❦ Count the breaths from one to ten, then begin again.

❦ Notice the stillness at the changeover points at the end of the inhalation or the exhalation.

❦ Let an image arise that evokes a feeling of wholeness, joy and peace; perhaps a beautiful natural scene of mountains, the sea, a tree, the sun, a child or an inspirational figure and breathe this image into your heart.

FIVE MEDITATION STEPS

You can memorize these steps, have a friend read to you, or make a tape for yourself. Sitting comfortably but upright, feel your weight on the chair or cushion and relax into it. Imagine breathing in and out through your navel, taking a few deep breaths to settle in. Let your attention gather at a point at the base of your spine, imagine it as a point of energy. Notice what sensations you feel there.

1 Move your attention to the crown of the head, imagine a point of energy there. Notice what sensations you feel. Feel these two points align, connected by a line of light, inside the body near the spine. Allow energy to move freely between these two points.

2 Let your attention come to rest at a point of balance along this line, deep within you, at the centre of your being.

3 From this centre of your being, imagine the line of light extending downward through your legs and feet, relaxing the toes and sinking into the earth. Breathing out, let all tension and fatigue run down this line into the earth.

4 Breathing in, imagine drawing up, through the soles of your feet, fresh, transformed earth energy. Allow it to fill your whole body from the feet up to the crown of your head, bringing a feeling of being supported and cradled by the solidity of the earth. Return your attention and your breathing to the centre of your being. Imagine the line of light rising to the crown of your head and above, out into the clear blue sky, to the heavens. Breathe in fresh air.

5 Allow light and clearness from the heavens to radiate down the line of light to fill the whole body. Breathe into the centre of your being and feel the two energies, from the earth and the sky, mingling. From this centre let your attention be on your breath moving in and out (using one of the focuses suggested above).

PSYCHOTHERAPY

The basis of psychotherapy is the natural desire of someone with problems to want to talk to someone else about them, and it is often called the talking therapy. Practitioners generally refer to the people they see as clients rather than patients, to emphasize that it is not just for sick people but for anyone with problems. There are a number of schools of thought about the processes involved in psychotherapy, and the techniques range from simple supportive counselling to complex psychoanalytical theories about the underlying feelings behind current problems, and how to release them.

At its most basic level, psychotherapy is the creation of a space for somebody to air their problems in a caring, non-judgemental and confidential atmosphere. This is almost an extension of a chat with a good friend, and the skill of the therapist lies not so much in what they might say, but in acting as a support for the client to unburden whatever is troubling the mind at the time. This kind of caring listening is often a part of the "treatment" given by many different skilled natural therapists.

Much of psychotherapy builds upon this passive listening, with somewhat more active interjections to point out areas of evasion, inconsistency or neglected issues. This helps people to break out of negative or destructive thought-patterns, to develop a better sense of their own identity, and to be happier in relationships.

Therapy can be short- or long-term. With relatively simple problems, for example, a phobia or single-issue problem, techniques such as behavioural or cognitive therapy may be used. These aim to change behaviour and attitude by respectively facing people with the feared experience or object, or getting them to try acting and thinking in a more positive way, in order to overcome the fear or anxiety. Such disciplines can be quite directive, with clients initially following instructions. Often, however, such apparently simple problems have deeper causes and a more long-term approach such as analysis may be beneficial.

Psychoanalysis is a distinctive, long-term approach, requiring a considerable period of training to become a practitioner, who therefore may be considered something of a specialist. The father of psychoanalysis was Sigmund Freud,

ABOVE: Sigmund Freud, the father of psychoanalysis, whose research revolutionized the way humans regard themselves.

the Austrian psychiatrist who developed theories of human experience that related psychological problems to our early childhood relationships with our parents. Dreams, fears and desires, both conscious and unconscious, and suppressed emotions are all investigated as factors in present problems. One of Freud's most brilliant pupils, Carl Jung, developed his own theories based upon archetypal symbols and myths, rather than childhood traumas, and numerous others have since added their own ideas to this complex field.

Thoughts and feelings are particularly significant in psychoanalysis, while other approaches also look at behaviour. Gestalt therapy, for instance, which was developed in the US by Fritz Perls in the 1950s, seeks to place a client's symptoms within the wider context of normal emotional responses; literally, the whole is greater than the sum of the parts. Changes in behaviour can affect feelings and thoughts, and vice versa. Trying to choose a suitable psychotherapist can therefore be something of a minefield for those who are unaware of the differences between the various schools. In the first place, decide how much change you want. Do you want to resolve a short-term problem, or undertake a complete overhaul of your attitudes and lifestyle?

Perhaps more than in any other therapy, the relationship between the client and the therapist is of great significance in psychotherapy and some time needs to elapse to build up confidence and rapport. Since people often gravitate towards therapies that suit their own personality, there can be a case for looking wider and experimenting a little – if you tend to be a thinker and good at intellectualizing problems, an approach that uses this technique may maintain this rather narrow view, so that a bodywork approach may be what you need; and vice versa of course.

ABOVE AND BELOW: A psychotherapist will listen to what you have to say with a non-judgemental approach. Their detatched interest is very important, allowing you to explain feelings which would be difficult to express to friends or relations who are unable to maintain the same objectivity.

AUTOGENICS

Autogenics is a system of relaxation exercises developed in the late 1920s and 1930s by a German psychiatrist and neurologist, Dr Johannes Schultz. He used hypnotherapy on many of his patients and became aware of the great benefits they gained from the deep state of relaxation brought about under hypnosis. This led him to try to devise a set of exercises to enable people to induce a state of relaxation themselves – the word autogenic means self-originated, or coming from within.

The aim of these exercises is to help switch off the part of the nervous system that produces the "fight or flight" response to stress, and to switch on the relaxation mechanisms. There are essentially six exercises, each focusing on a different sensation, and they may be carried out either lying down or sitting in one of two different ways. No special equipment is required, just the time and space to allow relaxation. The simplicity and effectiveness of autogenics have led to it spreading throughout Europe and America and even to Japan.

Autogenic training is normally carried out by a practitioner with a group of people, with the exercises being learned over several weeks. A feature of the training process can be so-called autogenic discharges, temporary sensations or emotions that can be quite intense and are often followed by a feeling of greater energy. These do not happen to everyone, but are one reason for training with a qualified practitioner, who can explain what they mean.

In a training session these sensations are enhanced and strengthened by the silent repetition of certain phrases, which, when carried out on a regular basis, can have remarkable effects in relieving stress and fatigue symptoms. The release of long-standing stresses can be the reason for the autogenic discharge phenomena.

In a group training situation, an autogenic trainer will probably focus on the first of the above exercises – inducing heaviness and relaxation – for a few weeks so that everyone is confident at performing the exercise. Most autogenic trainers encourage their group members to keep detailed diaries of home practice, and the weekly sessions may begin with a discussion of how everyone has got on in

ABOVE: *While concentrating on relaxing the body, stress and fatigue are dispelled.*

the previous week. This also allows for any individual adjustments that may need to be made to a member's programme.

Initially, repetition of these exercises at home should be just for a couple of minutes, perhaps repeated twice a day; during the course of the sessions, the trainer may well suggest that you increase the length of home exercises to around 15 minutes, two to three times a day. It is important that you fit your exercises into your daily routine so that they become part of your life.

Around 3,000 scientific articles have been published

AUTOGENIC EXERCISE

The following is a very basic exercise which can be used as a relaxation technique, using the principles of autogenics to relieve stress:

1 Focus your attention on feelings of heaviness and relaxation in the neck, shoulders and limbs.

2 Develop an awareness of a growing sensation of warmth in the limbs.

3 Concentrate on the heartbeat, and help to regulate it.

4 Build an awareness of your breathing patterns.

5 Create a feeling of warmth in your abdomen.

6 Create a sensation of coolness across the forehead.

describing the beneficial effects of autogenics, although no one can say for certain how the therapy works. Stress-related disorders such as stomach ulcers, migraine, asthma and so on can be improved by these simple exercises. Autogenics are a good example of how mental, emotional and physical health are inextricably intertwined. Repressed emotions or stresses may be responsible for later physical disorders, and this training can help to break this pattern and release the trapped feelings.

The above training exercise can be practised in various places and situations, such as at work, on the train or sitting in a park in your lunch hour. It needs no special clothing or adoption of difficult and awkward positions, and is sometimes compared to learning to drive. First, make yourself comfortable behind the wheel; start off calmly and slowly without any jerks or jolts; next change gear – or alter your physical and mental states – and finally come to a smooth, safe halt. The exercises above are designed to relieve stress and help the body cure itself. For further exploration into autogenics you should consult a practitioner who will give you a brief check-up to make sure the training is suitable for you. Some patients will only be treated under appropriate medical supervision and modified treatment is given to asthmatics, diabetics, pregnant women and epileptics. Therapists claim that autogenic training can help with a variety of ailments such as AIDS, irritable bowel syndrome, depression and eczema. Many practitioners of autogenics are professionals already involved in healthcare, such as doctors, psychotherapists and psychologists. This probably reflects the depth of research into autogenic training, and has meant that apart from private autogenic practitioners, autogenics may be available through hospitals or general physicians.

HEALING

Healing is based upon the concept that there is more to life than the purely physical; what that something more is depends on your religious or philosophical beliefs. A term that is commonly used is the spirit, although energy is another frequently used expression. For many healers this energy flows from God, or gods in other religions, but nearly all healers agree that this non-physical quality pervades the universe, and is the source of life. Healers claim to have an ability to channel this energy and help it stimulate our own self-healing energies.

For thousands of years healers have practised a number of non-physical methods of focusing attention and healing energy upon people. The most popular method is by the laying on of hands, either directly on to a diseased or affected area of the body or generally over the person receiving heal-

ing. Since there is often a religious element in the beliefs of the healer, or the society in which healers practise, the laying on of hands has often been restricted. In many states in the US, healing is still technically illegal unless you are a church minister, which has led to many people becoming ministers of unusual churches in order to practise. In the UK, it is only within the last 20 years or so that doctors have been able to co-operate with healers without the risk of being struck off the medical register.

There have, nevertheless, been several instances when the benefits of the laying on of hands were recognized within conventional medicine. For example, the former professor

BELOW: The image of healing hands is a powerful one and appears in religions around the world as a symbol of love and care.

of nursing at New York University, Dr Dolores Krieger, ran a course in "therapeutic touch" (essentially healing by another name) as part of the nurses' training. This proved popular with nurses and patients, and showed not only psychological and emotional benefits for the patients, but quantifiable improvements in health.

In the 1980s two lecturers in physiology, Dr David Hodges and Dr Tony Scofield, of London University, conducted controlled experiments to test the curative powers of a psychic healer and medium. This healer claimed he could take cress seeds whose ability to grow had been diminished by a soaking in salt water, and make them well again. The healer held half of the seeds in his hand and directed his healing energy at them. The treated and untreated seeds were then laid on wet tissue paper and left in the lab for a week.

The results were that the "healed" seeds grew significantly faster than the unhealed seeds, leading Dr Hodges and Dr Scofield to conclude that a healing power had enabled the sick seeds to throw off ill-effects and grow normally. This experiment went some way to contradict some medical experts who dismiss the work of healers with the theory of "spontaneous remission" in which the body temporarily heals itself, or auto-suggestion, whereby patients heal themselves by self-hypnosis.

Some healers operate directly within a religious context, giving "faith healing", often in mass gatherings. While healers would acknowledge that faith, either in the healer or in the process, is an important element, it is not generally regarded as essential. Indeed, it is also important that you retain your common sense when seeking a healer. In the last 20 years or so a fair amount of research has started to

BELOW: Healing is now becoming a more accepted part of modern medicine, with some general practices employing a healer.

ABOVE: Some healers transmit their healing powers by placing their hands on the patient's aura rather than directly on the body.

accumulate, showing that healers have some ability to affect physical processes by immaterial means. For example, the healer Matthew Manner has carried out many controlled experiments in both the US and the UK with interesting results on cancer cells, and work at the Universities of New York, Wisconsin and Minnesota indicate the benefits of "therapeutic touch". Nevertheless, healing is less amenable to scrutiny than some other therapies, and the possibilities for fraud, or at least misrepresentation, are thus greater.

Despite occasional sensationalized media reports of instant "miracle cures", most healers would say that healing is generally a gradual, slow process. Although, as mentioned above, healers do not as a rule emphasize the need for any faith on the part of the person receiving healing, they would encourage self-healing attempts and above all a positive attitude – the desire to get better. This encouragement of self-help empowerment is a useful guideline to bear in mind when seeing a healer for the first time; if the healer insists on sole responsibility for helping you, to the exclusion of all other treatments, then you are well-advised to look elsewhere.

Most good practitioners of natural medicine probably have some healing abilities, which may be especially evident if they practise a hands-on therapy – for example, massage. Healers concentrate on focusing this healing energy, sometimes with amazing results. Even where there is little or no change in their physical symptoms or illness, many people report that they feel stronger, calmer and more able to cope with their illness after a healing session.

BODYWORK

◆─▭◦◘─◆

What is the special importance of bodywork? Simply, it provides the most immediate way to affect another person, to reassure and relax them, to help to reduce pain, influence our ability to build relationships, and even fight off disease. Touch is an absolutely primal, vital requirement that is sadly neglected in many of our

societies. The continuing rise in the popularity of bodywork therapies shows how much this need is still there.

In the last 30 years researchers have started to look at the therapeutic effects of touch, and have shown that not only does regular physical contact lower anxiety levels and enhance the quality of life, but it affects physiological processes, too, ranging from lowered blood pressure, and even less arteriosclerosis, to reduced brain cell deterioration and memory loss with ageing. Musculoskeletal disorders are most often helped by manipulative or other physical treatments, and both pain levels and pain tolerance can often be aided with the help of bodywork therapies.

As if that were not enough, many therapies such as massage are also very enjoyable treatments to receive, and some techniques can be adapted for use at home, helping the giver too. A famous study in the 1960s looked at frequency of touch by couples in cafés around the world; in South America it was 180 times an hour, in the US twice an hour and in England never, so there is much room for improvement.

ABOVE: Professional massage is widely available at natural health centres.

OPPOSITE: Self-massage is often unconscious and with some practice can become part of our daily routine.

MASSAGE

ORIGINS AND DEVELOPMENT

Massage can fairly claim to be the oldest form of healing in existence. The use of touch to relieve aching muscles, to give comfort or to express love is as old as humankind, and is something humans share with animals as an instinctive way of bonding and sharing. As a stress-reliever it is probably without equal, and every culture throughout history has used massage in some form or other (every language, ancient or modern, has a word for massage).

Written records mentioning massage, or rubbing as it was known in former times, date back some 5,000 years, with the most ancient Chinese medical texts advocating stroking the limbs to "protect against colds, keep the organs supple and prevent minor ailments". In India, the Ayurvedic scriptures, which date back nearly 4,000 years, also recommend rubbing and shampooing the body to keep it healthy and promote healing, and there has been an unbroken tradition of using massage since that time; most Indian mothers are taught to massage their newborn babies, and later the children are taught to massage their parents.

BELOW: Before you begin a massage session prepare some clean, warm towels, some cushions and the oils you will use.

ABOVE: One of the best ways to relax with a partner is to give each other a soothing massage at the end of a stressful day.

In ancient Greece, the practice of rubbing up the limbs, or anatripsis, was highly recommended for treating fatigue, sports or war injury and illness. Hippocrates, the so-called "father" of medicine, writing in the fifth century BC, stated that the physician must be "experienced in many things but assuredly rubbing", and suggested that the way to health was to have a scented bath and an oiled massage each day. Medical centres, or gymnasia, nearly always included massage schools within them.

The Romans were equally enthusiastic about the benefits of massage, incorporating it into a daily routine in their spas, alongside hot and cold baths. One of the most famous Roman physicians, Galen, wrote several books on massage, exercise and health in the second century AD, and classified many types of strokes for use in different ailments. A good masseur was highly regarded.

Massage continued to be popular and respected in Europe after the Romans had left, although their elaborate bathing and massage facilities fell into disrepair. With the rise in more puritanical aspects of Christianity, however, the needs of the body were felt to be in some way sinful and massage became rather neglected.

From the time of the Renaissance, when classical medicine and philosophy were once again in favour, massage was revived and respected again; the French doctor Ambroise Paré, who was physician to no fewer than four French kings, used massage a great deal in his practice. Other cultures had always continued to value massage – Captain Cook wrote in his diaries how he was cured of sciatic pains in Tahiti by being massaged from head to foot by several women at once.

The most influential figure in renewing interest in massage during the nineteenth century was the Swedish gymnast, Per Henrik Ling (1776–1839). Ling studied the human body

in activity and rest, and laid the foundations for modern gymnastics. He developed a system of medical gymnastics, exercises for the joints, and massage, based upon ancient techniques, which led to a Crown appointment and the formation of an institute of massage. His classification of strokes and their effects forms the basis of most Western massage today, and brisker styles of massage are often called Swedish massage.

The latest development of massage happened during the 1960s and 1970s, especially in the US, where personal growth centres – most notably the Esalen Institute – adapted massage into a holistic approach that looked at releasing trapped emotional issues and creating overall health and balance rather than simply easing tired muscles or aching limbs. The American massage therapist George Downing was an early writer on this holistic view of massage, and many schools now teach the subject within this framework.

BELOW: Massaging your partner builds up trust and a feeling of ease, as you show your care for each other using touch.

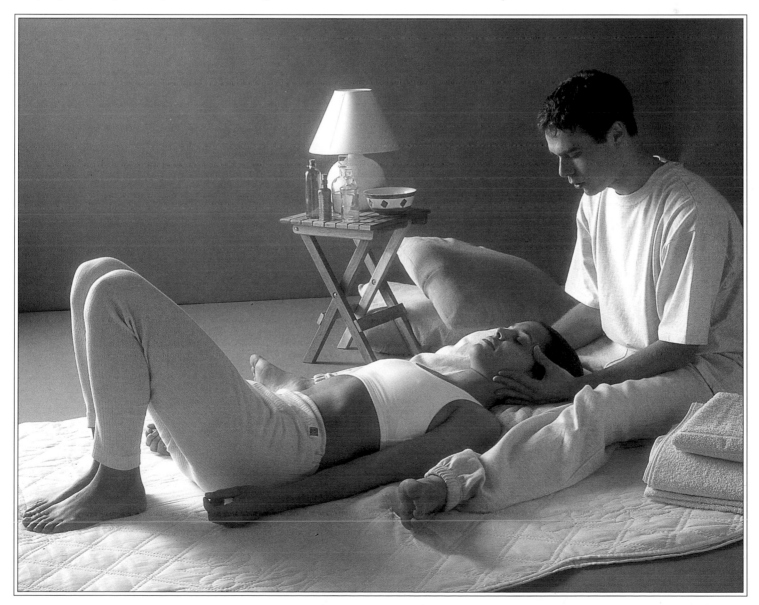

PREVENTIVE MASSAGE

One of the most positive aspects of massage is that you do not need to wait until you have an ailment or injury to receive massage; it is a pleasurable and therapeutic treatment at any time (with few contra-indications), and regular massage is one of the best ways to avoid stress-related illnesses or injury from high levels of exercise and sport. Massage is not appropriate to use where there is an acute infection, feverish condition or inflammation, and care needs to be taken with anyone with heart conditions, so the first rule should be: if in doubt, don't. The suggested strokes outlined below are generally safe, but are not a substitute for professional treatment if needed. They are intended for use in preventing ill-health, not in treating it, and as a means of reducing stress and tension, for yourself and for others.

SELF-MASSAGE

Although often thought of as something you need two people for, massage on yourself is also beneficial and can be done in odd moments during the day. In fact, without perhaps consciously realizing it, every time you rub a tense spot on your shoulder or ease a tight muscle on your forehead you are giving yourself a mini-massage. Use the following techniques throughout the day and you will feel less tired and tense at the end of it.

SHOULDERS AND FACE

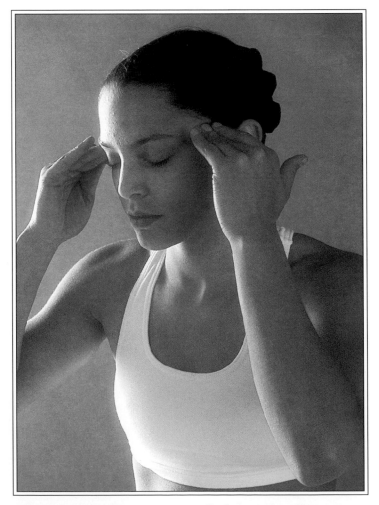

1 A lot of tension can build up in the areas of the shoulders and neck. A regular massage is very helpful, not only giving physical benefits but also breaking up the day and allowing your mind to rest. Squeeze and knead one shoulder firmly with the opposite hand, then change sides and repeat.

2 Try using your fingertips in small, slow circles all over your face, starting at the chin and steadily working upwards. If your shoulders ache from lifting your arms, just pause and rest before starting again, or do this stroke lying on your back on the floor.

HAND MASSAGE

Our hands are one of the most overworked parts of our bodies and will benefit enormously from self-massage throughout the day. People who work with their hands in a repetitive way such as keyboard operators should practise regular hand massage. Hands are also, of course, a vital massage tool and need to be taken care of. Swap hands with each massage technique as you do the following routine.

1 To release stored tensions and improve circulation, start by squeezing between each finger in turn with the thumb and index finger of the other hand.

2 Stretch the fingers by interlocking them and gently pulling them downwards. It is not the intention to "crack" the fingers but to stretch the tendons.

3 Make a rolling movement on each finger, working from the knuckle to the fingertip with firm pressure from the fingers and thumb of each hand.

4 Finally, with the thumb, make a firm circling motion on the palm of the other hand. This both squeezes and stretches taut, contracted muscles and should be a fairly deep action: if done too lightly, it just feels ticklish.

REVITALIZING ARM AND NECK MASSAGE

Even when we are not using our arms in a particularly physical way, tiredness induces aching limbs so that we feel physically drained. Use this quick self-massage routine to renew your energy levels during a busy day and prevent any build up of aches and pains.

1 Do a kneading action on the arms, working rapidly from the wrist to the shoulder and back with a firm, squeezing movement. Do this more quickly and briskly than usual in massage, to invigorate each arm and shoulder in turn, rather than soothe and relax the muscles.

2 Swiftly rub up the outside of each arm using small movements to really stimulate the circulation. Repeat in an upwards direction each time.

3 With the fingers and thumb of one hand, firmly squeeze the neck muscles with a circular motion.

4 Shrug your shoulders and bring them up close to your ears, hold the position for a few seconds.

5 Relax the shoulders down and feel the tension ebb away. Repeat the exercise two more times.

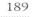

LEG MASSAGE

This massage is as beneficial to those of us with a sedentary average day as it is for the more physically active. Many of us spend far too long each day standing still, or barely moving around, leading to tired, aching limbs, swollen ankles or cramp. A quick leg massage at the end of the day can work wonders in reducing aches and sluggish blood flow. You could also use this routine in the morning to ease any stiffness. Start on the thighs, so that any fluid retention in the calves will have somewhere to go as the upper leg relaxes.

1 Using both hands, knead one thigh at a time, by squeezing between the fingers and thumb; squeeze with each hand alternately for the best effect. Repeat on the other thigh.

2 Do a similar action around both the knees, but using just the fingers for a lighter effect and working in smaller circles, again squeeze with each hand alternately.

3 Bend the leg and with your thumbs, work up the back of the calf with a circular kneading action. Repeat a few times, each time working from the ankle up the leg.

4 With the outside of the hands, lightly hack on the front of each thigh, using a very rapid, almost flicking motion. Keep this action gentle.

5 Stroke the length of your leg with the fingertips of both hands, from the ankle to the thigh to help blood flow back towards the heart.

MASSAGE WITH A PARTNER

Massaging your partner can be a wonderful way of sharing and giving, helping the relationship as well as easing tensions and preventing stress problems. Preparation is important in order to help release tired, aching muscles and create an overall experience. If you are massaging someone on the floor, use a mattress, quilt or cushions to make a comfortable surface. Cover with a sheet or towels to prevent oil staining your furnishings. Make sure that the room is warm and preferably with softer lighting to help your partner relax.

Aromatic essential oils can be used, but do use a good vegetable oil, such as sweet almond, and avoid thick, sticky mineral oils. The movements suggested below cover the major areas of muscle tension – use as many of them as you need. At the end of the massage, make sure your partner is comfortably wrapped in warm towels and given time to relax and enjoy the full benefit of the massage. Daily massage may not be practical for most people today, but even an occasional one has excellent health benefits.

When giving massage, remember to keep yourself feeling comfortable; breathe freely, try to keep a good posture and let your hands stay as relaxed as possible. If you need extra pressure in any movement, lean in with your whole body and use some of its weight, rather than tensing your fingers. Giving massage can be therapeutic too, and often leaves the giver refreshed and hungry! Above all, enjoy massage, and if in doubt get professional treatment.

ABOVE AND LEFT: Ensure that your partner is comfortable with what you are doing and the pressure you are using is at the right level – by keeping in touch.

BACK MASSAGE

One of the most reliable ways to relax and unwind – you may find the person being massaged drifts off to sleep – a back massage releases much of the tension we accumulate through the day. Make sure there are no draughts in the room and that your partner is warm and comfortable before you begin. Your oils should be ready and close to hand before you begin so that you don't have to interrupt after you have begun the session. Remember to warm your hands first.

1 Starting on the back, use a smooth, stroking movement downwards with the thumbs on either side of the spine (not pressing on the bones, just outside them) and then take the hands to the side and glide back up the shoulders. Repeat several times.

2 Then, from a kneeling position at your partner's side, use the whole of your hands and a smooth stroking movement to pull up steadily, one hand at a time, working all the way up and down one side of your partner's back a few times. Repeat from the other side.

3 Squeeze the muscles from one hand to the other, to knead the muscles of the back and shoulder and release deep-seated muscle tension. Make sure you knead generously rather than using a pinching movement. Repeat on the other side.

4 Stretch the back, using your forearms to glide in opposite directions. Try to keep a constant, steady pressure, lift off the arms when they reach the neck and buttocks, return to the centre of the back and repeat a few times.

LEGS

This is the perfect massage for the end of a day spent on your feet. It will release those tired aches and pains and leave you feeling relaxed. Do not use any pressure with these movements over varicose veins; if you do anything, just stroke over them lightly towards the heart.

1 Moving down to the back of the legs, knead and squeeze the calf muscles.

2 Do not put any pressure on the area behind the knee, but glide over this and knead the back of the thigh.

3 Then stroke all the way up the leg, hand over hand, to improve lymph and venous blood flow. Repeat these movements several times, always moving in an upwards direction. Repeat on the other leg.

4 On the front of the legs, kneading of the front of the thighs is helpful, but the front of the lower leg should be avoided as the shin bone is too prominent for this movement. Stroke all the way up the front of the leg and thigh, much as on the back of the leg. Repeat these movements on the other leg.

ABDOMEN MASSAGE

This should be a very gentle action, using a stroking movement and not applying any pressure. Don't do this straight after a heavy meal.

1 On the abdomen, use very slow circling movements in a clockwise direction to aid the digestive process. Make sure your partner is comfortable and relaxed with this movement.

2 Adjust the depth of pressure to your partner's comfort; if done slowly, deeper pressure can be very relaxing but do not overdo it.

ARM AND HAND MASSAGE

When massaging hands remember that some people find light movements ticklish and irritating.

1 For the arms, stroke and gently squeeze down the arm, from the wrist to the armpit, while supporting the arm with your other hand. You may need to swap hands in order to work all round the arm.

2 Then, with your thumbs, firmly massage into the palm of your partner's hand, using small circles. Repeat these movements on the other arm and hand. Use firm pressure to avoid tickling and irritating movements.

FACE

A good head massage can leave the recipient looking quite different as the facial muscles relax and worry lines disappear – you may be able to make your partner look ten years younger in just a few minutes. To massage the face, sit on the floor with your legs open. The person being massaged should lie on their back with their head between your legs. You might like to sit on a cushion. If this position is difficult for you to maintain, sit against a wall or a chair. Ensure you are comfortable before you start, as the benefits of the massage will be lost if you have to move after you have begun.

1 The neck and face can be slowly massaged with small circles, using the fingers of both hands working symmetrically to cover all the tiny facial muscles.

2 Place the thumbs side-by-side on the centre of the forehead and stroke out to the temples, working in strips – smooth away any worry lines.

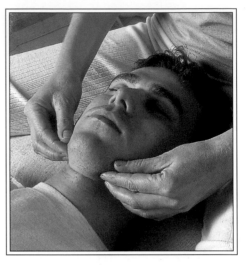

3 Take the chin between thumb and fingers and gently pinch your way out along the jaw, relaxing and releasing any tension.

FINISH

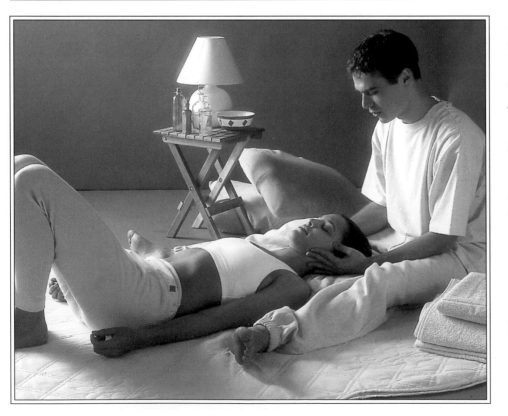

LEFT: *If you have worked through all these areas, or even if you choose just one – for example, the back – come to a finish slowly and just place your hands on your partner for a couple of minutes to complete the massage before leaving him or her to rest.*

MASSAGE TIPS

If you become tired or short of breath while you are massaging, rest and wait until you have recovered, maintaining contact by keeping one hand on your partner.

Don't wear tight fitting clothes or jewellery while you are massaging.

Make sure that your partner wraps up warmly after you have finished. Have a warmed dressing-gown or bathrobe ready for them to put on.

ROLFING

Rolfing is a system of working on the connective tissues of the body in order to correct imbalances in body posture and restore true alignment. It was founded and developed over some 40 years by Ida Rolf, an American bio-chemist who died in 1979 aged 84. She was familiar with yoga, osteopathy and other disciplines that might affect the body and health, but felt none of them adequately addressed the problem of restoring vitality and balance. She considered that it was necessary to ensure that the body was working in harmony with the force of gravity, and developed a technique which she originally termed "structural reintegration" to restore this harmony.

ABOVE: Rolfing can appear to be quite rough, as the connective tissue is manipulated through deep massage.

Ida Rolf gradually created a deep tissue form of massage, to work not so much on the muscles but on the connective tissues that surround muscles, bones and organs. This connective tissue can cover muscles like an envelope, when it is called fascia, or become thickened and bind muscles to bone, or a tendon. If it thickens and binds bone to bone, it is termed a ligament. As rolfers might say, if it fails to do any of these jobs, we call it a pain.

A common reaction of people to rolfing is that it hurts. The techniques can be rather painful at the time, as the practitioner seeks to remould the connective tissue to allow the body to come back into balance with the forces of gravity. Such pain should be only very temporary, however, and can be completely outweighed by the relief of chronic pain and discomfort from poor postural alignment after one or two rolfing sessions. As a general rule, rolfers work through the whole body in about ten sessions, steadily correcting postural faults in different areas through deep manipulative and massage movements.

The first session is essentially a diagnostic one, with the rolfer examining your structure, flexibility and posture, and perhaps taking photographs of how you hold yourself. Polaroids may be taken at the end to show what can be done even in one session. During the following two sessions the legs, shoulders, ribs and pelvis will be worked on to try to bring the body back into alignment with the forces of gravity. In the next sessions the practitioner works on the deeper muscles and tissues of the body, from the inside of the ankles, through thigh and pelvic musculature to the abdomen, back and neck. The final two or three sessions help to link all these areas together.

The whole process is essentially a process of learning about your body, and restoring it so that it can work more efficiently and with less strain. The deep work on the muscles and connective tissues can certainly cause discomfort from long-held tensions and stiffness, but generally this is replaced with a sense of the body becoming strong as the fibres are stretched back to their optimum length.

Since Ida Rolf's death, much of the training work has been carried on by the Rolf Institute in Boulder, Colorado, and practitioners from there have spread out through the US, Europe and beyond. Rolfing's emphasis on working with the connective tissue may indeed make it a painful process, but can have significant health benefits.

BELOW: Rolfing practitioners maintain that deep massage softens the collagen material and remoulds it back into a balanced state.

REFLEXOLOGY

The basic concept behind reflexology is that the whole body, indeed the whole person, is interconnected and that imbalances in one part of the body are reflected in changes elsewhere. There are probably some historical connections between the basis for reflexology and other systems, such as acupuncture or acupressure, and writings from ancient Egypt and Rome seem to describe healing points that correspond with reflex zones. It is certainly apparent that both the Incas and the Native Americans used forms of foot massage that are related to reflexology treatments. The latter may have been an influence on Dr William Fitzgerald whose observations and theories laid the foundations of modern reflexology.

Dr Fitzgerald was an American doctor, specializing in the ear, nose and throat area, who practised in the early part of the twentieth century in various hospitals in the US and England. Nobody is quite certain how he arrived at his ideas

BELOW: Reflexology can be practised at home for general relaxation and health but is no substitute for professional treatment which can reduce pain, improve the function of internal organs and also act as a diagnostic tool.

ABOVE: Reflexologists regard the feet as a map of the whole body so that by stimulating a particular point on the foot the therapist balances energy flow and can directly affect an internal organ or gland in the body.

but he discovered that pressure, or massage, on certain parts of the body helped to improve the functioning of internal organs, or else helped to reduce pain sensations. In 1913, he announced his findings, outlining his theory of interconnecting zones within the body – these can be visualized simply as ten vertical strips running the length of the body – with any problems arising in one of these zones being affected by the rest of that zone.

In 1917, Dr Fitzgerald, with his colleague Dr Edwin Bowers, published his ideas and the system of reflex zone therapy was established. It spread among doctors and others in the US, notably a Dr Riley who created a highly successful practice and expanded on the theories behind

SINUSES
TOP OF HEAD
PINEAL GLAND
PITUITARY GLAND
SINUSES
EYES
EARS
THYROID
LUNGS
SHOULDER
EYES
EARS
THYROID
LUNGS
SHOULDER
HEART
LIVER
STOMACH
SOLAR PLEXUS
STOMACH
SPLEEN
PANCREAS
ADRENALS
PANCREAS
SPLEEN
KIDNEY
KIDNEY
TRANSVERSE COLON
SPINE
ASCENDING COLON
SMALL INTESTINES
SPINE
DESCENDING COLON
BLADDER
HIP
BLADDER
SMALL INTESTINES
HIP
SCIATIC AREA
SCIATIC AREA

Right: A diagram of the reflexology zones of the soles of the feet. Other zones can be found at the sides and the top of the feet. It is important to have some training in reflexology before attempting to apply pressure to these points yourself.

reflexology. Dr Riley taught an assistant, Eunice Ingham, who popularized reflexology through a couple of influential books, *Stories the Feet Can Tell* and *Stories the Feet Have Told*. Unlike Dr Fitzgerald, who worked on various areas within the zones such as the hands, feet, lips, nose and ears, Eunice Ingham concentrated on the feet. She believed that since they contained points relating to all ten zones, they were of special significance in treatment.

Ingham's ideas about what reflexology did were rather simplistic, and are outdated nowadays, but they helped to focus treatment via the feet. She developed the theory that, with slower circulation to the extremities, tiny crystalline deposits occur around various nerve endings in the feet, much as silt forms in a river as the current slows. The reflexologist uses firm pressure to crush these little crystals and restore normal functioning. This theory is just one view of how reflexology works: no one has really come up with a comprehensive explanation and most practitioners today discuss its effects in terms of balancing energy flow (in similar fashion to Oriental systems of medicine).

Reflexology has expanded in popularity greatly across the world in the last 30 years. This is partly due to its relative simplicity as a non-invasive method of treatment, and partly from the plain fact that although nobody has successfully explained why it should work, it does. There have been some recent studies – for instance, one carried out by nurses at a hospital in Manchester, England – which demonstrated the benefits of reflexology in reducing the symptoms of stress, and increasing numbers of natural therapists are recognizing its value.

Reflexology is of considerable benefit in stress-related ailments, in reducing pain and in improving the functioning of internal organs; it also has some usefulness as a diagnostic aid, as tender reflex points can help to locate areas of dysfunction. Gentle, generalized foot massage techniques are suitable for home use too, to maintain good health, although they are not a substitute for professional treatment.

Stretching and loosening the feet will in itself improve local circulation and help general relaxation. Using steady, fairly firm pressure, you may locate tender spots on the feet. These should be treated with great gentleness and should not be pressed too hard or for too long, as this can produce a strong reaction in the affected area of the body. The thumbs are normally used, although fingers may be more useful in some places. Any tenderness at the end of the massage can be eased by soothing or rubbing the feet afterwards.

FOOT MASSAGE WITH A PARTNER

Arrange for your partner to be warm and comfortable; sitting on a chair with a section for the feet that can be raised, or lying on a bed may be appropriate. Ideally, your partner's feet should be almost up to the level of your shoulders. Make sure that you too are comfortable before beginning so that you do not have to alter your position. Oil can be used for foot massage, but the direct pressure technique does work better without it, so that your hands do not slip.

1 Initially, simply make contact with your partner's feet, by curving your hands over the top of them just a few inches away. This is called "greeting the feet" and its steady contact can be very relaxing and reassuring in itself. Our feet carry us around all day, with really very little protest, but tensions do build up in them and stretching movements can help to revitalize us very quickly, without the need of detailed treatment on specific reflexology points.

2 Massage each toe in turn using your thumb, then flex and extend them gently. Gently twist the foot sideways to stretch all the muscles.

3 Holding the top of the foot with one hand and cupping the heel in your other hand, use the top hand to flex and extend the whole foot, steadily, to loosen up all the joints.

4 If your partner is tired and exhausted, the feet and indeed the whole system can be reinvigorated by hitting the inside edge of the foot lightly with the side of your hands. Only use this movement if someone needs to be woken up.

5 Then ease out tensions in the lateral arch of the foot by holding the foot with both hands, one on each side, and stretching across the top of the foot in a movement rather like breaking open a crusty bread roll.

7 To finish hold the feet by resting your hands gently on top of them for a few minutes and slowly breaking contact, helping your partner to unwind completely.

6 A final and very helpful relaxing pressure can be given on the reflex points that relate to the solar plexus. This is often called the brain of the abdomen, and is a huge collection of nerve fibres that controls the digestive organs. The points on the feet are located between the big toe and the next toe, just below the large pad beneath the big toe; pressing both feet at the same time is more effective.

BENEFITS OF REFLEXOLOGY

Reflexology has been used to treat a number of common ailments including back pain, digestive problems, migraine, menstrual problems, sinus problems and general stress and tension. It has also been used for more serious ailments such as heart disorders and multiple sclerosis. It is also thought that a reflexologist can sometimes detect an impending illness and give preventive treatment, if appropriate, or advise the patient to see a specialist. By having regular treatment, perhaps every month or so, good health may be maintained and early warning signs spotted. Reflexology can have quite powerful effects and is therefore better avoided by pregnant women or people with arthritis, osteoporosis or heart and thyroid disorders. As a home therapy, however, reflexology massage should be restricted to a gentle relaxation method. You can try these simple movements on yourself, and if this is difficult the same effects can be produced by massaging the corresponding points on your hand.

CHIROPRACTIC

Chiropractic is a well-established system of treatment and, alongside osteopathy, is respected as one of the major forms of manipulative therapy. It is based upon the premise that structure affects function, and in particular that displacement of the structure of the spine can cause pressure on nerves which in turn affect other parts of the body. In the US it is extremely popular, with around 50,000 chiropractors in practice, and it is also widespread in Australia. In the UK there are currently more osteopaths than chiropractors, but both are accepted by the medical profession.

In 1895, in Iowa, a self-taught "magnetic healer" named Daniel David Palmer treated his office janitor, who had become deaf after bending over and feeling a click in his back. Palmer discovered a slight misalignment of the man's spine and manipulated the bones to restore true alignment; this led to the hearing being restored. Subsequently, Palmer went on to found a school of chiropractic – the word derives from two Greek words meaning practical use of the hand.

Chiropractors use a variety of manual adjustment techniques to help correct faulty alignment, and following a thorough physical examination, plus questioning about your general health, are likely to take X-rays to establish precisely what is happening to your skeleton. Manipulation is then carried out to give normal movement back to any affected joints, and you will probably be re-examined to make sure that the joints are now moving more freely. In chronic or severe cases, a series of treatments may be necessary.

The vast majority of people seeking chiropractic treatment suffer from some kind of musculoskeletal pain, especially in the neck or lower back. A common injury caused by car accidents is whiplash, where the head and neck are abruptly jerked, and chiropractors can often correct the trauma caused to the structures. Frequent headaches may also be a reason for a visit to a chiropractor, and relief is often reported from the manipulative adjustments.

Although some chiropractors restrict themselves completely to spinal adjustments, many practitioners, especially in the US, may give advice on exercise and nutrition, and even prescribe dietary supplements. This is similar to some schools of training in osteopathy which combine advice with naturopathy for all-round health benefits. The manipulative treatments have been the subject of some research, and in American, English and New Zealand studies, for instance, chiropractic has been shown to be one of the most effective forms of treatment for musculoskeletal problems.

The differences between chiropractic and osteopathy are largely historical, and both systems accept modern physiological ideas, mainly differing in the specific techniques used to achieve similar aims. That chiropractic treatment is covered by Medicare, Medicaid and most health insurance schemes in the US, and some in the UK, is a sure sign that the manipulative therapies have established their credentials.

ABOVE: *Chiropractic often involves a sudden movement which results in a "clicking" sound as the bones are realigned.*

ABOVE: *Backache is often linked to an injury sustained earlier in life and can be easily and effectively cured by chiropractic.*

ABOVE: *The practitioner sometimes uses his or her body weight to realign the bones, which can be alarming but is perfectly safe.*

CRANIO-SACRAL THERAPY

Cranio-sacral therapy has grown out of an osteopathic background, and an increasing number of osteopaths are including or even specializing in cranial osteopathic techniques. Cranio-sacral therapy is also taught and practised by other therapists (with some disapproval from osteopathic circles); probably the most fundamental quality needed from a practitioner is great sensitivity of touch.

Its origins date back to an American osteopathic physician, William Garner Sutherland, practising in the early years of the twentieth century. He developed the theory that the skull, which consists of eight bones joined by fine sutures, was able to expand and contract marginally, and did so in response to the rhythmic flow of

ABOVE: The cranium and its fluids are mobilized in cranio-sacral therapy.

cerebro-spinal fluid within the brain and spinal column. As this fluid wells up within the ventricles, deep inside the brain, it affects the membranes supporting the brain and in turn increases pressure on the cranium itself.

Dr Sutherland carried out experiments on himself, using various contraptions to stop his skull moving, with many startling results on his physical health and behaviour. This

led him to advocate very gentle manipulative movements, to mobilize the cranio-sacral rhythmic flow of fluid and allow this expansion/contraction to occur naturally and without any impediment. He theorized that any blow or trauma, from birth onwards, could impair this system, and lead to ill-health of many kinds.

Sutherland's theories were largely dismissed by orthodox medicine in his time; but modern medical research, notably at Michigan State University, has demonstrated that much of what Sutherland suggested has a good scientific basis.

Cranial techniques can be of particular benefit to young children, and this is an expanding field. One of the first people to work with Sutherland was a pediatrician, Dr Beryl Arbuckle, who became world-famous for her work with cerebral palsy sufferers. What is less known is that her osteopathic approach was almost entirely cranial. The Osteopathic Centre for Children in London also uses cranial work to a large, and successful, extent.

Conditions where cranial techniques may prove valuable include headaches, pains originating in the tempero-mandibular (jaw) joint, and recurrent ear and sinus infections in children. These examples may not seem surprising, but this therapy may also benefit children who have had birth traumas, brain injuries, or developmental and behavioural problems such as hyperactivity. Indeed, children can sometimes respond dramatically quickly to cranial work.

The rather unconventional theories behind cranio-sacral therapy, and the considerable sensitivity required from the practitioner, are probably the main obstacles to it becoming more widespread. The touch of a therapist is very light and yet quite profound changes are reported, and this can be disconcerting for some people. Apart from cranial osteopaths, most people who train in cranio-sacral therapy tend to be bodywork practitioners already, with high levels of palpatory ability as well as professional therapeutic skills, and their numbers are slowly but definitely growing.

BELOW: One of the gentlest therapies, cranio-sacral therapy can alleviate headaches and sinus pain, especially in children.

OSTEOPATHY

Osteopathy is one of the two major systems of manipulative therapy, together with chiropractic. Its origins date back to the nineteenth century, but it has philosophical connections right back to the Hippocratic school of medical thought in the fourth century BC. It was founded by an American doctor, Andrew Taylor Still, in 1874, after several years of trying to find a better way of treating his patients than bleeding and purging. He based his ideas on the ancient notion that the body can cure itself, and on the concept of the need for the structure of the body to be correctly aligned in order to release our innate self-healing power.

Although we stand upright our anatomy is still basically that of a creature which moves on all fours, and there is a constant strain on the whole framework. Still recognized that the effect of gravity is particularly severe on the spine, the vertebrae and the cushioning discs between them. Still's earlier training as an engineer helped him in his assessment of the problems that could result from misalignment of the patient's skeletal structure, and his philosophical outlook emphasized the interconnectedness of the body and its self-healing potential.

Still therefore developed the use of manipulative techniques to treat not just the spine but the whole body. Structure and function were seen as interdependent, and attention to the former would improve the latter. In 1892, he founded the first school of osteopathy, in Missouri. One of his students, John Littlejohn, subsequently founded the British School of Osteopathy in 1917. In the US, osteopaths are also medically trained, and represent some five per cent of American doctors; in the UK they considerably outnumber chiropractors, and have recently been granted State Registration as a recognized and statutorily regulated profession.

Osteopathic treatments will involve a detailed case his-

ABOVE: Many hospitals and general practices now employ an osteopath to support conventional treatments.

tory of your general health, as well as particulars of any accidents/injuries and the current problem, and then a complete physical examination to assess the range and freedom of movement of the body. Manipulative techniques, perhaps accompanied by some deep neuro-muscular massage, may be used to help to restore normal structural balance and functioning.

A number of specific techniques have been developed over the last hundred years or so, ranging from gentle, repeated movements of joints to increase their mobility, to quick thrust movements which rapidly guide the joint through its normal range. These latter manipulations can often cause the characteristic clicking noise that many people experience during a session. They may also temporarily irritate surrounding tissues and give some extra discomfort until the area settles down again.

A fairly recent development within some schools of osteopathy has been the use of cranial-osteopathic treatment. This involves very gentle movements to help the flow of cerebro-spinal fluid, a lymph-like fluid which moves rhythmically around the brain and spinal cord, bathing and nourishing the nerve tissues. Any impediment in this rhythm is seen as creating imbalance within the body, with subsequent ill-health (see also *Cranio-sacral Therapy*). Cranial-osteopathic treatments are especially helpful for infants – say, after a difficult birth – and in London, for example, there is an osteopathic hospital centre for children that uses these gentle methods in such circumstances.

Since osteopaths in America may also be family doctors, and in the UK they are not only State Registered but are starting to work in doctors' surgeries or even hospitals, osteopathy has become well integrated into conventional medicine; however, not all doctors accept that it is anything more than just a "back treatment".

ALEXANDER TECHNIQUE

The Alexander Technique is a method of training in posture, body movement and positioning. It was originally devised by Frederick Alexander, an Australian actor, around the turn of the twentieth century. He found that when he was giving an important Shakespearean speech on stage, his voice continually faltered. The only advice given to him was to rest his voice, which only helped until the next large role. Eventually, he set about studying exactly how he was using his body by watching himself in a mirror, and discovered that he tensed his body when performing. The effort of projecting his voice made him bring his head down, restricting his vocal cords and impairing deep breathing or voice control.

Over a period of time Alexander slowly adapted the way he held his body when acting on stage, and overcame this "startle reflex pattern" as he called it. Gradually he developed the idea that body use – how we hold ourselves, move and so forth – can affect the functioning of our internal organs and overall health. He started to teach his methods of body realignment, moving to London in 1904 and subsequently going to the US gaining widespread recognition.

The techniques he devised are based upon the principle of extending the spine, allowing it to reach its optimal length, and generally to redeploy the body's entire muscular system. Exercises are thus geared to restoring natural posture and ease of movement, with minimal muscular effort. A common phrase used to describe the ideal movement is, "the head leads, the spine follows."

Animals and young children usually move naturally, with a lengthened spine and a sense of poise. Unfortunately, we often acquire bad habits as we get older, and additional stresses can lead to imbalanced and excessive muscular effort in movement. If chronic tensions build up, the neck and back muscles contract, leading to rounded shoulders, a lowered head and an arched back, which causes further tension and so the problem gets worse and worse. Alexander teachers seek to help re-educate us to change these patterns and regain positive, easy body use.

Alexander schools have often been associated

FAR LEFT AND ABOVE: *The basic principle of Alexander's ideal posture is to keep your body in a straight line.*

with drama or music establishments, echoing the man's background, but the techniques are suitable for all kinds of occupations. Improvements in posture can be accompanied by health benefits such as greater mental alertness, better sleep, increased resistance to stress and enhanced performance of physical tasks. The techniques are learned from a teacher, in the form of lessons rather than treatment sessions, and may initially involve simple actions such as sitting down and getting up from a chair or walking to and fro, with corrective advice on how to use the body more efficiently.

Self-help measures may be of benefit in the first instance; copying Alexander's example and looking closely at your posture in the mirror might be valuable in identifying obvious imbalances. However, since bad habits can be difficult to change, or even spot sometimes, a series of lessons from a teacher is likely to be the most helpful way to correct these.

The Alexander technique is not a cure-all, but improvements in the way we hold and use our bodies can improve many people's overall health and movement.

EASTERN APPROACHES

The traditional Oriental view of health is quite different from the reductionist standpoint of modern, technological medicine in the West. In Eastern philosophy, illness is placed in the context of a holistic approach to life, and in particular the concept of an energy-based system. From the idea of a universal energy, or the highest level of spirituality, down to the lowest forms of life, much of Eastern ideology is an energetic one, with all parts of the human body interconnected and infused with a vital energy, and all life-forms similarly interdependent on an exchange of energies.

These concepts have led to the development of traditional therapeutic systems, such as acupuncture in China, shiatsu or acupressure in Japan, and yoga in India. Some of these are more suited to professional treatment of ailments, or imbalances in energy flow as they would be described, while practices such as yoga are very suitable for everyday life, in order to *prevent* illness as well as to promote self-development.

Modern medicine in many Far Eastern countries is now often an amalgam of conventional Western medicines alongside traditional approaches; they are quite happy to utilize the best of both worlds, and this is perhaps a useful pointer to the rest of us. Acute, severe illness may be treated with hi-tech medicine, but a more holistic approach can remedy most health problems.

ABOVE: Yoga is one of the most ancient ways of releasing the mind.

OPPOSITE: Acupuncture, once practised only in the East, is now available throughout the world.

SHIATSU

Shiatsu is a contemporary therapy with its roots in Oriental traditional medicine. It is sometimes described as Japanese physiotherapy since it is primarily a physically based "bodywork" system of treatment. The actual treatment approach and philosophy is similar to acupuncture in its usage of the meridians (energy channels) and *tsubo* (pressure points) as well as diagnostic methods, but without the use of needles. Unlike most other forms of bodywork, in shiatsu the receiver remains clothed for the treatment and this is often a consideration for patients.

The word "shiatsu" is Japanese and literally means "finger pressure". The application of pressure is the underlying principle of shiatsu. This pressure can be applied using not only your fingers, but also the palms of your hands, thumbs, elbows or knees, depending on the amount of stimulation required and which body area is treated. Stretching exercises and other corrective techniques will also be included in the treatment with the intention of creating flexibility and balance in the body, both physically and energetically.

Shiatsu works on the flow of energy or *qi* that circulates through our bodies in specific energy channels or meridians. Essentially, we all have a "life force" or "life energy" which created our physical structure and regulates physical, emotional, mental and spiritual stability. This life force, called *qi* in Chinese and *ki* in Japanese, maintains a homeostatic balance in your body.

The flow of *qi* can be disturbed either through external trauma, such as an injury, or internal trauma such as depression or stress. This is when symptoms like aches and pain start to occur and we start to experience a state of "dis-ease". In shiatsu the physical touch is used to assess the distribution of *qi* throughout the body and to try to correct any imbalances accordingly.

Touch is the essence of shiatsu and a wonderful means of communicating our love and compassion for others in a very direct way. Touch can be of very different quality, ranging from aggressive, abusive and mechanical to more nurturing, caring and intuitive. We all need to be touched in some way and shiatsu helps to fulfil this need. The caring touch used in shiatsu will help to trigger the self-healing process within.

LEFT: *The essence of shiatsu is touch. The practitioner will build up a relationship of trust and care with the patient.*

SHIATSU AT HOME

The exercises in this chapter give two routines, one which you can do on yourself and one with a partner. You may find that during or at the end of these routines you feel slight mood changes. Other reactions experienced after a professional treatment include cold or mild flu symptoms which disappear after a day or so. Do not attempt any shiatsu techniques other than the following exercises without consulting a trained practitioner.

THE HISTORY AND PHILOSOPHY

Oriental medicine developed out of a need to maintain good health and prevent illness. Therapies such as acupuncture, herbalism, moxibustion (the burning of the mugwort herb on the skin) and *amma* (Chinese massage) developed in different geographical areas according to lifestyle and cultural considerations. In the earliest recorded writing on Chinese medicine, *The Yellow Emperor's Canon of Internal Medicine*, written over 2,000 years ago, the Yellow Emperor asked the master of Oriental medicine why there were so many methods to treat one illness and why each method was effective. The master replied that environment was the main reason for using different approaches. In the east where the people lived close to the sea, tended to eat more fish and protein and suffered skin diseases, acupuncture developed as an effective treatment. In the west, where there are mountains and deserts, the people tended to be fat and eat too much animal protein. This caused problems with their internal organs which were best remedied by herbal medicine. In the cold northern mountainous regions, moxibustion was most effective in driving out respiratory disorders associated with the climate, such as coughing and mucus. In the flat central regions, the people developed symptoms of general weakness which was most effectively treated with *amma* and corrective exercises.

Amma (*anma* in Japanese) has been used for centuries to deal with many common ailments, aches and pains as well as treating more serious "dis eases". New influences from traditional Eastern medicine and Western science have gradually shaped it into what is today called shiatsu. There are several main styles of shiatsu found in the West: barefoot shiatsu, macrobiotic shiatsu, Namikoshi style, Ohashiatsu, Shiatsu-Do and Zen shiatsu. These are all valid and effective therapies using the basic shiatsu principles but with differing emphasis placed on techniques or philosophy. In Japan there are more than 87,000 registered shiatsu practitioners. This fact alone goes some way towards demonstrating its effectiveness in the prevention and treatment of disease.

QI – YOUR LIFE FORCE

Shiatsu acts on the subtle anatomy of the body described as *qi* in Chinese or *ki* in Japanese. The concept of *qi* might be a bit difficult to grasp at first as it is so little recognized in Western society, but everyone can learn how to perceive *qi* and appreciate its effects. *Qi* is a fundamental idea to Oriental medical thinking and is considered as our "life essence" which maintains and nurtures our physical body

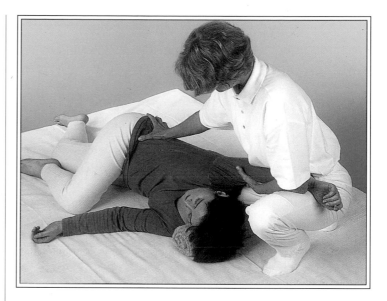

ABOVE: Here the practitioner stretches the gall bladder meridian and opens the rib cage.

and therefore also affects our mind and spirit. *Qi* is everywhere. It moves and changes quickly from moment to moment and can easily be replenished on a day-to-day basis. The human body is a field of continually moving energy, circulating through cells, tissues, muscles and internal organs.

The concept of *qi* was introduced to the West through acupuncture and the Chinese martial art of T'ai Chi Chuan. The Chinese word *qi* translates as "breaths". A Japanese dictionary defines *qi* as mind, spirit, or heart and lists hundreds of expressions which use the word *qi*, most of them ordinary ways of talking about human moods, attitudes, or character. For example, *genki* means "source of *qi*" or health.

It is much easier to demonstrate *qi* than to try to measure or contain it and there are a variety of exercises you can do to get in touch with *qi* and feel its affect on your body. *Qi* is a real force, made up of electric, magnetic, infrasonic and infra-red vibrations, which can be intuitively perceived and mentally directed. Like air that we breathe and depend on for our life and water that we take into our bodies, *qi* is the very source of our vitality. It is the force within us which gives us initiative, which drives and inspires us to move forward in life. When the *qi* leaves us, we die. According to the ancient philosophers, life and death is nothing but an aggravation and dispersal of *qi*:

"*Qi* produces the human body just as water becomes ice. As water freezes into ice, so *qi* coagulates to form the human body. When ice melts, it becomes water. When a person dies, he or she becomes spirit (*shen*) again. It is called spirit, just as melted ice changes its name to water."

WANG CHONG, AD 27–97

THE MERIDIAN LINES

LUNG:
Official in charge of jurisdiction.

The lungs govern *qi* and respiration and in particular are in charge of inhaling air. Intake of fresh *qi* from the environment which is fundamental for building up resistance against external intrusions.

Elimination of gases through the process of exhalation.

Openness and positivity.

LARGE INTESTINE:
Official generating elimination and exchange.

Helps the function of the lungs. Elimination of waste products from food and drink and stagnated *qi*. Transmission.

The ability to let go.

SPLEEN:
Official in charge of storage.

Transformation and nourishment. Spleen corresponds to the function of the pancreas in Western terms and governs general digestion including saliva and gastric bile; secretions from the small intestines; reproductive hormones related to the breasts and ovaries.

Maintains the health of the flesh, the connective soft tissue and the muscle.

Self-image is affected strongly by the spleen function and the desire to help others is apparent. Self-confidence.

STOMACH:
Official in charge of the granary or food store.

The stomach is responsible for receiving and processing ingested food and fluids.

Information for mental and physical nourishment.

Well grounded, centred and reliable.

HEART:
Minister of the monarch and has insight and understanding.

Governs blood and blood vessels.

Houses the mind and our emotions. The heart functions as the mechanism that adapts and integrates external stimuli to the body's internal environment.

Awareness and communication. Joyful.

SMALL INTESTINE:
Official in charge of the treasury who converts food into energy.

The quality of the blood and tissue reflects the condition of the small intestine. Anxiety, emotional excitement or nervous shock can adversely affect the energy of the small intestine.

Emotional stability and calmness.

KIDNEY:
Official who does energetic work.

Provides and stores fundamental *qi* for all other organs and governs birth, growth, reproduction and development.

Nourishes the spine, the bones and the brain.

Vitality, direction and will-power.

BLADDER:
Official in charge of storage of the overflow and fluid secretions.

Purification and regulation.

Gives courage and ability to move forward in life.

HEART GOVERNOR:
Official of joy and pleasure.

Protector of the heart and closely related to emotional responses.

Related to central circulation.

Influences relationships with others.

TRIPLE HEATER:
Official who plans construction.

Transportation of energy, blood and heat to the peripheral parts of the body.

Helpful and emotionally interactive.

LIVER:
Official in charge of planning.

Storage of blood.

Ensures free flow of *qi* throughout the body.

Creative and full of ideas.

GALL BLADDER:
Official with good judgement and decisions.

Stores bile produced by the liver and distributes it to the small intestine.

Practical application of ideas and decision-making.

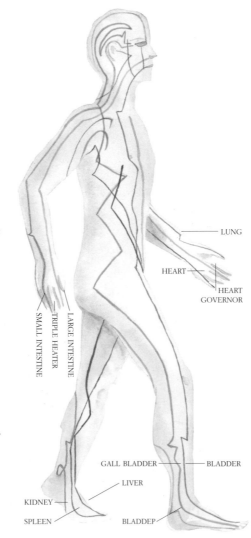

LEFT: Shiatsu works on the body's natural meridians, shown in this diagram. A shiatsu practitioner will work on these lines to promote balance and harmony.

THE MERIDIAN SYSTEM

Each of the twelve organs is linked with a meridian or channel of energy, named according to the internal organ it affects. The meridians connect all the different body parts with each other and like rivers of energy, ensure proper nurturing of *qi* or life force throughout your whole being. When you are healthy, the flow of *qi* proceeds unimpeded, like the water in a free-running river, and energy is well distributed throughout the meridian pathways. When the river, or meridian, is blocked for some reason, the *qi* is prevented from reaching the specific area it is supposed to nurture and cells, tissue or organs will suffer from lack of it.

The area or internal organ/system connected to this meridian will enter a state of "dis-ease", or a condition of stress. In the early stages the symptoms might be minor, perhaps just a nagging pain or discomfort. This is your body telling you that something is wrong.

Any type of "disease" is a sign that the energy within the meridian system is out of balance. When a meridian is blocked, one part of the body is getting too much *qi* and enters a state of excess, while another part is getting too little and becomes deficient in *qi*. This will result in one organ becoming overactive while another organ will become underactive and may be fatigued. If you do not listen to what your body is telling you at this stage, the symptoms might worsen and become more serious – from here degeneration of the system and body begins.

Along the meridians you will find more highly charged energy points, which are called pressure points in English or *tsubo* in Japanese. This is where the *qi* is most easily affected and stimulating different *tsubo* will correct the energy imbalance. By using different shiatsu techniques, such as pressure, stretching, rubbing and corrective exercises, you will be able to release the blockages, "open" the meridian and recharge yourself.

All the meridians either start or end in the hands or the feet and connect internally to the organ whose condition they reflect. Refer to the meridian line illustration for the pathways of the different meridians over the surface of the body and to the table for the functions of the meridians. In Oriental medicine, the organs are thought of in a conceptual sense, with official duties as in a government. When the different "officials" work together and co-operate, there is peace and harmony in the land (body). If there is disagreement or disorganization between the different departments, imbalances start to occur.

A further eight extraordinary meridians known as vessels also carry energy through our bodies. The two most important in their influence as regards shiatsu are the governing vessel and the conception vessel. These vessels are responsible for the control and regulation of the energy circulating throughout the meridian system and any necessary adjustments are made to them when excesses or deficiencies in the energy system occur.

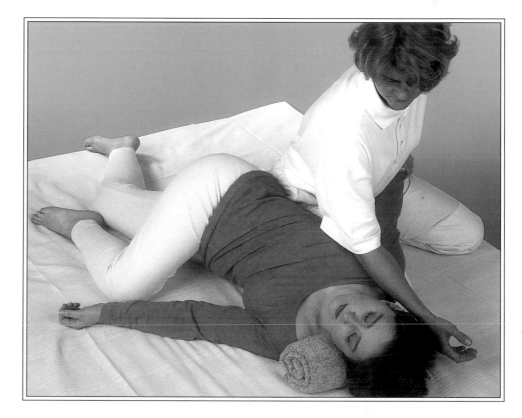

RIGHT: *The side position is a classic position used in shiatsu; here the practitioner half kneels beside the patient and opens the chest by gently stretching the lung meridian in the arm.*

SHIATSU WITH A PRACTITIONER

A shiatsu session usually lasts for about an hour with the actual treatment taking between 35 and 45 minutes.

In the first session the shiatsu practitioner will ask you many questions about your state of health, your lifestyle, any symptoms, likes and dislikes you may have, to build up your case history. An assessment based on Oriental diagnosis will be compiled. Apart from this oral diagnosis, your practitioner will use visual diagnosis, looking at posture, movement and facial diagnostic areas; and touch diagnosis, feeling the body and the different meridians for areas of excess and deficiency. As touch is the most essential aspect of shiatsu, this diagnosis continues throughout the whole treatment, your practitioner gaining new information about you as the sessions proceed.

You will usually remain clothed during treatment, but your practitioner may need to examine skin surfaces for discolorations and/or swelling at some stage. As the treatment will involve stretches and different movements for you to practise in between sessions, it is advisable to wear loose, comfortable clothing, preferably of cotton. Avoid receiving shiatsu after you have eaten. Digestion will draw energy to the abdomen and disturb your practitioner in reading the energetic movements in your meridian system. There should be as little outside disturbance as possible to maintain the balancing effects of the treatment. It is also suggested therefore that you refrain from consuming any alcohol on the day

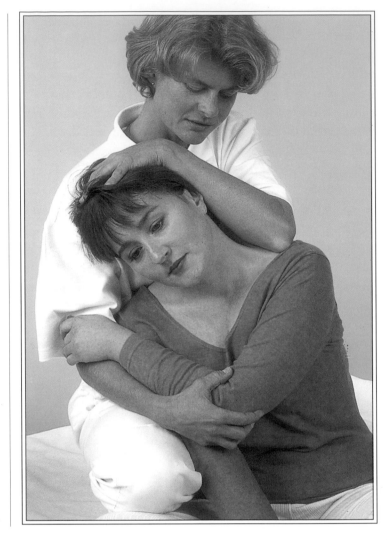

ABOVE: *The sitting position is one of the different positions used in a shiatsu treatment. In a supportive way the practitioner is treating the trapezius muscle, affecting the large intestine and gall bladder meridian on top of the shoulder.*

LEFT: *All meridians – or energy channels – either start or end in the fingers and toes.*

before your treatment as well as the actual day and avoid strenuous exercise following your shiatsu session.

HOW MANY SESSIONS?

A course of treatment usually involves four to eight sessions, preferably on a weekly basis. This depends on the nature of the problem. A long-term imbalance might need more treatments, while a couple of sessions for an acute disturbance might be sufficient. Remember that shiatsu is also a preventive therapy, aiding the maintenance of good health, so you do not need to be unwell to receive treatments. This is why many clients continue their shiatsu sessions, after the initial course of treatments, every month or two for their general health and well-being.

BELOW: Here the practitioner is treating the bladder meridian in the back of the leg, using the knee.

EFFECTS AFTER YOUR SHIATSU TREATMENT

The immediate effect of treatments differs with each individual. Depending on your state of health, your symptoms and how accustomed you are to receiving bodywork, you will have different reactions after your shiatsu treatments. A sense of well-being is common.

Because of the deep relaxation that usually occurs and the stimulus to the major body systems, you may have some healing reactions. Some people feel cold or flu-like symptoms, aches and pains, or headaches after the first treatment. These symptoms will only last for a day or so and usually subside with each subsequent treatment. It is important to remember that any such effects you may experience are positive signs from your body telling you it is making an attempt to correct its own condition in a natural way. These are signs of elimination and the beginning of the healing process.

Here are some simple shiatsu techniques which you can perform on a partner. This is an ideal way to release tension
without putting too much strain on the body. You may feel
sleepy afterwards. Keep your touch gentle.

1 Gently place your hands on your partner's shoulders. Take
a moment to tune into her energy. There may be tension in
the area to begin with. Squeeze the trapezius muscle – the
muscles of the shoulder and neck – using your thumbs and
fingers in a rhythmic kneading action.

2 With the little finger side of your hand, gently hack across
the shoulders and neck in a rhythmic motion. Gradually your
partner's muscles will relax and you can increase the intensity
and power of the hacking. Keep checking if this feels
comfortable for your partner.

3 Kneel at your partner's side supporting
the back with your leg. Place one hand
on the forehead and encourage the
partner to relax the head into your hand.
With the fingers and thumb of the other
hand, gently squeeze the neck muscles.

4 Kneel behind your partner and place
your forearms on the shoulders with
your palms facing to the floor. Lean into
your forearms using your body to apply
equal gentle pressure on to your
partner's shoulders.

5 Ask your partner to breathe deeply.
On the out breath, roll your arms across
the shoulder, from the neck towards the
shoulder joint, ending up with your
palms facing up. Lift your arms up and
repeat several times.

PRONE POSITION

1 Using the palms of your hands, press down gently on your partner's back. Start at the top of the back in between the shoulders and gradually work downwards. Apply the pressure as your partner breathes out. Keep your elbows straight. Repeat three times.

2 Measure two fingers' breadth from the centre of the spine to locate the bladder meridian. Use your thumbs and apply gentle pressure all the way down the back, working gradually from the top to the bottom.

3 For the upper part of the back, kneel or crouch at your partner's head. Using your thumbs, apply pressure to the bladder meridian. Hold this gentle pressure for a few seconds.

COMPLETION

To complete the session, lie your partner down on the back. Rest your hand on the stomach. This is called the Hara in the Orient, and is thought of as the vital centre of ourselves. In this position "tune in" to your partner's breathing. Stay in this position for a few moments until you can sense that your partner is relaxed and peaceful, then slowly move your hand away and gently dissolve the contact.

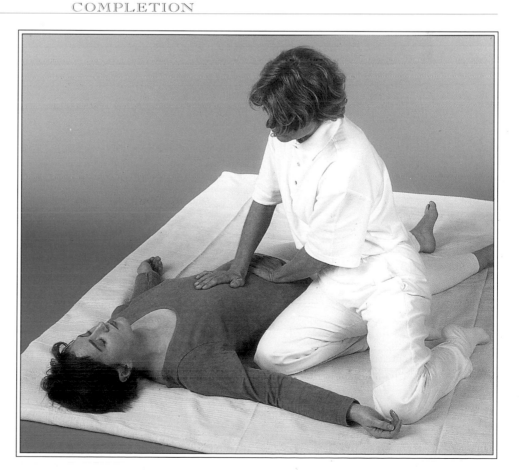

MERIDIAN STIMULATION

The following DoIn (a form of shiatsu) exercises are designed to improve, maintain and develop your general physical, mental and emotional health and well-being.

The exercises can be practised by anyone maintaining a normal daily life, at any time without any special effort. The DoIn exercises will open up the energy channels, release any blockages and facilitate the free flow of *qi* along the meridians, thus improving the circulation of energy throughout the whole body. You will feel invigorated and energized after performing the exercises, and it is recommended that you do them upon rising in the morning, or whenever you are feeling low and generally under par.

Although any part of the series of exercises can be practised independently, it is best to perform the whole sequence at one time to achieve the maximum benefit. Keep a natural posture and breathe normally throughout the exercises and try to maintain an empty mind, clear from any disturbing thoughts and feelings. Keep your focus on the exercise and feel the effect it has on your body. As you become accustomed to the routine, it will be easier to follow and you will find it takes even less time to complete.

1 Prepare yourself by gently shaking your body. Shake your arms and hands. Lift your shoulders up to your ears as you breathe in; let them relax on exhaling. Repeat a few times.

2 One at a time, gently shake each of your legs and feet. Then sit down in a chair or on a cushion on the floor, keeping your back straight. Keeping an upright posture allows a good energy flow.

HEAD

1 Clench both hands loosely and, with your wrists loose, start to tap the top of your head gently. Work your way slowly all around your head, covering the sides, front and back. Adjust the percussion pressure as needed. This exercise will wake up your brain and stimulate blood circulation which will be beneficial for your hair growth and hair quality.

2 Pull your fingers through your hair, gently stimulating the meridians running across the top and side of your head (bladder and gall-bladder).

3 Place your fingers on either side of the mid-line of your skull and apply pressure with your fingertips to the bladder meridian, working from the forehead to the back of your neck. Then move your fingers down to just above the ears and apply pressure. Repeat this sequence three times.

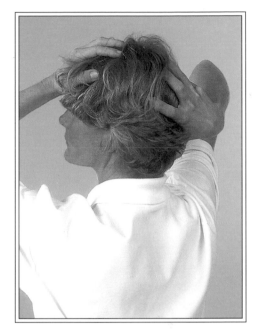

1 Now move your attention to the back of your neck. Bend your head down and using one hand, place your palm across the back of your neck and gently massage it using a squeezing motion.

2 Lift your chin slightly and with your thumbs, press either side of the base of the skull, supporting your head with your fingers. The pressure should be directed up against the skull.

3 Use one thumb to stimulate the skull's mid-base, while the other hand supports your forehead, tipping the head slightly up and back. Vibrate your thumb gently as you apply pressure, then release. Repeat three to five times.

FACE

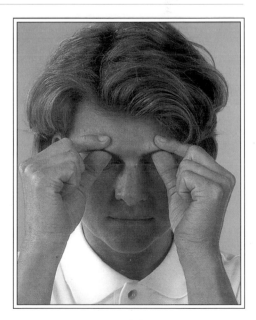

1 Apply both hands to your cheeks and using the palms gently rub your cheeks in an up-and-down motion until the skin becomes warm.

2 Bring your palms to your eyes, covering them and warming the area around the eyes. This stimulates blood circulation in the area and will be beneficial for tired eyes.

3 Using your index finger and thumb, squeeze your eyebrows starting from the centre line and moving laterally, three times.

▶

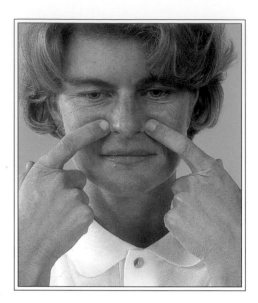

4 With an index finger and thumb, pinch the bridge of the nose and the corners of the eyes. This point is called "eye's clarity". It opens and brightens the eyes and clears vision and will be especially helpful if the eyes are tired.

5 Clench your fingers and apply your thumbs to the sides of your nose. Stroke down the side of your nose quickly at the same time as you breathe in. This will help to clear your sinuses and release any stagnation of mucus.

6 Use your index fingers to stimulate either side of the nose.

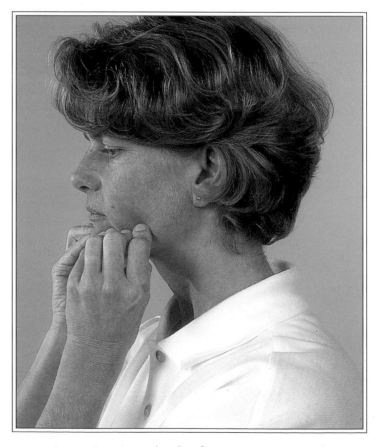

7 Using the four fingers of both hands, apply pressure around the mouth. This area of your face reflects the digestive-system and these exercises will activate the production of saliva and strengthen the system.

8 Using your thumbs and index fingers, squeeze your lower jaw. Repeat three to five times. This will stimulate the glands which are directly related to the ears, saliva and lymph so that they function properly.

EARS

1 Move your hands to your ears and massage them gently, using your index fingers and thumbs. Your ears relate to your kidneys and these exercises will improve mental balance as well as kidney and excretory functions. First rub the peripheral ridge of the ear in order to activate circulation; then rub the middle ridge and finally move to the inner ridges and indentations.

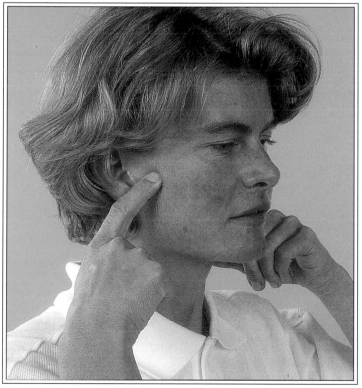

2 Squeeze your ear lobes and then, with the palms of your hands, vigorously rub the whole of both ears, up and down, until they become warm.

3 If you have a ringing in the ears, apply gentle pressure to the point in front of the middle of the ear.

SHOULDERS AND ARMS

1 Using your left hand to support the right elbow, with a loose fist tap across the top of your left shoulder with your right hand and, as far as you can, reach over your shoulder-blade.

2 Release the elbow, straighten your left arm in front of you, open up your palm and tap down the inside of your arm from the shoulder to the open hand. This will stimulate the energy flow of the lung, heart governor and heart meridians.

3 Turn your arm over and tap up the back of your arm, from the hand back to the shoulder again. This will stimulate the meridians on the back of your arm, namely the large intestine, triple burner and small intestine. Repeat three times.

HANDS

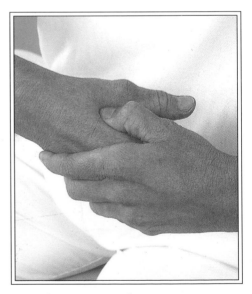

1 Use your right hand to work your left, massaging the centre of your palm gently with your right thumb. The point here is called "palace of anxiety", heart governor 8, and is good for relieving general tension.

2 Rotate and massage the joints of each finger using your right index finger and thumb. This is a great way to release any tension in your hands and helps to prevent arthritis as well as improving flexibility in the joints.

3 Apply pressure in between your thumb and finger. This point will help to relieve headaches, constipation or diarrhoea. It is a point sometimes used to expedite labour; therefore it should not be stimulated during pregnancy.

CHEST AND ABDOMEN

1 Open up your chest by tapping across it with loose fists, above and around your breasts and across the ribs. This will stimulate your lungs and enhance and strengthen your respiratory system.

2 Take a deep breath in as you throw your arms up over your head. Repeat the tapping. This is good for releasing tension in your chest and supporting you in expressing your thoughts and feelings.

3 Proceed down towards your abdomen and with open hands tap around your abdomen gently in a clockwise direction, going down on the left and up on the right side. This follows the flow of circulation and digestion.

4 Place one hand on top of the other and make the same circular motion around your abdomen for a minute.

BACK

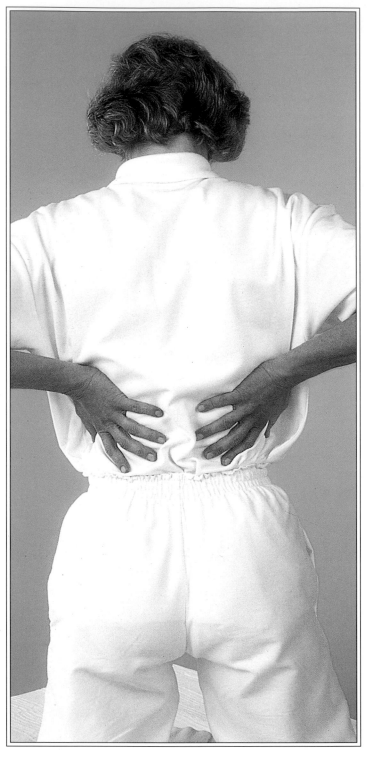

1 Place your hands on your back, just below the rib cage. This is the area of your kidneys. Start to rub the area slowly until you feel some warmth building up under your hands. This stimulates your kidney energy responsible for your vitality and also for warming your body.

2 Stand up with your feet shoulder-width apart. Bend forward slightly and tap your lower back gently using your loose fists. Reach up as far as possible and move down to the lower part of your spine, your hips and the muscles of your buttocks. Releasing tension in this area will stimulate your digestive and elimination organs.

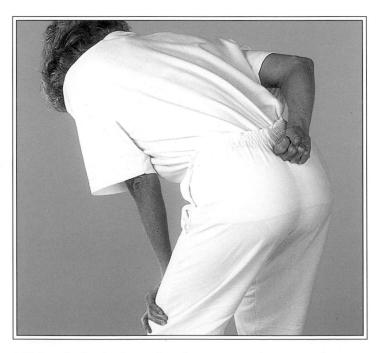

3 Using the back of your hand, tap across the sacrum bone at the base of your spine. This activates your nervous system and sends energy vibrations up the spine to your brain. Tapping the coccyx also decongests the sinuses, so breathe deeply through the nose when practising this exercise.

LEGS AND FEET

1 Stand with your feet wider apart. Keeping your knees slightly bent, start tapping with your fists down the outside of your legs from the hips to your ankles. This is where your gall-bladder meridian is located.

2 Now tap up the inside of your legs from the ankle to the groin area, stimulating your liver and spleen meridians. Use the palms of your hand rather than a fist if you prefer.

3 Then tap down the back of your legs following the flow of energy in your bladder meridian, from your buttocks to your heels. Come up the inside of your legs again.

4 Tap down the front of your legs, slightly outside the big quadriceps muscle. Tap all the way down to the front of your ankles and then come up the inside of your legs. Repeat this whole sequence three times.

5 Along the stomach meridian there is a good point for general well-being, on the outside of your leg, below your knee. Apply gentle pressure for a few seconds.

6 Remain seated on the floor, hold your foot and make a circular movement at the ankle to free up joint mobility.

▶

7 Tap the sole of the foot, with a loose fist, then massage the whole foot with both hands.

8 Hold your hands under the bottom of your foot and use your thumbs to rub downward along the top of your foot, in between each metatarsal bone to your toes.

9 Massage the web between each toe and then massage the toe joints gently. The point between the big toe and the second toe is good for abdominal cramps: do not use during pregnancy.

10 Come to the sole of your foot and apply pressure to this point with your thumb. This will have a revitalizing effect upon your body and stimulate energy flow.

11 Use your thumbs to massage the area under the ankle bone. This area, spleen 6, located four fingers' width up from the inside ankle bone, is a great point to use for any menstrual disorders.

12 Give the whole foot a good rub. Then grab hold of your ankle with both hands and shake out your foot. Now repeat this whole sequence with your other foot.

COMPLETION

1 After having worked your body, stroke your meridians gently. First stand up with your feet apart. Take a deep breath in and lift your arms up.

2 As you breathe out, bend your arms and place your hands on your head. Stroke down the back of your head to your neck.

3 Bring your hands as high up as possible underneath the shoulder-blades and stroke down the whole of your back, buttocks and legs.

4 Open your legs and come up the inside of your legs to the groin area. Proceed up the front over your abdomen and up to your chest.

5 Stroke out to the sides and open up your chest. Open your arms to the sides and then repeat the whole completion sequence again, three to five times.

MAKKO HO

The makko ho exercises originated in Japan and were developed to improve the flow of energy or *qi* in our bodies. They are widely used in the shiatsu world as a self-healing technique for practitioners and clients alike. Each exercise works on a specific pair of meridians, enhancing their function, and the full sequence of six exercises covers the whole body and its organs.

In makko ho you will find references in the text to the five Chinese elements of earth, fire, water, wood and metal. These elements are used in Oriental medicine for diagnosis, and even in the West we use expressions such as "he's all fired-up", or "she's very wooden" (meaning very stiff).

Where you find an element mentioned, try to think of its quality – the warmth and vitality of fire, the clear purifying aspect of free-flowing water, the strength and flexibility of wood, the firmness of the earth, the fine quality of air at the top of a mountain. The qualities of air are included in the metal element. Use your imagination and you will discover the elemental qualities in yourself.

When carried out regularly and with correct attention, the exercises serve as an excellent self-diagnostic tool and also enable people to improve not only the function of their organs but also their emotional and psychological states, which relate to and are governed by their meridians.

ABOVE: When practising makko ho exercises, focus your attention on your breathing and on the way it changes.

ATTITUDE AND BREATHING

While carrying out the makko ho exercises it is important to note that they will be less effective if their form is merely copied – even though the body will be well stretched. The true benefits of these exercises will be properly discovered by exploring them with the right level of attention.

The whole point of the makko ho exercises is to really feel into them and to use your breath to bring an awareness to the changing sensations in your body as you move through them.

Breathing is the vital focus which enables you to work with your body's limitations and to encourage change in its habitual functioning. Throughout the exercises be aware of the qualities of each breath that you take.

As you breathe in, the body fills up with air and expands and there is a natural increased tension as everything stretches. You can then observe how your body responds to this increased tension. Do you feel that there is any kind of irritation or resistance in your body tissues, or do you feel that they are enjoying the extra stretch – delighting in it, feeling alive and vibrant?

Observe how your mind or emotions respond to the tension. Are you happy and feeling good, or are you feeling angry or sorry for yourself? Note these and any other responses but try not to get trapped in them. Remember to be aware that the exercises and the breathing are enabling you to become more deeply in touch with yourself.

As you breathe out, the body is letting go of air and some waste products, with a physical relaxation in the body tissues. Observe how this affects you. Is there a feeling of relief in your body? How do you feel? Do you feel calmer and more at peace, or sad and experiencing some difficulty in surrendering to the exhaled breath?

At first, when you do the exercises you may find it difficult to think this way, but when you focus your attention on your breathing, you can really begin to discover something about yourself, your body and your reactions to the ever-changing qualities of the inhaled and exhaled breath.

THE PRACTICE OF MAKKO HO EXERCISES

Ideally the makko ho exercises should be practised at least once every day. It is beneficial to practise them on waking in the morning, to ease out the stiffness of sleep gently and to prepare for the day. They may also be done in the evening to refresh oneself after work, or before going to bed to enhance sleep.

It is important to carry out the exercises in the order they are given because this follows the natural flow of energy through the body and its organs. When the *qi*, or life force, is not flowing properly through the body, it becomes stuck or stagnant somewhere and this might lead to disease and illness in time. These exercises will act on the body to disperse the blockages and help the energy to flow unimpeded where it needs to go – nurturing the areas that are depleted

BELOW: It is important in makko ho to ease to your own personal limit gently, without forcing anything. Be kind to yourself.

and undernourished and rebalancing your body as a whole.

In order to enhance your body's healing potential through the makko ho exercises and to deepen your understanding of yourself, you should carry out the whole sequence of exercises three times, together with a specific, self-healing phase where you work on two exercises of your own choice.

The optimum practice of the makko ho exercises used here is as follows:

1 Follow the exact sequence of the six exercises as described in detail below. Take your time using your breath and focused attention and do each exercise three times before moving on to the next one. This first series helps to stretch the physical body and disperse tension.

2 Repeat the whole sequence and this time bring more awareness to how you feel in your mind and body as you breathe through the exercises. Note which exercise you feel really comfortable with and would like to stay in for a long time; and which you strongly dislike or have most resistance to.

3 Self-healing phase:

(i) Choose the exercise that you liked best and do it once slowly and stay in the position, breathing and relaxing into it and feeling nurtured by it. By focusing in this way you help to draw energy gently to where it is needed and this will affect your mind and emotions as well as your body. When you feel ready, come slowly out of the position and pause.

(ii) The second choice you now make helps to balance your overall energy pattern. Choose the exercise you least liked, the one in which you felt very tense or irritable. Work more quickly with this one, without straining, and repeat it again and again using the exhaled breath to help you release tension, until you begin to feel tired or easier with the exercise. This method will help to disperse excess energy where it was blocked or sticking, thus allowing a freer flow again.

4 Repeat the whole sequence of exercises once more and note any changes in yourself, in your sensations or attitude as you move through them.

5 Rest on the floor for a few minutes to allow your body to assimilate and settle after the exercises. Breathe gently and deeply without straining and relax.

LUNGS AND LARGE INTESTINE

The lung and large intestine meridians are concerned with exchange of air and elimination of waste products. They represent the metal element which is connected with the air, breathing, boundaries and the emotion of grief. Be especially aware of the breath and the qualities of taking in and letting go in this exercise. Remember to keep observing your sensations and feelings. This exercise will help with breathing problems and regulate elimination.

1 Stand with feet shoulder-width apart, toes turned slightly inwards, and feel your connection to the earth. Link your thumbs behind your back and check that your jaw is relaxed.

2 Breathe in, feeling the breath fill your body and lungs. Breathe out, straightening your arms, open the chest and lean slightly backwards.

3 Breathe out, bending forward with your back, arms and legs straight. Keep this position for three breaths. On the third exhaled breath, return to your original position. Repeat twice more.

SPLEEN AND STOMACH

The spleen and stomach meridians represent the earth element which is concerned with digestion and nourishment. Be aware of your connection to the earth and the support it gives your body in this exercise.

1 Kneel between your feet with your buttocks resting on the floor and your knees close together. If this is not possible, sit on a small cushion. On an exhaled breath gradually lean backwards, easing your body down by supporting yourself with your arms, and then elbows. Do **not** strain your knees or back, if you experience discomfort do not push. Use your breath to relax.

2 Ease down to the floor, without straining, keeping your knees close together on the floor. Stretch both arms over your head, interlock your fingers and stretch. Breathe deeply three times in this position, be aware of the movement of the belly as you breathe, your connection to the earth and the nourishment received through the breath.

3 On the third exhaled breath ease out of the position and bend forward to ease out the lower back. Repeat twice more.

ALTERNATIVE SPLEEN/STOMACH EXERCISE

If you are unable to kneel you may try this alternative sequence. Stand with your feet together and feel your connection to the earth. Lift your left foot and clasp it behind you. Breathe out and draw the leg upwards behind you, keeping the knee close to the other leg. Hold and feel the stretch. On the third exhaled breath release the stretch and place your foot on the ground.

Repeat twice more, then carry out the sequence with the other leg.

HEART AND SMALL INTESTINE

The heart and small intestine meridians represent the qualities of assimilation of food and integration of external stimuli and emotions in the body. Representing the fire element, they promote warm-heartedness and joy in our lives. Be aware of an alive warmth and increased circulation in this exercise.

1 Sit on the floor, place the soles of your feet together, hold them and draw them close to your body. Breathe in, feeling a warm expansion in your body.

2 On the exhaled breath, draw your body down, bending your elbows and easing your knees towards the floor. Do not strain your hips. Keep your back straight. Breathe fully three times in position, feeling expansion in your back and observe how you feel. On the third exhaled breath, return to the original position. Repeat twice more.

BLADDER AND KIDNEYS

The bladder and kidney meridians relate the water element and qualities of fluidity and easy flow in our lives. Connected to the nervous system, they may become stressed, leading to a fearful state of mind and rigidity in the body.

During this exercise concentrate on welcoming the qualities of easy-flowing, purifying water. Imagine it is gently washing over you like a wave, cleansing you and easing away any fears, tension and distress.

1 Sit upright with your feet parallel, hip-width apart, pointing upwards at a 90° angle to the floor, or towards your head. This will keep your knees straight.

2 On the inhaled breath, draw your arms up above your head, palms facing each other. Keep your back straight.

3 Breathe out and ease forward, bending from the hips, arms forward, parallel to the legs. Look ahead. Ease farther forward on another breath. On the third breath, release the position.

TRIPLE HEATER AND HEART PROTECTOR

The triple heater and heart protector meridians relate to the fire element in its quieter aspect, like a gentle candle flame. They have a protective function in the body on the physical

level of immunity and temperature control, and also emotionally – helping us to cope with the knocks and crises in life, especially with regard to relationships.

1 Sit, cross-legged, with one or both feet on your thighs. Cross your arms and rest your hands on your thighs, palms facing upwards, fingers together. Do not strain your knees, if you are not comfortable simply cross your legs.

2 Breathe in feeling a warm expansion. On the exhaled breath slide your hands out sideways from the body, keeping your palms flat and horizontal. Bring your body forward, without collapsing.

3 As you breathe three times, feel a warm protection within you. On the third exhaled breath return to the original position. Repeat twice, then cross your legs and arms over the other way and continue three more times.

LIVER AND GALL-BLADDER

The liver and gall-bladder meridians relate to the wood element and the tree's qualities of strength and flexibility when it is healthy. Try to feel these qualities in yourself, if your body feels stiff, you may be frustrated or angry.

1 Sit upright with your right leg outstretched and flat on the floor; the foot is vertical to keep the knee straight. Tuck your left foot into the body. Breathe in, feeling an alive quality.

2 On the exhaled breath lean sideways over your right leg grasping your big toe if possible, keeping your leg straight, and easing your body downwards. Do not strain. Keep your chest open and your left arm close to your ear. Feel a strong stretch to the side of your body. Look upwards. Do not collapse your chest or bring your raised arm in front of your face. Breathe three times. Release on the third exhaled breath. Repeat three times.

3 Return to the upright position and then change sides with your left leg stretched out and your right foot in. Breathe in. On the exhaled breath lean sideways as before, this time to the left. Breathe three times. Repeat three times.

FINISHING EXERCISE

1 After you have completed the whole sequence (ideally three times plus the specific self-healing phase), lie flat on the floor with your eyes closed and just breathe gently for a few minutes, allowing everything to settle in your body.

2 You may be aware of tingling sensations as your inner energy responds to your makko ho exercise session. Another finishing position is lying flat on the floor with your knees up. Breathe into your stomach and relax.

FURTHER PRACTICE

Human nature being what it is, it is inevitable that resistances to doing these exercises will occur at some stage. You are encouraged to note your resistances and continue the exercises anyway and not to give up in the first week, before you really begin to feel the benefits of the makko ho exercises. While acknowledging the hectic pace of our lives, it can always be possible to carry out at least one sequence of exercises per day. Obviously the more time and energy you give to yourself, the greater the benefits will be. Enjoy your exploration and be well.

YOGA

The word yoga is by now well known outside India. In fact, over the last four decades it has quietly and steadily taken root in Western culture and language. Yet if you ask a number of people what yoga is, you are likely to get many different responses. These responses are sometimes contradictory. However, yoga can be summarized into the following three possibilities or approaches.

1 YOGA AS POWER

First, yoga can be explained as a means to attain a degree of power or control over the body and mind. Yoga links the body and the mind through intense physical and mental effort. For instance, through rigorous physical practices a state of concentration is developed and maintained which is used to hold power over the body and the breath. Within this approach, such control is often seen as a prerequisite to the body and mind becoming free of disturbances and distractions. This power arises out of three areas of personal development:

i) Mastery of the body through physical postures;

ii) Control of the breath through breathing techniques;

iii) The ability to concentrate through mental techniques.

This intense effort produces energy and control that is available for whatever purpose suits one's direction in life. Many people could usefully enjoy more power over certain areas of their lives. The question is whether they are prepared to put in some effort to reach this point.

In the words of a yoga teacher from long ago: "Yoga is the means by which that which was not attained

RIGHT: Yoga is a process by which you grow in self-understanding.

earlier is now attained." This approach is known as the yoga of energy and will. As such, this aspect of yoga is an art and offers a fascinating field to explore. It appeals to many people searching for power in and over their lives. However, this approach is only a means towards a more important goal.

2 YOGA AS MEDITATION

Here the concern is more with the mystery of life rather than the mastery of life and yoga is a means for meditation with self-inquiry as the primary focus. "Who am I?" is the question that acts as a map for an inner journey into your mind. It is a quest to touch and be touched by the "soulful" quality of being that resides within a person. In this approach, yoga is a tool for a movement towards a deeper relationship with your sense of soul, by searching both into and beyond what you experience as the everyday self. It is a journey of discovery, exploring and ultimately going beyond attitudes that, for better or for worse, have shaped your life, work and relationships.

Yoga is a skill by which you seek to sustain awareness and clarity in spite of the vagaries of everyday life. The quality of this awareness engenders a freshness within which actions are less affected by the usual attitudes and habits. In other words, there is more choice over how you respond or react. In those situations where your reaction would have been automatic, there are now different possibilities.

Yoga is a process by which you grow in your understanding of yourself. From this you come to realize that you can change those aspects of yourself that are unhelpful on your journey through life. This means first recognizing the qualities that hinder your personal growth – an important, if not always comfortable, stage in the journey. Second, having reflected on how you are rather than who you are, you go on to discover that there exists within you a resource with the potential to transform these undesirable aspects. From this you can take steps towards living more creatively. Here again a teacher is important as a guide for advice and suggestions on practices to support the process of growth into an understanding of how you are and ultimately who you are. To quote another saying from the teachings on meditation: "Before I can be nobody, I must first be somebody." This approach is known as the yoga of reflection and discovery.

3 YOGA AS THERAPY

Here, yoga, as both a restorative and preventive, is applied as a therapy to help people with emotional problems or poor health. Here the approach needs to be very different for each person. One person's potential to change his or her situation will be affected by his or her problem, while another person's problem will be affected by his or her potential to change his or her situation.

According to traditional Indian medicine, becoming known in the West as Ayurveda, those diseases that are chronic and cannot be resolved by medicine alone can be helped by using yoga practices. Old yoga texts also talk about the benefits of certain postures and breathing techniques in the treatment of disease.

Using these ideas, it is possible, primarily within a one-to-one relationship, to introduce personalized yoga practices. These practices can both respect the problems or disease in the individual and support his or her intention to influence the way he or she is affected in similar situations in the future.

However, most people experience the dominance of their old ways when confronted with familiar situations. They would like to change but the old patterns are powerful and resist alternatives. It even seems that sometimes what they would really like to do is to carry on exactly as before but without the troublesome symptoms which accompany their lifestyle. To ignore or block these symptoms through

continual suppression will ultimately prove a futile path.

The process of one's inner intelligence is such that it will let one know what needs looking at with increasingly strident messages. This means that the steps to ignore these messages must also intensify. Better to co-operate with yourself before you are forced to by a more serious consequence.

In this respect, yoga as a therapy also presumes that you are willing to accept some responsibility within your situation. Here, with the support of a teacher, you can introduce and work towards sustaining creative changes in your lifestyle. This may also include, as well as specific practices, a review of those relationships which exacerbate your problems. This approach is known as the yoga of rejuvenation and prevention.

YOGA PRACTICES IN THERAPY

The above three aspects of yoga – therapy, power and meditation – are mutually supportive in helping to maintain physical health, psychological vitality and spiritual purpose within the commitments of daily life, work and relationships. The guiding principle is to see the person rather than the problem or disease and to accept that more than a pre-ordained technique is involved. Because of his or her lifestyle, a person may be experiencing certain problems or illnesses. It is also presumed that the situation has become such that the person is willing to explore alternatives to develop a more harmonious relationship between his or her inner nature and outer lifestyle.

Above: At the end of a yoga session you will feel warm, relaxed and alert. Take time to feel these benefits, and to collect your thoughts before you get up.

CHOOSING APPROPRIATE ASANA OR POSTURES

A good starting-point from which to explore yoga is the physical body and the practice of postures which will generate an improvement in the overall function of the system rather than just the form of the body. In yoga these body postures are called "asana" and although many different positions are possible, only a few are required in the area of therapy. Here are six different positions which are not too far from those used in everyday life.

1 A simple starting posture, especially useful if tired. On an inhale, raise your arms, keeping your shoulders relaxed. On the exhale, lower the hands on to the thighs.

2 A similar movement but taken from a standing position. Keep your elbows relaxed, concentrate on allowing the neck to stay tension-free.

3 Another standing posture, this time a more challenging position to stimulate and invigorate. The posture's focus is in the chest and upper back.

4 A typical kneeling posture, adaptable as either a preparatory movement for other more demanding postures, or a posture for beginners.

5 A kneeling-forward bend is valuable where the back and legs are stiff and as a counterposture to more demanding postures. A good pose for beginners.

6 A lying posture is helpful for rest and relaxation as well as recovery between more demanding postures. A useful pose for all situations and all levels of experience.

MOVEMENT IN ASANA PRECEDES STAYING

The first requirement when using yoga to work with the body within a therapeutic situation is to encourage a creative flow of energy throughout the system. For this, the notion of repeatedly moving into and out of a posture is emphasized rather than holding a posture for a certain amount of time. Here are two sets of repeated movements to try out. When you have developed an ease of practice, the concept of staying and focusing on a particular area can then be considered.

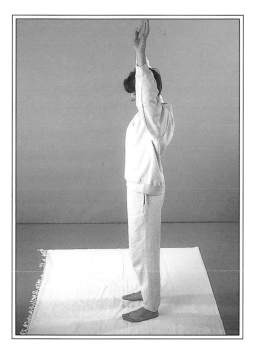

1 Stand with your feet slightly apart and your arms above your head.

1 Lie on your back with your knees bent and your feet flat on the floor. Keep your arms by your sides with the palms facing to the floor. Keep your breathing steady.

2 Using a slow, unhurried movement, bend at the waist and touch the floor either side of your feet. Bend your legs if you need to. Return to the standing position and repeat.

2 Move your arms so that they are above your head but still resting on the ground, palms facing upwards. Slowly lift your body, with the weight on your feet and shoulders, so that your pelvis is off the ground. Hold for a few seconds, then slowly return to the first position. Repeat.

BREATHING AS AN INTEGRAL PART OF MOVEMENT

To assist in creating a smooth, flowing movement, conscious breathing is added to the movement. This assists a sense of involvement, acts as a measure for anticipating stress and offers a sense of harmony in linking breath, body and mind. Within postures, except when resting, always breathe through the nostrils rather than the mouth. Beginners may find it takes practice to develop correct breathing. Co-ordinate the speed of the movement with the length of your breath. Forward bending or closing movements are generally done with an exhalation, backward bending or opening movements generally with an inhalation.

A ROLE FOR THE MIND IN PRACTICE
These yoga practices need a certain quality of mental concentration, to help steady the body and focus the mind. To help in linking your faculties, you have the rhythm of the movement plus the harmony of the breath to engage your mind. There are also other techniques, such as working with the eyes closed, or counting the length of the breath. As you become more proficient, try these techniques to increase the benefit of the exercises.

1 Lie on your stomach, face down, with your legs relaxed and slightly apart. Breathe in and allow your chest to lift, keeping your shoulders relaxed.

2 Come up as far as you can without straining. Breathe in, wait for a second, and then allow the exhale to bring you slowly back to the starting position. Repeat four to six times.

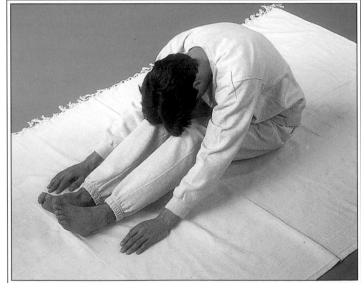

1 Now change your position and sit with your legs extended out in front of you and your knees slightly bent. Breathe in as you lift your arms above your head, keeping the shoulders relaxed. As you breathe out, bend forwards over your knees.

2 As you reach the limit of the exhale, allow your head and shoulders to relax with your hands resting on the ground. Begin to breathe in again, lifting the arms off the ground and sitting up until you have reached the starting position. Start the next exhale and repeat the movement.

ADAPTING THE POSTURE TO THE PERSON

It is also important that the posture is adapted to the person and not the person to the posture. If necessary, the basic posture should be modified to allow access to the form. The bodies of many students, especially in a therapy situation, are limited by age, weight or stiffness.

In yoga terms, the spine is the mainstay of your being at many levels. Therefore anything you do with posture needs to influence your spine, and any adaptations of the postures need to be applied with this in mind. Here are two more postures with alternative adaptations.

▲ 1 In its traditional form this posture involves feet being together and the inner arms pressed against the ears. An extreme form for the young or very fit.

2 An adaptation offering a more appropriate form for beginners: keep your shoulders relaxed and your chest open to allow free breathing.

◄ 1 A strong, standing position known as the "warrior" demands flexibility and strength to maintain. Position your legs in a wide stride with your arms stretched to the limit.

▶ 2 In a modified position the stress on the legs is reduced: your shoulders should be relaxed allowing for easy breathing.

PUTTING THESE PRINCIPLES TOGETHER

These principles introduce the basic guidelines that accompany your first steps into practice. Perhaps it would be helpful at this point to try an experiment aimed at pulling together these different ideas into a personal experience.

Sit comfortably on a chair with your spine erect and unsupported and your hands resting palms down on your thighs. Now go through the following exercises, repeating each set four times only. The actual exercises simply involve raising and lowering the arms. Each set of movements will, however, add a further level of engagement with the intention of deepening your involvement. Here you are inviting an experience of the way that you need to work if yoga is to be effective as a therapy. Focus on the smoothness and length of the breath and the flow of the movements.

2 Raise and lower your arms in a forward direction. Repeat this movement four times. Then rest in the first position. Repeat the exercise but this time lower your arms as you breathe out through the nostrils, raising your arms to any breathing pattern you wish. Do this four times.

3 Repeat the exercise. This time raise your arms on the inhalation and lower your arms on the exhalation. Again, breathe through the nostrils rather than the mouth. Now raise and lower your arms as before but consciously lengthen the exhalation while keeping it smooth as you lower your arms.

1 Sit on a chair with your spine erect and unsupported and your feet flat on the floor in line with your knees and slightly apart. Rest your hands on your knees with your palms facing downwards.

4 Repeat the process but this time work with your eyes closed. Remember to keep your attention focused on the smoothness and length of the breath as well as the flow of the movements.

YOGA IS A RELATIONSHIP

The above principles link together to offer possibilities that enhance your relationship with yourself through your practice. This opens the possibility that a deepening of your practice comes not from adding more difficult postures but from refining your relationship with what you already have. Life is already full of pressures to go for the newest model, to bring more in from the outside rather than concentrating on bringing more out from the inside. So you need to take care that you do not become an avid consumer of a new posture or new technique purely for the sake of it.

Yoga is a relationship within which you commit yourself to depth of involvement rather than breadth of involvement. In that sense, yoga is no different from how any relationship with someone or something you care for and wish to spend time with should be. From this relationship you can eventually start to experience the fruits that arise from the time, care, work and attention. Keep the following words of a teacher from long ago in your mind as you adapt yoga to suit your particular needs:

"Yoga is known through practice.
Practice itself leads to Yoga. One who cares for their practice for a long time tastes the fruits."

PRACTICE 1

A simple practice sequence follows which aims at reducing stress generally, and in particular tension headaches which often accompany it. The practice uses postures with breathing techniques and a simple visualization and is helpful where the emphasis is on generally relaxing and lessening accumulated stress.

1 Standing with your feet slightly apart, allow your body to settle. Focus on deepening your breathing. When it is full and steady, raise your arms as you breathe in.

2 The speed of this movement is decided by your breath. Finish the inhale with your arms above your head, shoulders relaxed. Bring your arms down as you breathe out. Repeat eight times.

1 Stand with your feet about 60–90cm (2–3ft) apart with the back foot at an angle and the leg straight. As you breathe in, raise your arms while pushing the front knee forwards with the back leg braced.

2 Complete the inhale with your arms raised and your chest open. Wait a few seconds, then start to breathe out, lowering the arms and straightening the front leg. Repeat this sequence eight times.

1 Kneel up with your legs slightly apart and your feet relaxed. As you breathe in, raise your arms, keeping the shoulders loose and your chest open. As you breathe out, bend forward, keeping your back rounded.

2 Continue to breathe out until your hands are on the ground and your shoulders relaxed. Wait a few seconds then breathe in while lifting your arms and then your back. Repeat eight times.

3 To finish, lie on your back with your feet apart and your arms slightly away from your sides. Allow your breathing to settle and then slow it down while softening your body, as if you were melting into the floor. Relax in this position for about two to three minutes.

PRACTICE 2

The second practice sequence concentrates on alleviating the symptoms of accumulative stress which might occur after many hours working at a keyboard or computer screen. This practice serves both as a curative of aches and pains, and as a preventive to help in minimizing any build-up of tension in the head, neck and shoulder areas.

1 Sit on a chair with your feet apart and your spine erect. Rest your hands on your thighs. Keeping your eyes closed, imagine that you are focusing on a point on the floor in front of you. Maintain this internal focus for a few minutes, breathing gently, before relaxing.

2 As you slowly breathe in, gently and slowly raise your head while keeping your shoulders relaxed. As you breathe out, again gently and slowly, lower your head without allowing your back to slump. Repeat this movement eight times.

3 From the same sitting position, slowly breathe in and raise one hand to touch your forehead, while at the same time raising your head. As you breathe out, lower your hand and head. Repeat eight times, alternating hands.

4 This time, raise both hands at the same time as you breathe in and lower both as you breathe out. Repeat this sequence eight times.

5 Now rest your hands on your thighs while you turn your head from side to side with each breath. As you breathe out, slowly turn your head to the left; as you breathe in, bring your head back to the centre, repeat to the right. Repeat this sequence eight times.

6 Still with your hands on your thighs, take a breath. As you breathe out, raise your hands, bringing your palms over your eyes. Breathe once, then as you breathe in again return your hands to your thighs. Repeat four times.

7 Lie on the floor, let your breathing settle and your body soften. Focus your attention on any tightness in your body and use your exhale to release it. After two minutes, rest for a minute or so.

FINAL THOUGHTS

Some of the possibilities that underpin yoga through practice have been introduced above. The practice of yoga as power, meditation and therapy has been considered. Each aspect, although having its own approach and focus, complements and offers the practitioner a holistic model for the development of body, mind and well-being.

In the West today therapy is the starting point that most often brings people to yoga. The use of yoga as therapy has been approached from the viewpoint of the person rather than the problem. It is not appropriate in considering yoga practice to "lump" people together as back-pain sufferers or migraine sufferers. It is true to say there are some common characteristics within various problems, but then so there are in all areas of people's lives. People live together in groups determined by commonalities and yet each person is unique. This is what needs to be considered when proposing practices for individuals: "Teach what is inside you, not as it applies to you yourself but as it applies to the other."

With this as a priority, some basic principles common for anybody wishing to practice yoga were considered. Such concepts offer an intelligent means to enter into the spirit of the practice with the least disturbance to what is, in the field of therapy, already an unhealthy body and mind. These principles are also offered as a way to deepen your relationship with yoga. Through that link you will discover something new about yourselves. From the view of yoga, this means that the way things affect you can change and you can influence the process of change and its consequences. From here, two different practices, designed to support two students who, confronted with the same problem, turned out to have very different needs, were proposed.

RIGHT. Practise a little yoga every day for the best benefits.

FURTHER PRACTICE

If you wish to take your interest in yoga further, take lessons with a qualified yoga teacher, choosing one who concentrates on your particular interest. You should do a little each day rather than practise irregularly. Wear loose or stretchy clothing when practising and use a mat or folded blanket on the floor. Don't practise yoga with a full bladder or bowels, and wait at least three hours after a heavy meal. Take a shower after a practice session to complete the relaxation and refreshment.

Yoga is a journey to be experienced. However, that journey not only requires patience and perseverance, but also enthusiasm and confidence. In this respect, as in any relationship between people, it is necessary to consider priorities. To students interested in undertaking a home practice, two suggestions are offered.

First, think of yoga as a new book. Before you try to fit this book into what is probably an overcrowded bookshelf, take a decision to remove an existing book to make room for the new one. Do not, however, try to remove a large book and make unrealistic adjustments in the space on your shelf. Instead, take out a slim volume and this way, create realistic space without yoga becoming another pressure.

This leads on to the second suggestion. Life is often divided into agendas, two of which are headed "chore" and "reward". Try to keep some room on the latter list for your practice in the same way that you would greet an old friend. Take time in their company and return to your everyday life rejuvenated and better able to embrace your surroundings.

MOXIBUSTION

The practice of acupuncture has become quite wide-spread in the West, and indeed throughout the world in the past 25 years or so. Most people are aware that it is an ancient Chinese system of healing that involves the use of fine needles inserted into the body at specific points to achieve a particular therapeutic effect. Acupuncture has a long lineage; indeed, many of the principles of diagnosis and treatment were laid down in the *Huangdi Neijing* (or *Yellow Emperor's Canon of Medicine*) – the earliest Chinese medical text extant, dating from 500–300 BC. The origins of acupuncture probably go back much further.

Acupuncture's underlying principle is that of vital force (or *qi*) animating mind and body. For various complex reasons the flow and distribution of *qi* can become unbalanced or out of harmony, and the aim of acupuncture is to determine the pattern and underlying causes of this disharmony and rectify it by needling particular points on the body.

Less well-known than acupuncture is moxibustion, an integral part of Chinese medicine and most commonly practised in conjunction with acupuncture. In moxibustion, a small quantity of the moxa herb (or mugwort – *Artemisia vulgaris*) is burned on the end of an acupuncture needle (while the needle is in position) or in the form of a small stick or cone placed directly on the skin (usually being removed

BELOW: Acupuncture needles, moxibustion sticks and the moxa herb are all used in the practice of moxibustion.

RIGHT: The meridian lines used in both acupuncture and moxibustion.

before the skin is burned). Moxa can be used in its own right or to augment the effect of the needles; its use is indicated where the body's energies need warming or tonifying, or to help move stagnation of the *qi*.

The use of needles for self-treatment is clearly inappropriate but the use of moxa in the form of the moxa stick can be very effective in the area of health promotion and maintenance. In particular, it is useful for its general tonic effect, especially for the middle-aged or elderly. Its application can be wonderfully soothing and relaxing for mind and body, and this alone is of great benefit to health in general. **There are, however, some contraindications for the use of moxa:**

- During pregnancy.
- With people with hypertension (high blood pressure).
- On any rashes, especially if the skin is broken.
- During acute illness in general but in particular if this involves feeling heat or fullness anywhere in the body, a raised temperature or any inflammation.
- In cases where the inhalation of smoke is an irritant (the moxa stick gives off herbal-smelling smoke).
- On any sensitive part of the body such as the face.

A few people may not enjoy sessions involving the use of moxa or respond well afterwards. There may be a number of reasons for this: for example, their energy may already be "over-heated". As a general rule, it is best not to use moxa again if any symptoms seem worse after its use.

HOW TO USE THE MOXA STICK

For mild moxibustion the moxa stick provides the most convenient means for self-application. About an inch or so of the stick will be used in any one session.

The stick is best lit from a candle; this takes about half a minute and it is helpful to blow on the lighted end occasionally to improve combustion. It is also quite useful to remove about 2.5 cm (1 in) of the outer layer of paper (but *not* the inner layer), since this helps the stick to burn more evenly. During a session, the ash will occasionally have to be tapped off into an ashtray. While burning, the stick imparts rather a strong-smelling herbal smoke, which is quite pleasant, but some ventilation is recommended.

After a session, it is essential to ensure that the stick is properly extinguished. It is rarely sufficient merely to "stub" the lighted end out – it tends to start burning again. The best way is to cut off the lighted end with a sharp knife, then dampen the end, being careful, of course, not to get water on to the unburned section of the stick, which should then be stored in a dry place for further use.

APPLICATION OF THE MOXA STICK

The application of moxa should be a very relaxing and pleasurable experience; you should stop if it does not feel so. The sensation of warmth emanating from the stick on to the skin should not be so great as to be uncomfortable. The distance that the stick is held from the skin will vary from person to person and from point to point. About 2.5cm (1in) from the skin is a rough average. As the stick is held near the skin, the sensation of warmth will gradually increase; the stick is pulled away before the sensation of heat becomes uncomfortable and after a few seconds the stick can be brought nearer the skin again. This "dabbing" action backwards and forwards with the stick is repeated a number of times, until the skin feels hot and slightly pink and the sensation of warmth feels as if it has penetrated the body. Another easier and perhaps more relaxing method of using the stick is to find a distance from the skin that allows the sensation of warmth to build up to a comfortable level that can be maintained for a period of time without having to "dab" the stick.

There is no fixed rule as to how long to spend using the moxa stick during a session. The session should last as long as it takes to allow the selected point or points to become quite warm, and the skin slightly pink with the feeling that the heat has penetrated. On average, this might be about a minute or two for each point, but sometimes longer. If all the points mentioned in the step sequence were used together, the session should take about 10–20 minutes. It is very important not to overheat a point as there is a very slight chance this might lead to the skin blistering after the session. This will not happen if the application is gentle.

The number of sessions or their frequency can also vary. It is recommended, however, that the sessions should not be more than twice weekly, with breaks of one or two weeks every month or so. There is no advantage in using moxa over an indefinite period and it is desirable to have regular breaks. Provided the sessions feel pleasant, relaxing and beneficial, many of the points mentioned here can be regularly warmed with moxa for a limited period. Be aware of the contraindications, however.

How to use the Moxa Stick

1 Light the moxa stick with a candle, holding the tip in the flame until it is smoking steadily. Blow on the lighted end to encourage combustion.

2 When you have finished the session, cut off the lighted end of the moxa stick with a sharp knife on to a board. Make sure it is completely cooled before you store it.

SOME RECOMMENDED POINTS

Some points which are suitable for you to practise at home are illustrated here. Remember to take care not to hold sticks for more than a minute or two at a time over each point. Keep asking your partner if they are comfortable: they should feel a pleasant warmth and no more. Before you apply the stick, draw small circles on the correct points of the body with a pen to ensure that you will focus it on the right spot.

1 Stomach 36 (*zusanli* – "leg three miles"). You will find this point just underneath the knee.

2 Large Intestine 10 (*shousanli* – "arm three miles"). This point is located just above the elbow joint.

3 Directing Vessel Points: REN 4, the first of three points located on the stomach, just below the ribs.

4 REN 6, the second stomach point is found just below the navel.

5 REN 8 is found halfway between the navel and the pubic bone.

6 Using the moxa stick on areas of the body is one of the most effective uses for mild moxibustion. It is appropriate for areas which feel chronically cold, weak, stiff or achy, including joints. It is not generally recommended in cases of acute pain. To apply, simply hold the moxa stick above a general area of the body – for example the lower back – for a few seconds for a general feeling of warmth and well-being.

AROMATHERAPY

The pure essences of aromatic plants have been prized for thousands of years for their health-giving properties and heady scents. This section of the book takes an in-depth look at the ancient art of aromatherapy which has been refined through many centuries. Each individual essential oil is described in full detail; its origins and its therapeutic effects and uses are revealed. After a detailed look at the many qualities of essential oils, you can learn how to harness their therapeutic powers through massage, beauty treatments and perfuming your home, to enhance every aspect of your life. These potent, volatile essences are nature's gift to mind and body.

AN ANCIENT ART

The value of natural plant oils has been recognized for more than 6,000 years, for their healing, cleansing, preservative and mood-enhancing properties, as well as for the sheer pleasure of their fragrances. Today, these properties are being rediscovered as we look to the wisdom of past eras and civilizations to restore the balance that has been lost in modern-day life. Stress, pollution, unhealthy diet, hectic but sedentary lifestyles – all these factors have adverse effects on our bodies and spirits. The art of aromatherapy harnesses the potent pure essences of aromatic plants, flowers and resins, to work on the most powerful of senses – smell and touch – to restore the harmony of body and mind.

SECRETS OF THE OILS DISCOVERED

The origins of aromatherapy can be traced through the religious, medical and social practices of all the major civilizations. It is likely that the Chinese were the first to discover the remarkable medicinal powers of plants around 4500 BC. However, it is the Egyptians who must take the credit for recognizing and fully exploiting the physical and spiritual properties of aromatic essences. From hieroglyphs and paintings we know that aromatic preparations were used as offerings to the gods. Furthermore, the natural antiseptic and antibacterial properties of essential oils and resins, particularly cedarwood and frankincense, made them ideal for the purpose of preserving corpses in preparation for the next world. The discovery of remarkably well-preserved mummies up to 5,000 years after their preparation is a tribute to the embalmer's art.

By around 3000 BC priests who had been using the oils in religious ceremonies and embalming rites became aware of the usefulness of their properties for the living, too. Closely guarding their secrets, they became the healers of their time, mixing and prescribing "magic" medicinal potions. Use of essential oils gradually permeated all levels of society as cosmetics and perfumes became widespread.

From Hippocrates we know the Greeks had some awareness of the therapeutic properties of the oils and their value as sedatives and stimulants was certainly recognized. The Greeks and Romans used aromatics widely in rituals and ceremonies and the oils played an important role in the rise in popularity of baths and massage and body-culture generally. However, with the fall of the Roman Empire the use of essential oils died out in Europe.

LEFT: *The personal use of perfume was widespread in ancient Greece and Rome. The Roman girl in this portrait (from around AD 350) carries a small pot of aromatics.*

RIGHT: *From the tomb of the Noble Senedjem, ancient Egypt. The cones of unguent worn on the heads melted in the heat, waxing and scenting the hair and body.*

This Milesian container for perfumed oils is fashioned in the form of a Siren, a sea nymph of Greek mythology. It dates from around 525 BC, when Miletus was one of the principal Ionian seaports.

The art flourished elsewhere, though, particularly in Arabia, where Avicenna first distilled rose essence in around AD 1000. Arabia became the world's centre for production of perfume, importing raw materials from Egypt, India, Tibet and China, and trading their products internationally.

With the Crusaders the art of perfumery was reintroduced to Europe around the twelfth century. Records show that aromatics were used as protection against the plague and the lower incidence of death among perfumiers suggests they were to some degree effective. The fifteenth century saw the rise of the great European perfumiers, and their wares were widely used to disguise body smells and ward off sickness. By the seventeenth century the aphrodisiac properties were well recognized, and with the work of herbalists, such as Culpeper, the therapeutic properties also started to be recorded, laying the foundation for modern aromatherapy.

THE MODERN RENAISSANCE

The term "Aromathérapie" was first used in 1928 by a French chemist, René-Maurice Gattefossé, to describe the therapeutic action of aromatic plant essences. His work was taken up by Dr Jean Valnet who found the essences' remarkable regenerative and antiseptic properties effective for healing the wounds of World War II soldiers.

The application of aromatherapy to beauty therapy and health care was pioneered by Marguerite Maury in her influential book, *The Secret of Life and Youth*. She also developed the method of applying the oils through massage.

Today there is a world-wide revival in the art of aromatherapy and contemporary research is beginning to understand the scientific foundations of the oils' properties and applications, discovered by trial and error over thousands of years.

ESSENTIAL OILS

The vital element in any aromatherapy treatment is the pure essential oil. The oils are very different from the heavy oils we use for cooking; they are concentrated essences, much lighter than water and highly flammable. They evaporate quickly, so they are usually mixed with other ingredients to trap their effectiveness. Because they are so concentrated, essential oils are measured in drops.

ESSENCE

This is a natural living substance: the "living" element of a plant which is captured and capsuled. It is a delicate operation. For instance, certain petals and leaves must be picked at exactly the right moment, or the quality of the oil is affected. Only the purest essences are used in aromatherapy so that the therapeutic properties are maximized and the effects are predictable.

Essential oils are extracted from an array of plant sources – petals, leaves, seeds, nut kernels, bark, stalks, flower heads and gums and resins from trees. Apart from their sensuous vapours, which provide the fragrance in many perfumes, they can be used in the bath, smoothed over the body, and used in the myriad ways described in this book.

Because of their small molecular structure, essential oils can penetrate the skin more effectively than vegetable oils, which only lie on the surface. Used medicinally over the centuries, essential oils have now become an established "alternative" natural therapy which can assist in the treatment of almost every type of ache and pain, as well as smoothing away the stress and strains of modern life.

HOW THEY WORK

Essential oils are composed of tiny molecules which are easily dissolved in alcohol, emulsifiers and, particularly, fats. This allows them to penetrate the skin easily and work into the body by mixing with the fatty tissue.

As these highly volatile essences evaporate they are also inhaled, thus entering the body via the millions of sensitive cells that line the nasal passages. These send messages straight to the brain, and affect the emotions by working on the limbic system, which also controls the major functions of the body. Thus, in an aromatherapy treatment the essential oils are able to enhance both your physical and psychological well-being at the same time.

Each oil has a distinct chemical composition which determines its fragrance, colour, volatility and, of course, the ways in which it affects the system, giving each oil its unique set of beneficial properties.

METHODS OF EXTRACTION

DISTILLATION

The Egyptians stored their raw materials in large clay or alabaster pots. Water was added and the pots heated so that steam rose and was pushed through a cotton cloth in the neck of the jar. This soaked up the essential oil which was then squeezed and pressed out into a collection vessel. The same principle remains in use today as high-pressure steam is passed over the leaves or flowers in a sophisticated still often using a vacuum, so that the essential oils within them

MAIN PICTURE: Field of lavender, Drome, southern France. French lavender produces the finest quality oil, with a fruitier and sweeter aroma than English lavender, which has a camphorous undertone. It takes one tonne (one ton) of plants to yield about 9 kg (20 lb) of essential oil.

INSET TOP: Egyptian relief showing perfume-making, from the fourth century BC. The large alabaster pot (a "linge") was filled with flowers, herbs and water, and then heated. The aromatic vapours would saturate a cloth stretched across the pot's opening.

INSET BELOW: Art meets science in the skills of the perfumier, blending a subtle new fragrance from the hundreds of essential oils at his disposal.

vaporize. When the steam carrying the essential oil passes through a cooling system, the oil condenses and can be separated easily from the water.

MACERATION

Flowers are soaked in hot oil to break down the cells, releasing their fragrance into the oil which is then purified and the aromatics extracted.

ENFLEURAGE

This is the method by which flower essences, such as jasmine, neroli and rose, which are more delicate and difficult to obtain, are extracted. Flowers or petals are crushed between wooden-framed, glass trays smeared with a greasy animal fat until the fat is saturated with their perfume.

PRESSING

This is a method of squeezing out essential oils from the rinds and peel of fruit, such as orange and lemon, into a sponge.

QUALITY CONTROL

Once the flowers and plants are harvested they are usually processed and stored quickly to preserve the freshness. Climate, soil and altitude can all affect the character of an oil. French lavender, for example, is famous for its rich aroma but, like wine, the quality can vary from year to year.

Always buy pure and natural essential oils as synthetic clones or adulterated oils do not act on the body in the same way and many of the beneficial properties are lost. The best quality oils may be expensive but they are always worth the extra cost.

USING ESSENTIAL OILS

You can soak and splash in them, feed your skin, sensually smooth them all over, or simply breathe in their wonderful aromas. The pleasure and versatility of aromatic oils make them one of nature's kindest gifts. There are many ways of dispersing their fragrance and utilizing their therapeutic properties.

INHALATION

Steam inhalation is an excellent method for treating respiratory problems, colds and so forth, but should not be used by asthmatics. Add 6–12 drops to a bowl of steaming hot water. Place a towel over your head and breathe deeply. This is also a great way of deep-cleansing the face.

THERAPEUTIC MASSAGE

This is the classic aromatherapy treatment, triggering the body's natural healing process by using lymphatic massage and essential oils to stimulate the flow of blood and lymph fluid. The aromas also act upon the emotional centre in the brain (the "limbic" system) which governs the way we feel.

For massage use a 1–3 per cent solution of essential oil to base oil.

FRAGRANCERS

These attractive pots, also known as diffusers or vaporizers, are simple to use. Fill the top china bowl with water and add a few drops of essential oil. The candle in the pot underneath heats the water, slowly releasing the natural

Decorative fragrancers for diffusing essential oils.

fragrance of the oil into the room.

Stand the burner on a plate or tile, not on plastic surfaces. Depending on the size of the room, 3–6 drops of essential oil are sufficient. It is also possible to buy battery-driven fan vaporizers which blow air through oil-impregnated pads, which can be changed to suit the mood.

BATHS

Run hand-hot water and then add 5–10 drops of the essential oil to suit your mood. Close the door, keep in the vapours, and soak for 15 minutes. For sensitive skin it is better to dilute the oil

in a base oil first, like sweet almond, apricot or peach kernel. Essential oils can mark plastic baths if they are not dispersed thoroughly. Wipe the bath straight after use.

FOOT BATH

Refresh tired feet by adding 4–5 drops of peppermint, rosemary and thyme to a large bowl of hot water. Soothe with lavender.

HAND BATH

Soothe chapped skin by soaking in a bowl of warm water (not hot) with 3–4 drops of patchouli or comfrey before a manicure.

SHOWER

After soaping or gelling, rinse well. Dip a wet sponge in an oil mix of your choice, squeeze and rub over your whole body while under a warm jet spray.

SAUNA

Add 2 drops of eucalyptus or pine oil per 330 ml (½ pint) water and throw over the coals to evaporate. These are great cleansers and detoxifiers.

JACUZZI OR HOT TUB

Relax by adding 10–15 drops of sandalwood, geranium or ylang-ylang, or simply bubble over with the stimulating effects of pine, rosemary and neroli.

ROOM SPRAYS

To make a room spray blend 10 drops of essential oil in 100 ml (7 tbs) water. A preservative of 15 ml (1 tbsp) vodka or pure alcohol can be added to the solution but this is optional. Shake well before filling the sprayer.

PILLOW TALK

Perfume your pillow with 2–3 drops of oil. Choose a relaxing oil to unwind or one for insomnia if you have sleep problems. For a different mood, try an aphrodisiac like ylang-ylang or be extravagant and use rose or jasmine, the two most expensive pure oils.

PERFUMES

The finest perfumes are traditionally blended from pure essential oils, particularly the flower extracts, though these days synthetic aromas tend to be used for cheaper perfumes. The art of the perfumier is subtle and skilled, and difficult to emulate at home as it is hard to find a medium to use as a substitute for alcohol. If you have a favourite oil or blend of essences you can use it all over in a body oil (3 per cent solution), or make a very concentrated blend (25 per cent) to dab behind ears, knees and on wrists and temples.

POMANDERS

Hang porous corked bottles in the wardrobe. The essential oil is absorbed by the clay and released slowly. Fill with the fragrance of your choice: try melissa or bergamot, or cedarwood to keep away moths.

POT POURRI

Add a few drops of an appropriate flowery or spicy essential oil to refresh tired pot pourri, or make your own.

HANDKERCHIEF

The most portable way of using essential oils. Add 3–4 drops to a handkerchief. Useful for treating colds or headaches, or for clearing your head at work.

FROM THE TOP: perfume bottle, pot pourri and oil lamp.

HUMIDIFIERS

You can add your favourite oil to the water of a humidifier or improvise by adding 5 drops of essential oil to a small bowl of water placed on top of a radiator.

RING BURNERS

Use the heat from light bulbs to release perfumed oils. Small ring burners, usually made of porcelain or aluminium, sit over the top of the bulb. Add a few drops of essential oil, and the heat from the bulb will gently vaporize the essential oil.

WOOD FIRES

Sprinkle drops of cypress, cedarwood, pine or sandalwood over the logs to be used about an hour before lighting the fire and then burn them to release your favourite aroma.

SCENTED CANDLES

Wax candles can be bought ready-impregnated with essential oils and are a delightful way of fragrancing a room. Or you can add a few drops of essential oil to an oil lamp for the same effect.

COMPRESSES

Soak a clean cotton cloth (such as a face flannel, handkerchief or small towel) in 160 ml (¼ pint) warm water with 5–10 drops of essential oil. Squeeze out and lay across the area to be treated. Cover and leave until cold. A useful method for sprains, bruising, headaches (place the compress across the forehead) and hot flushes.

BODY AND FACIAL OILS

These can be used on a daily basis to nourish the skin. Use a 1 per cent blend of essential oil to carrier oil for the face and a 3 per cent blend for the body for an effective treatment.

BLENDING AND STORING

❦ ❦

Essential oils are the basis for all traditional aromatherapy. Each has a particular fragrance and properties and the art of blending them harmoniously combines the skills of perfumier and pharmacist. Although two essences may have a similar smell or property they may not necessarily mix well together. One essence can overpower the other. For example, frankincense and ginger, both heavy smelling essences, give an overpowering, unpleasant smell when combined, whereas lavender and rosemary happily marry together. In general it is best to use a maximum of three oils in a blend so there is less chance of detracting from their individual qualities.

Assemble bottles of different sizes for storing appropriate quantities of blended oils. Funnels and droppers ensure accurate measurements and help prevent spillages.

THE ART OF BLENDING

Essential oils are highly volatile substances which should be handled, mixed and stored with care and used sparingly. Spillage of one particular oil can overpower a whole room and adversely affect young children and animals.

The power of aromatics is quite subtle. Never try to sniff or smell a pure essential oil straight from the bottle. Place a drop on the side of a glass and become a connoisseur: sniff, consider and take notes if you wish.

MIXING

Base oils play an important role in carrying and diluting highly concentrated essential oils, which are only used in small quantities measured in drops. These base oils dilute the pure essentials, inhibiting the evaporation rate and – since they spread evenly and easily over skin – encouraging quick absorption of the therapeutic oils into the skin.

When mixing, use a glass, porcelain or aluminium bottle and check that you have the correct amount of vegetable carrier oil before adding the recommended drops of essentials with a dropper or pipette for accurate measurements. Mix well and label the bottles clearly.

If you accidentally spill any, wipe up instantly with a paper tissue and dispose of it outside as the smell will be overpowering.

STORING

Dark glass bottles with stoppered caps are used to store essential oils. At home, keep them in a cool dark place, stand them upright, and always out of sight and touch of children. Never store essential oils in plastic bottles: both the oil and the bottle will perish. Oils will keep for at least a year if properly stored, although citrus oils may have a shorter life.

CARRIER OILS

Base oils are normally extracted from nuts or seeds and each has its own particular quality. Choosing the appropriate carrier oil will add considerably to the dynamic nature of a massage and can have specific benefits, such as helping to guard against heart disease or inflammatory diseases such as arthritis.

Sweet almond oil is probably the best all-purpose carrier oil because it is neutral and non-allergenic. It can even be used for massaging babies. Walnut acts as a co-ordinator and balances the nervous system; sesame is ideal for stretch marks; apricot kernel, peach kernel and evening primrose oils are all good for cell regeneration.

Walnut and evening primrose oil help alleviate menstrual problems, including pre-menstrual tension. Wheatgerm acts as an anti-oxidant and will preserve a mixture.

These oils are all rich in nutrients, and are ideal for most dry and sensitive skin types. The most important thing when buying these basics is to check that they have been naturally processed and not chemically treated. Cold-pressed is best.

AROMATICS

Aromatic oils extracted from flowers, fruits, leaves, barks, resins and roots have been used throughout the centuries for their healing properties and marvellous fragrances. Hundreds of essential oils are used today in such industries as food, cosmetics, pharmaceuticals and perfumery. Modern-day aromatherapy uses a much smaller selection, but the range of aromas and applications is nonetheless remarkable.

This section is a connoisseur's guide to thirty-five of the most popular, versatile and safe oils. Get to know their individual characters, their origins, their therapeutic values and discover your own favourites. Lavender, geranium and rosemary are excellent all-round oils and provide a good basis for any collection. Rose, though expensive, is also well worth the investment if you would like to explore the benefits and delights of aromatherapy.

BASIL
OCIMUM BASILICUM

Origins Basil was used in baths and body massage by ancient Greek nobles. The Egyptians used the aromatic fragrance in their offerings to the gods and also mixed it with essences of myrrh and incense to embalm bodies. In India it is believed to offer protection to the soul and is sacred to the Hindu gods Krishna and Vishnu.

Description Native of Africa and the Seychelles and now grown as a popular culinary herb in Europe, it can grow up to 90 cm (3 ft) in height and has small white flowers. The essence is distilled from the leaves and is a greenish-yellow with sweet green overtones.

Therapeutic effects Ideal as a nerve tonic, to lift fatigue, anxiety and depression. Also good for bronchitis, colds, fever, gout and indigestion, and reputed to soothe snake bites.

Uses Inhalation, baths and massage. It has both hot and cold qualities. When used in the bath or smoothed over the body it has an invigorating effect – great for sluggish skin and pepping up circulation. Combined with other oils such as thyme it also acts as a powerful antiseptic.

Cautionary note A powerful depressant if over-used. Also best to avoid during pregnancy.

BAY
PIMENTA RACEMOSA

Origins Roman emperors wore sprigs of bay, known as *Laurus nobilis* (Roman laurel), not only as a sign of wealth, but to ward off evil spirits. Greek priestesses chewed the leaves for their soporific effect, and after gastronomic banquets it was chewed as a breath freshener.

Description Popular as a culinary herb, bay is an attractive evergreen shrub whose shiny leathery leaves produce clusters of yellowish-green flowers in spring. The spicy-smelling oil is extracted from the leaves and is yellowish-brown in colour.

Therapeutic effects As a pulmonary antiseptic, it helps relieve bronchitis, colds and flu. Also used to aid digestion and sleep, to soothe rheumatic aches and pains, and as a general tonic.

Uses Inhalation, baths and massage. Widely used in perfume and exotic bath essences for its uplifting effects.

BENZOIN
STYRAX BENZOIN

Origins In the Far East the gum from the benzoin tree was one of the main ingredients used in incense to drive away evil spirits. The compound tincture is highly potent, pharmaceutically used in friar's balsam and as a fixative in perfume.

Description The benzoin tree is cultivated in Borneo, Java, Malaysia, Sumatra and Thailand. Like the rubber tree, its gum is taken from the bark by making a deep incision in the trunk. The gum is dark, with reddish-brown coloured streaks. These pigments contain the fatty oils which exude a delicious aroma similar to vanilla.

Therapeutic effects Valuable for treating urinary infections, it has a warming, relaxing, action suitable for respiratory conditions such as bronchitis, coughs and colds. Also effective for relieving skin conditions, and for gout.

Uses Inhalation, massage and in cough medicines. This is an energizing oil which can be used in one of two forms: simple tincture or compound – the former is not so toxic and is preferable for skin conditions.

BERGAMOT
CITRUS BERGAMIA

Origins Native to Morocco, it was not until bergamot rooted in Italy that its essential properties were recognized.

Description The bergamot tree belongs to the same family as the orange tree and the essential oil, as in most citrus varieties, is expressed from the fresh peel of the fruit. The oil is emerald green in colour, and smells spicier than lemon but with a similar, citrus quality. The odour is familiar from its use as a flavouring in Earl Grey tea.

Therapeutic effects Has a powerful uplifting and refreshing action. As an antiseptic it has proved effective in the treatment of mouth and skin infections, and sore throats. Can lower fever, and help with bronchitis and indigestion.

Uses Bergamot blends well with most essences and is a popular top note in perfumery. Along with neroli and lavender it is a main ingredient in eau-de-Cologne and is commonly used in toiletries to refresh and relax. In massage it can stimulate or soothe depending on the oils with which it is mixed.

Cautionary note In concentrations above 1 per cent it can irritate the skin. Also, even though it is sometimes added to commercial suntan agents to stimulate melanin production, it must never be used in home mixtures for tanning purposes.

CEDARWOOD
JUNIPERUS VIRGINIANA

Origins Cedarwood oil, similar to sandalwood, was used by the Egyptians in the embalming process. It was highly prized for its antiseptic properties and so became an important ingredient in cosmetics. Originally it was made from the beautiful Lebanon cedar, but, over-felled for furniture, this is now very scarce, and the red cedar is primarily used in its place.

Description The cedar is grown in North Africa and the US for its highly valued, fragrant wood. The clear, syrupy essential oil is extracted by steam distillation of waste woods. The odour of the oil is reminiscent of wooden pencils.

Therapeutic effects Used for skin complaints such as acne, alopecia, dandruff and eczema, and respiratory problems, especially bronchitis and catarrh. Also acts as a diuretic for help in urinary infections.

Uses Inhalation and massage. Increases sexual response. Blends well with cypress, juniper and rose.

Cautionary note Will irritate the skin in high concentrations.

CHAMOMILE
ALTERNATIVE SPELLING: CAMOMILE
ANTHEMIS NOBILIS

Origins The Egyptians thought this was a sacred flower and dedicated it to the Sun God. It was used in ritual ceremonies and medicinally to stop fits and fevers.

Description Chamomile species grow throughout Europe, North Africa and are often found growing wild. They have fine, feathery leaves with tiny white or yellow-centred daisy-like flowers. The pale blue oil is extracted from the flower and has a slightly apple fragrance which blends well with rose, geranium and lavender.

Therapeutic effects Particularly noted for its anti-inflammatory and sedative properties, it is excellent for childhood ailments (whether in children or adults!) from peevishness to earache. Also used for allergies, anaemia, burns, dermatitis, diarrhoea, fever, indigestion, insomnia, menstrual and menopausal problems, rheumatism, toothache and ulcers.

Uses Certain chamomile species are used for herbal infusions, but the oil is used in body, bath and hair products for its anti-allergenic properties. Use in dilute form for children.

CINNAMON
CINNAMOMUM ZEYLANICUM

Origins The Chinese believed that no remedy or treatment was complete without cinnamon. It is one of the oldest spices known – used by the Egyptians, Romans and Greeks, and it was also mentioned in the Old Testament.

Description Grown in the Far East, East Indies, and China, cinnamon has a distinctive hot, peppery aroma and taste. The twigs and leaves are picked and distilled to produce a sweet, pungent and bitter aromatic oil, which is a dark yellow-brown in colour. Its warm, spicy essence is often used in perfumery.

Therapeutic effects Useful for fatigue and depression, it is also a tonic for the respiratory and digestive systems, especially useful for coughs, colds, flu, stomach ache and diarrhoea. An aphrodisiac, it may also help impotence.

Uses Inhalation and massage. Burn to prevent the spread of flu virus, or add bark or oil to spice up a pot pourri. To relieve muscular spasms use in a compress or massage.

Cautionary note Use only in very low concentrations or under professional advice.

COMFREY
SYMPHTUM OFFICINALE

Origins Herbalist Nicholas Culpeper wrote in his medicinal scripts in the seventeenth century that this herb "helpeth those that spit blood or make a bloody urine". The root boiled in water or wine was drunk to help solve all internal problems, inwardly healing wounds, ulcers of the lungs and to help the flow of blood.

Description Normally grows wild near damp watersides. Comfrey has large hairy leaves which can irritate the skin if touched. The stalk grows to 90 cm (3 ft) high with pale purplish flowers. The leaves and roots are used in herbal decoctions but the oil is extracted from the leaves and stalks.

Therapeutic effects Containing allantoin, a cell regenerator, comfrey oil is particularly valuable for the treatment of wounds and skin disorders, including eczema, psoriasis, athlete's foot and torn muscles. Helpful, too, in treating stretch marks and for menopausal and menstrual problems.

Uses Massage and compresses.

CYPRESS
CUPRESSUS SEMPERVIRENS

Origins Egyptians used this wood to adorn their stone coffins along with using the oil for its medicinal properties. In France it is traditionally planted in graveyards.

Description A tall, conical, evergreen tree, it originated in the East but is popularly grown throughout the Mediterranean area, especially in Algeria and southern France. The essence is obtained by the distillation of the leaves, twigs and cones of the tree. Clear, pale yellow or green, it has a refreshing, spicy fragrance, reminiscent of pine-needles.

Therapeutic effects Most noted for its astringent and antispasmodic qualities, it can be used for circulatory conditions, colds, coughs, flu, haemorrhoids, menstrual and menopausal problems, varicose veins and whooping cough. It also acts as a sedative to soothe nervous tension.

Uses Inhalation, baths and massage. Use in compresses for swelling or rheumatism or in the bath as a muscular tonic. Its astringent properties make it suitable for use in cleansers for oily skin.

Cautionary note Not to be used by anyone who suffers from high blood pressure.

Eucalyptus
Eucalyptus globulus

Origins One of the tallest trees in the world, it originated in Australia and later grew in Tasmania, China, the US, Brazil and the Mediterranean. There are something like 200 species. The Aborigines may have been the first to use it medicinally.

Description The silvery, blue-green leaves produce a pale yellow oil which has a cool, camphorous smell. The fresh leaves give a rich yield of highly potent essence, one of the most versatile in aromatherapy.

Therapeutic effects The principal constituent of the oil is the antiseptic eucalyptol. Combined with its anti-inflammatory properties, eucalyptus oil is particularly helpful for asthma, bronchitis, flu, sinusitis, skin infections, rheumatism and sores. It can also reduce fever, is a strong diuretic, and its head-clearing qualities are well-known.

Uses Baths, inhalation and massage. It has a cooling effect on body temperature, reduces fever and is also a remedy for muscular/rheumatic aches and pains. It is widely used in cold and cough medicines and rubs. Use in the bath to relieve cystitis or on a handkerchief to clear the head.

Fennel
Foeniculum vulgare

Origins The ancient Greeks and Romans advocated the strongly flavoured fennel seeds to give them strength, to ward off evil spirits, kill fleas, and sweeten the breath.

Description These graceful perennial plants are found in Europe, often by the sea, and have delicate bright green feathery foliage. Their bright tufts of yellow flowers attract the bees. As a herb, the fresh leaves are particularly valued for fish dishes whereas the seeds, which smell like aniseed, are used in liquorice. The sweet oil, which has a similar smell, is extracted from the crushed seeds.

Therapeutic effects Noted as a diuretic, and a mild laxative, fennel has been found effective for colic, constipation, digestive problems, kidney stones, menopausal problems, nausea and obesity. It is also often helpful for increasing milk yield during breast feeding.

Uses Massage. The sweet aromatic oil is mainly used for flavouring medicines to help flatulence and indigestion. It is a constituent of gripe water, and can be infused in teas.

FRANKINCENSE
BOSWELLIA THURIFERA

Origins Frankincense (also known as olibanum) and myrrh were the first tree resins used as incense by the Egyptians. They were burned to clear the air in sickrooms and during religious ceremonies to drive away evil spirits. They ranked alongside precious stones as a valuable commodity and, according to the Bible, were offered by the three Kings to celebrate the birth of Jesus Christ. The gum comes from a small tree grown in Arabia, Africa, and China. It was first brought to Europe in the late seventeenth century.

Description To make the gum, a deep incision is made in the tree trunk where the resin exudes in tear-shaped globules which harden on contact with the air. The essence is spicy, with camphor undertones, but becomes lemony when mixed with myrrh.

Therapeutic effects Has an uplifting effect and aids concentration. Helpful as an expectorant in cases of bronchitis, coughs, colds and laryngitis. Reputed to preserve a youthful skin, eradicating wrinkles.

Uses Inhalation, baths and massage. Inhale to release catarrh, or relax with a few drops in a bath or body massage oil to warm, relax and meditate. It is often combined with myrrh, and blends well with essences such as basil and sandalwood.

GERANIUM
PELARGONIUM ADORANTISSIMUM

Origins The geranium originates in Africa and was not brought into Europe until 1690. It was used in ancient times as a remedy for tumours, burns and wounds.

Description Widely grown throughout Europe, it reaches around 60 cm (2 ft) in height. There are hundreds of different species cultivated for their pretty flowers, but only the aromatic pelargoniums (the ones that smell lemony when the leaves are pinched) give rich yields of the sweet yellowy-green essential oil. This is distilled from the leaves, stalks and flowers.

Therapeutic effects Unusually, it is both sedative and uplifting, and so invaluable for treating nervous tension and depression. Also used for circulatory and skin problems, especially wounds. Use in a footbath for chilblains.

Uses All uses. A popular ingredient in perfumes for its sweet, fresh, floral essence, the geranium is also therapeutically massaged or inhaled for its relaxing yet refreshing qualities. It can blend well with most other essential oils.

HYSSOP
HYSSOPUS OFFICINALIS

Origins Ancient alchemists used the powdered leaves and roots as a purgative and in ointments to spread over the stomach to combat worms. Small doses taken internally were mixed with honey to clean the mucous matter from the intestines or with crushed figs to loosen the bowels.

Description A small herbal perennial, hyssop has long stalks with narrow leaves and blue flowers. The oil, extracted from the leaves and flowering heads, is used in perfumes and liqueurs, including Chartreuse.

Therapeutic effects Hyssop is used for disorders of the cardiovascular system, and as it is both stimulating and sedative, it can regulate blood pressure whether high or low. It has powerful effects on the respiratory tract, for bronchitis, coughs and colds, and is also used for skin disorders.

Uses Massage and inhalation. It is also used in cough mixtures for bronchial conditions.

Cautionary note Use only in extremely small quantities. Do not use during pregnancy.

JASMINE
JASMINUM OFFICINALE

Origins An ancient favourite of the Arabs, Indians and Chinese, jasmine had a wide variety of uses including perfuming the body, scenting rooms and flavouring herbal teas. It was introduced from Persia to Europe in the sixteenth century.

Description The *Jasminum grandiflora* species is a small bush, native to the East Indies and Egypt and cultivated in southern France, Spain, Algeria, Morocco, India and Egypt. Its delicate white flowers produce a honey-sweet floral bouquet with fruity undertones. The deep red oil is produced by *enfleurage*, and has an intense rich, floral fragrance that is warm and exotic. It is one of the most important and expensive extracts, along with rose, used in perfumery.

Therapeutic effects Jasmine is a mood enhancer, lifting anxiety and depression. An aphrodisiac, it has a reputation for the treatment of both frigidity and impotence. It will also relieve menstrual cramps and is soothing to inflamed or irritated skin.

Uses Inhalation, bathing and massage will all exploit its warming and relaxing qualities. Also makes a delightful uplifting perfume or room fragrance.

JUNIPER
JUNIPERUS COMMUNIS

Origins Grown in North America, Asia, Africa and Europe, this small shrub with aromatic leaves and berries was popular as incense to burn in religious ceremonies and to purify the air and ward off the plague.

Description An evergreen bush with thick branches and narrow needle leaves, juniper produces small yellow flowers and small purplish-blue berries. Both the berries and leaves have a strong aromatic fragrance, similar to pine needles, but the oil is extracted from the berries by distillation, producing a pale yellow essence.

Therapeutic effects Diuretic and antiseptic, it is especially effective for the urinary tract and an excellent treatment for cystitis and water retention. Use for acne, colic, coughs, dermatitis, eczema, flatulence, rheumatism and skin ulcers.

Uses Inhalation, baths and massage. The oil is a great stimulator and, like cypress and pine, makes a refreshing bath oil. Massaged on the skin it stimulates the circulation.

LAVENDER
LAVANDULA OFFICINALIS

Origins Lavender comes from the Roman word "lavare" meaning to wash. It was one of most favoured aromatics used by the Romans in their daily bathing rituals. Both the Greeks and Romans burned lavender twigs as a room purifier to ward off the plague. It was brought to Europe by the Romans.

Description A shrubby plant with woody branches and long narrow leaves, it has purple-blue flowers on long spikes. After cutting, the plants are dried and steam-distilled. The essential oil is clear to pale yellow in colour with a strong aroma.

Therapeutic effects Its sedative and tonic effects make lavender a great balancer of the nervous and emotional systems. Excellent for migraine. As an antiseptic it can be used for many skin conditions and infections of the lungs, digestion and urinary tract. Extraordinarily versatile.

Uses Inhalation, baths, room spray, massage and most other uses. Use as a cold compress or place a few drops in boiling water and inhale for headaches and migraine. A warm towel wrap will soothe nervous exhaustion. A late-night lavender bath will help combat sleeplessness.

LEMON
CITRUS LIMONUM

Origins Early seafarers stocked up with fresh lemons before a long voyage to help prevent scurvy and to purify the ship's drinking water. Its astringent and antiseptic properties were fully appreciated in the first aid kit and used to treat cuts, bruises and insect stings.

Description The lemon tree, which has white-pink flowers and bright yellow fruits, is cultivated in most Mediterranean countries, Brazil, the US, Argentina, Israel and Africa. The pale yellow oil is expressed from the rind and peel of the fruit and has classically been used in perfume for its intense, sharp, citrus-fresh aroma. The essence becomes cloudy, and deteriorates over time, if not properly stored.

Therapeutic effects Lemon is highly antiseptic and astringent, and so is naturally used for skin complaints including boils, warts and verrucas. Also good for lowering blood pressure, colds, digestive problems, fever and gallstones.

Uses Inhalation, baths and massage. Lemon, as with most citrus oils, is a good cleanser inside and out. Use in skin-care preparations for oily skin. Evaporated in a fragrancer it will help colds and act as an insect repellent.

LEMONGRASS
CYMBOPOGON CITRATUS

Origins This sweet-scented grass was mainly used to season food in India, the African Congo, the Seychelles, Indonesia and Sri Lanka. Its main constituent, citral, was discovered to be a strong, cleansing antiseptic, and used to deodorize clothing and footwear. Dried leaves were burned to keep the mind alert.

Description Lemongrass is a tall-stemmed, grass-like tropical plant. Its oil is steam-distilled from the fresh or partly dried grasses, and has a refreshing, lemony smell. It is used in low-cost citrus soaps, perfumes and cleaning agents.

Therapeutic effects Through its anti-bacterial action, it is good for skin complaints, sore throats and respiratory problems. Also effective against headaches.

Uses Inhalation and massage. For the active work-out enthusiast, lemongrass is the ideal cooler and deodorizer. It can help alleviate athlete's foot and its refreshing fragrance acts as an energizer. Massaged or breathed in, it tones the heart and works on the digestive system. The oil will also repel insects.

MARJORAM
ORIGANUM MARJORANA

Origins The Greeks grew marjoram for use in their perfumes and herbal potions. They prescribed it as a medicinal antidote and to purge the system.

Description This popular perennial plant is one of the classic culinary herbs, and is grown world-wide. The amber-coloured essence is extracted by steam-distillation from the fresh and dried leaves and flowering tops. Its warm and slightly spicy aroma is often used in masculine fragrances.

Therapeutic effects A warming agent, able to relieve spasm, it is particularly valuable for treating the nervous system. Use for anxiety and insomnia, but also for arthritis, asthma, bronchitis, circulatory problems, constipation, headaches, menstrual problems, muscular strains and rheumatism.

Uses Inhalation and massage. It blends well with bergamot, lavender and rosemary. In bath and body oils it gives a warm, relaxing feeling. Steam-inhaled or smoothed over the sinuses and temples, it can relieve colds.

Cautionary note Do not use in early pregnancy. Do not use in high doses as it can have a narcotic effect and is also known to curb sexual drive.

MELISSA
MELISSA OFFICINALIS

Origins The Greeks and Arabs knew the properties of melissa and in the sixteenth century the Swiss physician Paracelsus hailed it as the "elixir of life".

Description Mostly a native of Europe, it is also cultivated in North America. Better known as sweet balm or lemon balm, it is a bushy perennial of the mint family. The aromatic oil smells like lemons and is extracted from the leaves by distillation.

Therapeutic effects Long known as an uplifting and calming cure for "melancholia", its tonic, antispasmodic properties make it effective too in the treatment of allergies, colds, diarrhoea, hypertension, menstrual problems, migraine and stress headaches, nausea and palpitations.

Uses Inhalation, baths and massage. The essential oil helps lower blood pressure and remove tension. Add 6 drops to the bath water. Melissa calms the body and mind, yet lifts the soul: an essential oil to dream with.

MYRRH
COMMIPHORA MYRRHA

Origins The Egyptians and the Greeks prized myrrh as a precious commodity. It was used by both civilizations in worshipping their gods, celebration rituals, cosmetics, perfumes and herbal treatments. The Egyptians combined it with frankincense for embalming and purification purposes.

Description A small tree, rather like a bush, myrrh is native in Arabia, Somalia, Ethiopia and other North African countries. Although the leaves are aromatic it is the resin which is distilled to produce the viscous, yellow essential oil. It has a warm, lightly spicy, sweet smell.

Therapeutic effects Anti-inflammatory and expectorant, myrrh will ease bronchitis, catarrh, coughs and colds. Good too for digestive problems, infections of the mouth and throat, and skin conditions.

Uses Inhalation and massage. It is used in pharmaceuticals and perfumery. In aromatherapy, because of its cooling effect, it blends well with camphor and lavender.

NEROLI
CITRUS AURANTIUM

Origins Neroli is believed to have been discovered by the Romans. In 1680 it was used to scent the bath water and gloves of Anna Maria Orsini, Princess of Nerola, who brought the fragrance into fashion amongst the Italian aristocracy.

Description Neroli oil is better known as orange blossom. It comes from the white blossoms of the bitter orange tree which originated in China but also grows in Egypt, Morocco, Algeria, the US, Italy and southern France. The pale yellow oil is expensive to produce since it takes approximately 1 tonne (1 ton) of flowers to extract just 1 kg (2 lb) of oil. These are hand-picked as they are just about to open and then distilled. Its powerful, wonderfully uplifting, floral fragrance is reminiscent of lilies and is extensively used in eau-de-Cologne.

Therapeutic effects An excellent sedative and anti-depressant, neroli counters anxiety, hysteria, shock and palpitations, and combats insomnia. It is helpful for dermatitis and dry skin, pre-menstrual tension and menopausal problems.

Uses Inhalation, baths and massage. Use in the bath or as a body oil to alleviate the symptoms of pre-menstrual tension and generally improve circulation, or just for the benefits of its delightful fragrance and relaxing properties.

ORANGE
CITRUS AURANTIUM (BITTER ORANGE)
CITRUS SINENSIS (SWEET ORANGE)

Origins China was the first home of the orange tree and the fragrant qualities of sweet and bitter orange oils have long been prized for culinary, cosmetic and medicinal use.

Description The sweet and the bitter oils are similar and both are extracted by cold pressing of fresh orange peel (it is only neroli oil which is extracted from the blossom). The bitter and sweet oils range from yellow to brown in colour and are used extensively for their fresh top notes in perfume.

Therapeutic effects Refreshing but sedative, orange is a tonic for anxiety and depression. It also stimulates the digestive system and is effective for constipation. Its antiseptic properties work well for mouth ulcers.

Uses Baths and massage. These essential oils, rich in Vitamin C, are used widely throughout the food and cosmetics industry in products ranging from bath and body oils to chocolate-orange confectionery.

PARSLEY
PETROSELINUM SATIVUM

Origins A lot of folklore surrounds the parsley plant. It was a medieval belief that it grew in the garden only if the man or woman of the house was "honest". When chewed, it would keep away the devil or, as later discovered, reduce bad breath.

Description Native to Asia Minor, it is now found all over the world. The common parsley is cultivated for its culinary uses and essential oil properties. The highest content of oil comes from the ripe seeds but the leaves are also used in distillation. It has a warm, herbaceous, spicy smell and is used in many herbal perfumes and cosmetic products.

Therapeutic effects A diuretic, useful for kidney and urinary problems and water retention. Also high in Vitamin A – essential for healthy hair, skin, teeth and eyes; and iron – for the blood and liver, and during menstruation and menopause.

Uses Massage. It blends well with fennel to help combat excessive water retention when massaged over the body. In conjunction with lemon and rosemary it can help clear toxins in the liver and kidneys. In general, a good oil to help calm the nervous system.

PATCHOULI
POGOSTEMON PATCHOULI

Origins Along with rose, jasmine, sandalwood and basil, patchouli was one of the favourite perfumes used in India, where shawls and blankets were impregnated with this rich oil. It is an aphrodisiac, and became very popular again in the 1960s for this reason.

Description The oil is extracted from the dried, fermented leaves of the small shrub and emits an intense, woody, sweet-spicy, balsamic odour. It improves with age and is used as a fixative in perfume.

Therapeutic effects Patchouli is an astringent, and is useful for scalp and skin conditions including dandruff, acne, eczema and scars. It has an uplifting effect for depression and anxiety, and can help alleviate fluid retention.

Uses Inhalation, baths and massage. Small quantities will have a stimulating effect; larger doses sedate. Often worn as a perfume and used for an exotic, sensual massage.

PEPPERMINT
MENTHA PIPERATA

Origins The Egyptians used this aromatic herb in flavouring wine and food and valued its menthol content. Culpeper recorded in the seventeenth century that it was the herb most useful for "complaints of the stomach, such as wind and vomiting, for which there are few remedies of greater efficacy".

Description The leaves of peppermint are shorter and broader than spearmint with larger spikes of purple flowers. A British classic, it has spread throughout the world. The almost colourless peppermint oil is distilled from the whole of the partially dried plant and has a strong refreshing fragrance.

Therapeutic effects Excellent for the digestion, as a decongestant, and for skin disorders. Use for colds, flu, flatulence, headaches, indigestion, nausea, toothache and sunburn.

Uses Inhalation, baths and massage. Peppermint oil is still used in gripe water to calm upset stomachs. A few drops on a handkerchief can alleviate headaches and symptoms of sea and travel sickness, as it is refreshing and invigorating. It makes an effective skin tonic or bath oil in the summer because of its cooling properties. Used in a footbath it can help sweaty, smelly or tired feet, or in a compress to relieve hot flushes.

Cautionary note For skin complaints do not use in a concentration of more than 1 per cent as it can cause irritation.

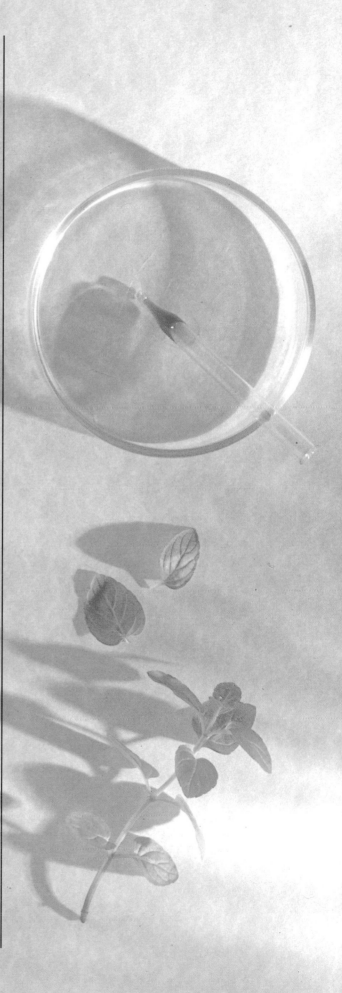

PINE
PINUS SYLVESTRIS

Origins The Scandinavians have traditionally used pine in the sauna or steam bath for its refreshing and antiseptic qualities.

Description This species of conifer grows wild all over Europe, North America and the former Soviet Union. General pine oil comes from the heart of the wood but the best essences are distilled from the pine needle. The oil has a fresh fragrance with a resinous woody undertone.

Therapeutic effects Acts as an antiseptic, and is particularly valuable for treating the respiratory tract, for bronchitis, catarrh, colds and sinusitis. Will also help relieve cystitis, arthritis and muscular aches and pains.

Uses Inhalation, baths and massage. Widely used to give coniferous fragrance in household products and in some masculine perfumes, this oil is popularly used throughout the cosmetics and pharmaceutical industries in balms, body rubs, soaps and bath oils. The oil can be used as an antiseptic deodorizer (add a few drops to freshen shoes) and in saunas or hot tubs for its invigorating steam.

ROSE
ROSA CENTIFOLIA, ROSA DAMASCENA

Origins The rose has been loved for its fragrance at least since Roman times, when it was used in garlands, scented baths and perfumes, often in ostentatious public displays. But the rose has its private uses too: Cleopatra reputedly carpeted her bedroom in rose petals to aid her seduction of Mark Antony.

Description The *Damascena* rose is cultivated in Bulgaria. The flowers are picked at dawn and the yellowy-brown oil is extracted within 24 hours. It takes approximately 5 tonnes (5 tons) of blossoms to produce just 1 kg (2 lb) of oil – not surprisingly one of the most expensive in the world. *Centifolia* roses, also yielding a richly fragrant oil, are cultivated in France, Algeria, Morocco and Egypt.

Therapeutic effects An aphrodisiac and mood enhancer, rose is a general tonic and fortifier, useful for circulatory problems, constipation, headaches and mental fatigue, menstrual and menopausal problems and skin disorders.

Uses Baths and massage. One of the least toxic of all essences, it is particularly good for older, drier, skins, and is useful for pot pourri or to perfume bed linens and underwear (add a few drops to the final rinse).

ROSEMARY
ROSMARINUS OFFICINALIS

Origins First favoured by the Egyptians, rosemary was popular with the Greeks and Romans who believed it symbolized love and death. During the plague it was burned in public places and worn around the neck for its antiseptic qualities.

Description A small shrub, it grows to around 90 cm (3 ft) high, with grey-green leaves and pale blue-white flowers. The clear oil is steam-distilled from the flowers and leaves, and has a powerful, warm, woody aroma.

Therapeutic effects A good stimulant, especially for the circulation and memory. Also helps alopecia, bronchitis, burns, colds, dandruff, diarrhoea, flatulence, headaches and obesity.

Uses Inhalation, baths and massage. Inhale from a handkerchief to clear headaches and fatigue. In massage it stimulates the lymphatic system.

Cautionary note Use in low concentration, as excessive doses may bring about epileptic fits or convulsions. Do not use in early pregnancy or if you have high blood pressure.

SAGE
SALVIA OFFICINALIS, *SALVIA SCLAREA* (CLARY SAGE)

Origins A sacred herb, its properties were used by the Egyptians to help cure infertility in women. The Chinese have used it medicinally for centuries.

Description The many varieties of common sage are all shrub-like herbs with rough, wrinkled leaves. The oil is distilled from the dried leaves and has a powerful, spicy fragrance with a hint of camphor.

Therapeutic effects A tonic, particularly renowned for regulating menstruation, it can also help relieve arthritis, bacterial infections, throat infections and water retention.

Clary sage (*Salvia sclarea*) is also used for its sedative and euphoric effects, and in treating insomnia, anxiety and depression, as well as menstrual and menopausal problems. It has a spicy fragrance, rather more floral than common sage.

Uses Bathing and massage. A sage bath helps muscular aches and the effects of prolonged stress or mental strain.

Cautionary note In high doses, sage can overstimulate and should be avoided by anyone who suffers from epilepsy. Both sage and clary sage should be avoided in early pregnancy.

SANDALWOOD
SANTALUM ALBUM

Origins In China, India and Egypt sandalwood was used in perfumes and cosmetics. It has also been prized by furniture makers, and in India many of the temples were built with this lovely wood. Worshippers also covered their bodies with its essence, along with rose, jasmine and narcissus.

Description The evergreen sandalwood tree grows to a height of up to 8 m (30 ft) in Indonesia, South East Asia and in particular East India. The syrupy, balsamic oil is extracted from the roughly chipped and powdered wood by steam distillation. It has a rich, warm, woody odour. It is used as a fixative in perfumes and gives the lingering classic base notes in many expensive fragrances.

Therapeutic effects Sandalwood's sedative properties are good for treating depression and tension. It is also an expectorant and antispasmodic; useful for bronchitis, coughs, nausea, cystitis and skin complaints. Regarded as an aphrodisiac.

Uses Inhalation and massage. Apply in a warm compress to revitalize dehydrated skin. Blends well with neroli and rose. Massage enhances its soothing effects.

TEA TREE
MELALEUCA ALTERNIFOLIA

Origins The antiseptic properties of the tea tree were discovered centuries ago by the Aborigines of Australia who used it medicinally for treating sunburn and many bacterial/fungal infections, from ringworm to athlete's foot. It was known as an antidote for venomous snake bites.

Description A native of Australia and Tasmania, it is often referred to as the swamp tree. It produces white hanging flowers on a long spike, but the pale green oil is extracted from the twigs and leaves, which have a strong aromatic odour. The oil itself has a camphorous smell, reminiscent of eucalyptus.

Therapeutic effects A strong disinfectant and antiseptic, it is ideal for skin complaints, including athlete's foot, burns, cold sores, mouth ulcers, verrucas, thrush and warts. Also effective for many respiratory complaints.

Uses Inhalation and baths. Tea tree can be used to kill fleas on pets but is more commonly used as a deodorizing/antiseptic foot bath. Dab on cold sores. Inhale to alleviate laryngitis and bronchitis. Diluted in water, it can be used as a mouthwash (not swallowed) to soothe ulcers.

THYME
THYMUS VULGARIS

Origins The ancient Egyptians incorporated the essential oil of thyme into their embalming fluids. The Greeks drank a herbal infusion of the leaves after banquets to aid digestion. Culpeper considered it a great lung strengthener and a remedy for shortness of breath.

Description This common low-growing wild herb has dark green leaves, woody stalks and small pink flowers. It is cultivated throughout the Mediterranean, Algeria, former Yugoslavia and in Egypt for culinary and pharmaceutical uses. The oil is extracted from the whole flowering herb by steam-distillation and has a pungent, sweet herbaceous smell. It is an important component in colognes and herbal perfumes.

Therapeutic effects Helps fatigue and anxiety, but best known as a natural antiseptic for treating coughs and infections of the respiratory tract. Good too for rheumatic aches and for skin problems such as sores and swellings.

Uses Massage and baths. When added to a bath, its invigorating effects help revive tired muscles.

YLANG-YLANG
CANANGA ODORATA

Origins A tropical tree, its first medicinal uses were to treat malaria, soothe insect bites and generally fight infections. Its antiseptic qualities were appreciated but it was also recognized as an aphrodisiac and a tonic to the nervous system. In the past, the flowers were mixed with coconut oil to perfume and condition the body and hair.

Description A native of Indonesia and the Philippines, the ylang-ylang tree reaches a height of 20 m (60 ft). The yellow flowers are freshly picked in the early morning and the oil extracted by steam-distillation. It has a narcotic, floral-sweet, jasmine-like aroma which adds warmth to perfumes.

Therapeutic effects A great relaxer (if used sparingly) and highly recommended for anxiety, depression, insomnia and frigidity. It also has benefits in treating high blood pressure and skin conditions.

Uses Baths and massage. This oil can soothe away all forms of stress when used as a bath oil or massaged onto the body. Its lasting fragrance is often used in facial and skin preparations, pot pourri and pomanders. It blends well with bergamot, melissa, sandalwood and jasmine.

OILS FOR COMMON PROBLEMS

KEY
R Relaxing oil
S Stimulating oil
U Uplifting oil

Some oils have more than one of these properties, tending to balance or normalize the emotions and bodily systems.

CAUTION

This chart is a general guide only. For the treatment of persistent problems, seek the advice of a qualified aromatherapist. Chronic conditions should be referred to a medical practitioner.

Never mix more than three oils in any one treatment as the synergistic effects are less predictable. Do not exceed the proportions of essential oil to carrier oil suggested in this book.

The following oils should not be used during pregnancy:
Basil • Bay • Clary Sage • Comfrey Fennel • Hyssop • Juniper Marjoram • Melissa • Myrrh Rosemary • Sage • Thyme

		Acne	Anxiety	Arthritis	Athlete's Foot	Blood pressure: High	Low	Body odour	Bronchitis	Cellulite	Colds/chills
Basil	R, U		❀						❀		❀
Bay	R			❀				❀	❀		
Benzoin	S			❀				❀	❀		❀
Bergamot	R, U	❀	❀								
Cedarwood	R	❀							❀		
Chamomile	R	❀	❀	❀							
Cinnamon	R							❀			❀
Comfrey	R				❀						
Cypress	R		❀					❀		❀	
Eucalyptus	S	❀		❀					❀		❀
Fennel	S										
Frankincense	R										❀
Geranium	R, U		❀								❀
Hyssop	R, S					❀	❀		❀		❀
Jasmine	R		❀								
Juniper	R, U	❀	❀							❀	
Lavender	R, U	❀	❀	❀	❀	❀		❀	❀		❀
Lemon	S	❀						❀			❀
Lemongrass	S	❀			❀			❀			
Marjoram	R		❀	❀		❀			❀		
Melissa	R, U		❀			❀					
Myrrh	S								❀		❀
Neroli	R		❀					❀			
Orange	U		❀			❀					
Parsley	S										
Patchouli	R	❀	❀		❀					❀	
Peppermint	S							❀	❀	❀	
Pine	S			❀					❀	❀	❀
Rose	R		❀	❀							
Rosemary	S							❀		❀	❀
Sage	S		❀	❀				❀	❀		
Clary Sage	R, S		❀			❀					
Sandalwood	R	❀	❀						❀		
Tea Tree	S				❀				❀		❀
Thyme	S		❀						❀		
Ylang-Ylang	R		❀			❀					

Chart of ailments (columns) and remedies (rows, unlabelled on this page). A flower symbol (❀) marks each recommended combination.

	Constipation	Cystitis	Dandruff	Depression	Diarrhoea	Eczema	Fainting	Flatulence	Haemorrhoids	Hayfever	Headache	Hormonal regulation	Indigestion	Influenza	Insomnia	Menopausal problems	Menstrual problems (general)	Irregular periods	Painful periods	Mental fatigue	Muscular aches	Nausea	Obesity	Pre-menstrual syndrome	Rheumatism	Sexual problems	Sinusitus	Stress	Throat infections	Travel sickness	Varicose veins	Warts	Water retention
1				❀		❀					❀		❀	❀			❀			❀		❀		❀									
2																									❀								
3		❀																															
4		❀		❀				❀																					❀				
5			❀			❀										❀								❀									
6	❀			❀	❀	❀	❀	❀			❀	❀	❀	❀		❀	❀	❀	❀	❀				❀	❀		❀						
7					❀									❀						❀		❀											
8						❀										❀				❀													
9	❀			❀	❀	❀			❀				❀	❀			❀		❀		❀	❀	❀	❀				❀					❀
10		❀			❀					❀	❀		❀							❀			❀		❀		❀		❀				
11	❀							❀								❀					❀	❀											
12															❀										❀								
13			❀	❀	❀	❀					❀				❀					❀				❀		❀	❀	❀					❀
14				❀	❀			❀					❀			❀	❀																
15				❀	❀														❀					❀									
16	❀	❀			❀	❀		❀					❀			❀	❀	❀	❀	❀		❀		❀	❀			❀			❀	❀	❀
17		❀	❀	❀	❀		❀				❀		❀		❀	❀	❀	❀		❀	❀		❀	❀	❀			❀			❀	❀	
18		❀		❀	❀			❀					❀		❀										❀				❀		❀		
19				❀							❀		❀												❀				❀				
20	❀										❀		❀		❀				❀		❀			❀		❀							
21				❀							❀	❀	❀		❀	❀	❀		❀						❀								
22					❀	❀			❀																			❀					
23				❀										❀	❀					❀	❀			❀	❀	❀							
24	❀			❀								❀	❀		❀																		
25		❀																															❀
26			❀	❀		❀																	❀			❀							
27				❀		❀	❀	❀		❀			❀								❀				❀				❀	❀			
28		❀												❀						❀	❀			❀		❀							❀
29	❀			❀				❀			❀				❀	❀	❀	❀	❀						❀			❀					
30	❀		❀	❀		❀	❀			❀		❀								❀	❀	❀	❀	❀	❀						❀		❀
31		❀		❀		❀										❀		❀	❀	❀	❀		❀	❀			❀	❀				❀
32				❀			❀												❀						❀			❀					
33			❀	❀		❀			❀																			❀			❀		
34				❀										❀															❀			❀	
35								❀								❀				❀				❀	❀								
36				❀																				❀									

THE ESSENTIAL MASSAGE

An aromatherapy massage using essential oils is a therapeutic treatment for both mind and body which works mainly on the nervous system. Aromatherapy is both holistic and practical in that it helps to protect the body's life-saving immune system and energize or stabilize emotions. It is often called the "sensual science" because it combines the powers of touch with the sense of smell. More effectively than any other massage, aromatherapy can either relax or stimulate the body and mind. The highly potent essential oils penetrate the body via the skin and are also inhaled as the massage progresses.

SETTING UP

Any massage is relaxing but you can enhance the experience by following a few simple steps to help create the right mood.

An aromatherapist uses a massage bench, but at home you can work comfortably on a cushioned floor or a futon (Japanese mattress). An ordinary bed is not really firm enough. Prepare the floor or surface with a large cotton sheet covered with a bath towel. You should also have to hand a pillow, a large wraparound towel for the body, and a warm blanket or even a hot-water bottle by the feet.

RELAXING YOUR PARTNER

Additional touches help to establish a calming atmosphere. You could fragrance the room with a burner, using a relaxing oil, and switch on some background music: play instrumental tracks, voices can be distracting.

The room temperature should be warm. Once the oils are gently massaged in, the whole body responds by slowing down and, although the skin may feel warm to touch, the body feels colder. It is important to keep your partner comfortable, so offer to cover parts that are not being worked on if you think your partner may be getting cold. Being at ease with one another is an important part of any treatment.

Choose a room which feels like a comfortable retreat: draw the curtains, switch on the heater and dim the lights. In aromatherapy, it is important to be able to switch off from everyday noises and that means the television, the telephone, or traffic zooming by, so close the window and shut off the rest of the world.

ABOUT THE TREATMENT

A complete aromatherapy massage takes just under an hour from top to toe. It is important to find out before massage about physical aches and pains, in particular back injuries, recent operations or whether the person you are massaging is in an "emotional" state of mind at the time.

GIVING THE MASSAGE

❧ Make sure you have read through the step-by-step instructions several times to familiarize yourself with the sequence. You do not want to keep stopping to refer to the book.

❧ Try the movements on your own body to get a sense of how the strokes should feel and how much pressure to use.

❧ Massage movements should be slow to help relaxation and eliminate tension which tightens the muscles.

❧ Remember that the movements should flow into each other. If you find you have missed out a step or gone on to the wrong part of the body, do not panic. Finish the part you are working on before going back to it, or leave it out altogether, rather than interrupting the flow of the massage.

❧ When you give the massage, make sure *you* are relaxed and comfortable, as well as the person being massaged, or you will transmit your own tensions to your partner and it will not be an effective massage.

❧ Try to maintain contact with your partner's body as much as possible; even as you move into a different position try to keep a hand on the body.

❧ When massaging different parts of the body keep the areas not being worked on covered with a large towel or blanket. The heat helps the body to absorb the oils and make the massage more therapeutic.

CHOOSING THE ESSENTIAL OIL

Aromatherapists never start a massage immediately. In order to provide the most effective treatment, the therapist has to ascertain the state of mind and body of the individual, and establish whether there are any specific problems to attend to. Is the problem physical? Is it mental? Is it a combination of both? To help them to treat a wide variety of complaints, aromatherapists have many oils at their disposal, but they never mix or use them until they have worked out a prescription for the receiver's individual needs.

Mixing the oils is a trained art, yet there are simple recipes you can use at home to deal with specific problems from muscular aches and pains to headaches and stress. With potent essential oils it is far better to use less, rather than more, so if in doubt, start the massage technique with a base oil like sweet almond and add 2 or 3 drops of just 1 essential oil. Lavender, rosemary and geranium are good all-purpose oils, or use chamomile for particularly sensitive skin.

APPLYING THE OILS

❧ Keep the oil in an easy dispenser or bowl so you do not have to worry about lids during the massage. But keep the oil covered in some way as essential oils will quickly evaporate.

❧ Always warm your hands before applying oils.

❧ Some therapists recommend warming the oil in your hands before applying it to the body as a courtesy to the recipient. Others advise against this on the grounds that it hastens evaporation of the essential oil and that the oil takes on your own energy rather than your partner's.

❧ If the part of the body you are working on is particularly hairy or the skin is very dry you will need to apply more oil.

❧ Keep your touch light and sensitive. Remember that your hands are the main channel of communication.

❧ If you become tired while masssaging, sit back for a minute but don't let your hands leave your partner's body as it is essential to maintain the continuity.

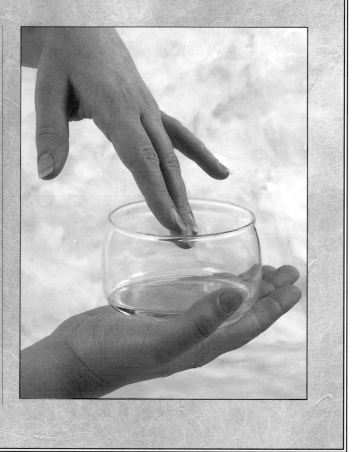

❧ If the recipient's back is stressed in any way, place a pillow under the knees when lying on the back, and under the pelvis when lying on the stomach.

❧ Wear loose, comfortable clothing to give the massage, so your movements are not hampered.

❧ If oil is accidentally spilt on clothing, dab off quickly with a tissue. It will soon evaporate, but it may leave a stain so rinse out clothing in warm soapy water.

❧ For complete relaxation avoid chatting during the massage: play music if you do not like silence. But do encourage feedback from your partner – you must be told if something does not feel good.

❧ Ensure that the person you are going to work on is given the following set of guidelines.

RECEIVING THE MASSAGE

Before the Massage

❧ Have a cool shower or wash before a massage. Do not soak in a hot bath, or the oils will immediately seep into the skin.

❧ Do not use an underarm deodorant or body spray before the treatment, as this will block the effect of the oils.

❧ Do not have a large meal just before an aromatherapy massage as the body's systems will have to work too hard at digesting to be thoroughly relaxed.

❧ Do not drink alcohol before a treatment.

❧ Do not have a massage if you have flu or a fever or any serious condition (see Caution, page 278). Wait until you are over the worst and then let an aromatherapy treatment help restore your system's balance.

After the Massage

❧ Drink a glass of still water immediately after a treatment.

❧ Lie still for at least five minutes before getting up.

❧ Do not bathe or shower for at least 12 hours after a treatment to allow the oils to be absorbed by the skin and begin the all-important work of detoxifying the body.

❧ Drink plenty of water for the rest of the day as the kidneys will be active in eliminating the toxins.

❧ Avoid alcohol for at least 12 hours after the treatment to give the body a chance to detoxify thoroughly.

THE MASSAGE STEP-BY-STEP

Following your assessment, select the oils you are going to use and blend 10–15 drops of your chosen oils with 4 tablespoons of base oil. The massage starts with your partner lying face down, with the back uncovered and the rest of the body covered with a towel or light blanket.

ESTABLISHING CONTACT

Take a few moments to create a bond of communication with your partner and to prepare yourself for the massage. Focus or "centre" yourself by becoming aware of your whole body and its role in giving the massage, and letting go of outside concerns to concentrate on the task in hand.

CAUTION

Aromatherapy is an holistic therapy in that it works on the person as a whole. Though it is an excellent way of treating minor ailments, stress and negative emotional states, it is not a substitute for conventional medical treatment. If symptoms persist, always consult a medical doctor.

Never attempt to treat the following conditions:

- cancer
- progressive neural disorders
- heart conditions
- advanced asthmatic conditions
- post-operative states
- severe varicose veins
- very high blood pressure
- epilepsy

For oils to avoid during pregnancy see Pregnancy Treatments on page 297.

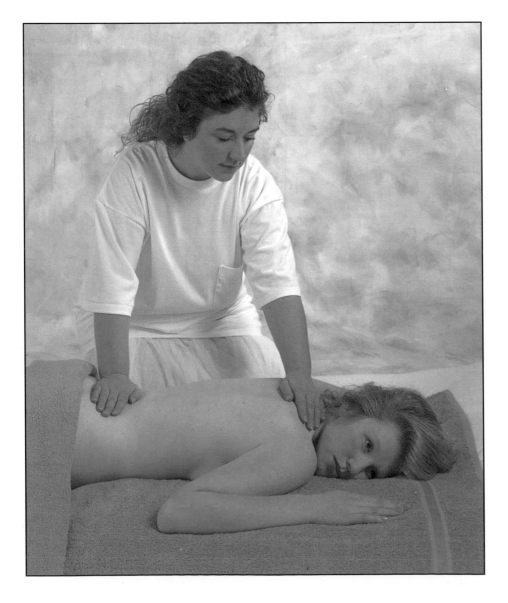

LEFT: *With your partner face down, rest one hand lightly at the base of the neck (the occipital bone) and place your other hand on the lower back (the sacral area). Hold the position for a count of 20, while you focus on your breathing and clear your mind. This is carried out with dry hands.*

THE LEG

EFFLEURAGE (SMOOTHING STROKE)

This is a smooth, sliding movement which soothes the skin and distributes the oil. Always worked in the direction of the heart, *effleurage* improves circulation, lymph flow and the function of the muscles. It is used between movements throughout the massage to provide continuity and to prepare a new area with oil.

ANKLE THUMBING

The ankles are an important centre of energy, and this movement helps to relieve congestion.

1 Seated to the side of your partner, begin with one hand at the heel, brushing in an upward, sweeping movement to the buttock ridge and sliding round to the thigh.

1 Sitting at your partner's feet, cradle one ankle gently with your hands, allowing the thumbs to sit naturally above the heel.

2 As the first hand comes round the thigh, place the other hand at the heel and brush with an upward sweep, ending at the back of the knee.

3 As the second hand comes off, cross the first hand over and begin the movement again from the heel up to the thigh.

Repeat the sequence about six or seven times, keeping the movements continuous and flowing, and then repeat on the other leg.

2 Keeping the rest of the hand still, apply a light pressure with the thumb as it brushes in an upward and outward movement.

3 Repeat with alternate thumbs, continuing in a rhythmic sequence for about 30 seconds.

FLUSHING

Flushing drains the lymph channels and stimulates the circulation. This movement should
not be used on anyone with severe varicose veins.

1 Sitting at your partner's feet, gently slide the thumbs up the middle of the leg, ending at the back of the knee.

2 Slowly bring the hands back down to the ankles by brushing down the sides of the calf muscle, taking care not to drag.

Repeat the movement five or six times.

KNEADING

Move back round to the side of the leg for this movement. It is particularly effective for
relieving tension at the back of the legs.

1 Place the hands gently on the calf, one at the top and one just above the ankle.

2 Grasp the calf muscle firmly with both hands and slide them toward the centre of the calf, lifting the muscle.

3 Using gentle pressure, knead the area by bringing the fingers and thumbs together and raising the muscle further.

Continue kneading for about 30 seconds.

WRINGING

1 Place the hands on opposite sides of the calf, just above the ankle. Gently glide the hands past each other so the heel of one hand is pushing away from you while the other hand is pulling.

2 Keep the thumb of the pulling hand raised so the thumbs do not collide as they pass each other each time.

3 The hands alternate the pushing and pulling as you work all the way up the calf and down again. The pressure should be firm but gentle.

Clear these movements by flushing through again from ankle to back of knee.

THUMBING THE KNEE

This is the same action as the thumbing performed at the ankle base. It is helpful for people who suffer from cold feet as it stimulates the circulation.

1 Cup the hands gently around the knee, allowing the thumbs to sit naturally on the fleshy part at the back of the knee.

2 With the same thumbing movement used on the ankles, brush one thumb upward and outward, covering the full width of the knee, and follow immediately with the opposite thumb.

FLUSHING

Flush through with the thumbs
together from the back of the knee
to the top of the thigh.

WRINGING

Wring the leg from the knee to the
top of the thigh with the same
action as used on the lower leg.

THIGH PUSH

This knuckling movement is very effective for breaking down cellulite, helping to
disperse the fatty tissue and improve the circulation.

1 With the supporting hand wrapped
around the wrist of the working hand
for stability, place the clenched fist
on the side of the thigh, just above
the knee.

2 Drag the fist slowly up the side of
the thigh toward the hip bone. This is
not a heavy action – all you need is a
little gentle pressure.

Repeat five or six times, working slightly different parts of the thigh each time.
Finish the leg massage by repeating the opening *effleurage* movement and then repeat all
the steps on the other leg.
Cover the legs with towels before proceeding to the next stage. An extra blanket or hot-
water bottle at the feet might also be appreciated.

BACK MASSAGE

The back carries a lot of strain and these relaxing movements are often the most appreciated part of the massage. Do not be tempted to use too much pressure: it is better to keep the strokes broad and flowing.

Seated to the side of your partner, apply oil evenly over the back with smooth upward strokes, following the direction of the lymph flow.

FIGURE-OF-EIGHT

This sequence loosens the tissue all over the back and helps to stimulate blood and lymph flow, and relieve tension.

You should be kneeling level with the buttocks, facing the head so that you can lean into the movement and reach the shoulders without straining.

1 To begin this large sweeping movement, place both hands on the lower back, just above the base of the spine, fingers pointing toward the head.

2 Slide both hands all the way up the sides of the spine to just below the base of the neck.

3 Move the hands out around the shoulders and in toward each other across the upper back.

4 As the hands pass each other, cross the right arm over the left and continue gliding.

5 With arms still crossed, reach down around the waist.

6 Pull the flesh up firmly around the waist and then gradually release the sides as the palms glide to the middle of the lower back and pass each other.

7 Continue the movement by sliding the palms out around the hips and complete the figure-of-eight by returning the hands to the starting position.

Repeat six times, always keeping the movements broad and flowing.

FANNING

This action works on the nerves along the spine and helps to disperse the fluid that accumulates in the back tissue as a result of tension. The effect is wonderfully relaxing.

1 Place one hand on the lower back, at the base of the spine. The fingers should be splayed open, with the index finger pointing to the side of the spine.

2 Fan the hand round in an upward and outward motion away from the spine. The other hand follows on the same side as the first completes the movement. Work all the way up the side of the spine, alternating hands.

Repeat the steps four or five times before moving round to work on the other side of the spine.

BUTTERFLY SHOULDERS

Before being given an aromatherapy massage, always wash off any anti-perspirant or deodorant. This is particularly important for this movement as it drains the lymph towards the major lymph glands in the armpits – the axillary glands. This movement relaxes the shoulder and disperses tension.

1 Place one hand at the bottom of the shoulder blade (scapula) with fingers splayed and the second hand poised to follow on the same side.

2 Brush the hand up and out in a smooth fanning movement. Follow with the second hand, work all around the shoulder blade and out over the shoulder, toward the armpit.

Repeat the whole movement four times, then work on the other shoulder.

FOREARM SWEEP

Kneeling at the side of your partner, turn the head away from you.

1 Place your forearm alongside the spine with your elbow just above the buttocks. Clasp the working hand with your other hand for support and stability.

2 Using the flat bone of the forearm (the ulna), slide all the way up the side of the spine to the top of the shoulder ridge.

Lift the arm off gently and repeat twice from the beginning.

Then turn your partner's head and work on the other side of the spine, using the opposite forearm.

DRAINING

Sit to the side of your partner, facing across the back.

1 With hands together and palms raised, place the fingertips at the side of the spine, just above the coccyx (tail bone).

2 Keeping the fingers together, pull them toward you down the side of the back.

Repeat the movement all the way up the spine, ending at the base of the neck so the final movement pulls across the shoulders toward the glands in the armpit.

Repeat with the other side of the spine. You can work the opposite side without changing your position by reaching across and brushing away from the spine, or you can move around your partner and repeat as above, if it feels more comfortable.

KNEADING THE NECK

This gentle *petrissage* movement releases tension and helps disperse the fatty deposits that can build up in this sensitive area.

Your partner should rest facing down with forehead on hands, so that you can work your fingers into the base of the neck. Smooth the hair away from the neck.

Resting one hand gently on the back of the head, use the other hand to pull up and knead the muscles in the base of the neck (the occipitals), rolling the muscle between the thumb and the other fingers.

FRONTAL MASSAGE

Help your partner to turn over onto their back, and ensure he or she is comfortable.
Provide cushions or rolled towels for any parts that need support, such as behind the legs
or neck. Cover the body up to the neck with a towel or blanket to keep your partner
warm.

SPINAL STRETCH

This movement is not suitable for people suffering from severe back problems, although
it helps relieve minor aches and stiffness.

  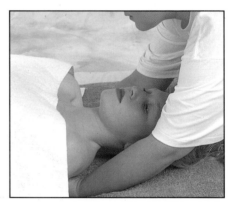

1 Seated at your partner's head, place the hands to the sides of the neck, palms up, with the middle fingers lifted, to prepare for the movement.

2 Slide the hands underneath the back, just between the shoulder blades so the middle fingers are pressing on either side of the spine.

3 Gently lift the torso so the rib cage rises, maintaining the pressure from the middle fingers.

4 Slowly pull your fingers up the sides of the spine. When you reach the top of the neck, hold for a count of 2 and then release. Repeat three times in all.

5 Finish the movement by cradling the head gently with both hands.

THE FACE

This treatment is a great boost to the circulation, and the complexion will improve with each treatment.

Seated at the head, prepare the face for the massage with a simple refreshing cleanser, using upward and outward strokes. Apply a small amount of facial oil to the face and neck with flowing movements.

TAKE CARE

Even when diluted, essential oils are extremely potent so work carefully around the eye area. If the oil accidentally makes contact with the eye, apply a few drops of pure sweet almond oil to dissipate it. Never wash the eyes with water.

FOREHEAD STROKE

1 Rest your thumbs on the centre of the forehead, just above the eyebrows, with the palms supporting the sides of the head. The stroke should be kept light and sensitive as the facial skin is very delicate.

2 Slowly draw the thumbs out toward the temples and down to the sides of the ears. Repeat the stroke several times, moving the starting position up a little each time until you reach the hairline.

DRAINING THE CHEEKS

This sequence of raking movements stimulates the lymphatic flow in the face, improving the complexion, clearing the sinuses and releasing tension.

1 Place the index fingers on either side of the nostrils and hold for a count of five.

2 Slide the fingers out and down to the ears. Lift the fingers and replace by the nostril. Sweep in a slightly narrower curve to reach the jawbone just below the ears.

3 Repeat with successively smaller curves, ending by tracing the laughter lines around the mouth, downward to the side of the chin.

CHIN MASSAGE

This not only tones the jawline, but also stimulates the energy points that govern the stomach and small intestine.

1 Place the thumbs on the chin, allowing the rest of the fingers to cradle the jaw.

2 Brush alternate thumbs down and outward, with a light stroke. Repeat the movement six or seven times with each thumb.

NECK SWEEP

This is an extremely soothing stroke which improves the tone of the muscles as well as flushing the neck.

1, 2 ABOVE and RIGHT: Apply a little facial oil to the neck, upper chest and shoulder areas using the flat of the hand. Gently brush down with the hand from the side of the ear out to the shoulder, using a broad sweeping stroke to cover the area.

3 Repeat the movement working around the front of the neck, down from the chin to the top of the chest, and then sweep from the other ear to the shoulder.

The sequence of sweeps around the whole neck should be repeated three times.

FANNING THE SHOULDERS

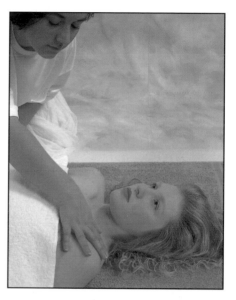

1 With fingers spread, brush with the flat of the hand across from the breastbone and out over the shoulders.

2 The second hand follows closely behind the first, so they are draining simultaneously toward the armpit.

Repeat twice before moving onto the other shoulder.

STOMACH AREA

ABDOMEN

1 LEFT: Apply a little oil evenly over the stomach. Place the palm of a hand on the centre of the abdomen.

2 Work the area with tender circular movements, always in a clockwise direction.

Repeat with the other palm. This movement aids digestion.

RIB CAGE SWEEP

This movement helps to cleanse the stomach and spleen by pushing the lymph away from these areas.

1 Starting with the outer edge of the hand placed at the centre of the rib cage, sweep away from you, following the line of the ribs with a long sweeping movement out to the waist.

2 As the first hand finishes the movement, the other hand follows on the same side.

Repeat the movement with both hands six or seven times and then move around the body to work the other side of the rib cage.

WAIST PULLS

1 Reach across your partner, placing a firm grip around the waist with one hand. Reinforce your grip by placing your other hand on top of the first hand.

2 Lift the waist by pulling your partner's body-weight toward you, then gently release while sliding the hands around the hipbone. This cleanses the liver and gall bladder.

3 Complete the movement by sliding the hands across and around the pelvis, draining toward the major glands in the groin. Be careful not to dig with the fingers as this is an extremely tender area. Keep the pressure light and even over the whole hand. This is particularly beneficial for women who suffer from menstrual problems.

Repeat five or six times before moving around to the other side of the body.

FRONT OF LEGS

EFFLEURAGE   LEG STRETCH

Apply oil to both legs using an *effleurage* movement working up from the ankles, as used on the back of the legs.

Repeat the *effleurage* strokes sequence several times to ensure an even distribution of oil.

Supporting the leg at the ankle and behind the knee, bend the leg up and place it in line with the shoulder.

Clasp the hands around the back of the knee. Ask your partner to inhale deeply, then pull the calf muscle toward you.

Hold for a slow count of 3. As your partner breathes out, release the pull on the calf.

Repeat the whole movement three times, then gently lay the leg down and repeat the stretch on the other leg.

ARMS AND HANDS

EFFLEURAGE

1 Seated to the side of your partner, move the arm slightly away from the body. Apply the oil by sweeping from just above the wrist, up to the shoulder and round.

2 As the first hand comes off the arm, the other hand starts at the wrist and sweeps upward to the gland sited in the elbow joint.

3 The first arm crosses the second as it reaches the elbow and again sweeps from wrist to shoulder.

Repeat six or seven times.

You can follow the *effleurage* with flushing to the inside of the arm, using the same movements performed on the leg, working from the wrist to the elbow. Before going on to the second arm, massage the hand of the first arm.

HAND MASSAGE

2 Pull back to the fingers, gently massaging the joints between your thumb and forefinger as you draw toward the tips. Finish with a slight pull to the finger to stretch it out.

1 Resting your partner's hand palm down over your own palm, use small brushing movements with your thumbs to work upward between the joints of the fingers toward the wrist.

3 Repeat with each finger, finishing with the thumb.

Now repeat the movements on the other arm and hand.

To finish the massage, cover your partner to the neck, check he or she is warm and comfortable, and leave to rest for a minimum of 5 minutes (up to 15 minutes is preferable). Upon returning, help your partner to sit up carefully and offer a glass of water.

PREGNANCY TREATMENTS

Pregnancy can be one of the most exciting and fulfilling times of a woman's life. The joy of bringing another human being into the world creates a tremendous feeling of contentment and anticipation, but it is also a time of great physical and emotional upheaval. Together with the ever-important trio of exercise, good diet and rest, essential oils can play an important role in helping a woman cope with the stresses of nine months of pregnancy, the pain of labour and post-natal recovery.

COMMON AILMENTS

Surging hormone levels and changes in your swelling body can bring a host of discomforts, many of which can be alleviated by aromatherapy treatments and other simple steps.

BACKACHE
The lower back region takes a lot of strain during pregnancy, and will benefit from a firm massage with 4 drops each of lavender and sandalwood in 30 ml (2 tbsp) base oil. 6 drops of lavender in the bath will help to soothe away the aches.

MORNING SICKNESS
Eat little and often during the day, avoiding junk food and heavy meals late at night. Choose fresh foods which are free from preservatives or chemicals. Try herbal tea infusions such as chamomile, peppermint or orange blossom, which are good for the digestion.

HEARTBURN
Avoid heavy meals and particularly rich, spicy foods. Peppermint tea infusions help, and you can rub the solar plexus with a blend of 2 drops each of lemon and peppermint essential oils in 15 ml (1 tbsp) of base oil.

Spoil yourself with the luxurious and relaxing scent of rose for body and facial oils, to keep your spirits up during pregnancy.

SORE BREASTS
These need extra care and attention during pregnancy as they expand. Use a gentle massage oil with rose and orange, 3 drops of each in 15 ml (1 tbsp) sweet almond oil; or if breasts are swollen, make a cool compress using rose water and place over the breasts while having an afternoon rest. Sweet almond oil on its own is excellent for sore, cracked nipples during breast-feeding. Never use pure essential oils on the breasts during this period as they can easily be transferred to the baby while feeding.

CONSTIPATION
Make sure your diet contains plenty of fresh and high fibre foods and drink plenty of still water. Tension can also be a contributory factor, so try a relaxing bath with 3 drops of lavender and 4 drops of rose. Massage your abdomen and the small of the back with a blend of 4 drops of chamomile or orange in 15 ml (1 tbsp) base oil.

SLEEP PROBLEMS
In the last few months of pregnancy, because of various discomforts it is often difficult to get a good night's sleep. A relaxing bath with neroli and rose is soothing, and you can add ylang-ylang for its calming, sedative effect – a maximum of 8 drops in total. Sprinkle 2 drops of rose or lavender on the edge of the pillowcase to help induce sleep.

STRETCH MARKS
When the stretched skin returns to the body's normal shape it can leave tiny jagged scars. A daily massage around the hips and expanding tummy, using 5 drops of lavender in 15 ml (1 tbsp) jojoba, wheatgerm or evening primrose oil, will help keep skin smooth and supple. Start around the fifth month of pregnancy and continue after the birth until you return to your normal weight.

SWOLLEN ANKLES

These can be reduced with a cool to warm footbath of benzoin, rose and orange. Add 2 drops of each directly to the bowl or mix with 15 ml (1 tbsp) base carrier oil such as sesame seed. Rest with feet raised on cushions or pillows.

VARICOSE VEINS

During pregnancy the blood flow to the legs is often slowed down, causing the veins to dilate. Mix 2 drops each of cypress, lemongrass and lavender with 30 ml (2 tbsp) apricot kernel base oil, and smooth gently over the legs for relief. If veins are prominent then one of the best oils for the circulation is geranium, though this should always be very dilute for use in pregnancy. Add 4 drops to the bath or to 15 ml (1 tbsp) carrier oil to massage the leg with upward movements. Do not work directly on the veins or apply too much pressure to the leg.

LABOUR

To create a relaxing atmosphere in the labour room, use a few drops of lavender in a fragrancer, or try rose, neroli or ylang-ylang to fortify you as the labour progresses. Any of these oils can be used in a massage blend for the lower back to help with contractions. If labour is progressing slowly, try marjoram as a massage oil or compress across the abdomen to stimulate contractions.

AFTER THE BIRTH

The "baby blues" often occur around the third or fourth day after childbirth, though some women can suffer a more severe form of post-natal depression for up to a year. A bath of jasmine and ylang-ylang will help you feel better, or use a body oil of chamomile, geranium and orange (5 drops to 30 ml (2 tbsp) sweet almond oil), which is a good mix

CAUTION

The following oils should be avoided during pregnancy (particularly the first five months) because of their strong diuretic properties or tendency to induce menstruation:

Basil • Bay • Clary Sage • Comfrey Fennel • Hyssop • Juniper Marjoram • Melissa • Myrrh Rosemary • Thyme • Sage

Use all essential oils in half the usual quantity during pregnancy and take extra care in handling them. Ensure that the oils you are using are pure essential oils, as adulterated blends or synthetic oils can sometimes have less predictable effects.

If you have a history of miscarriage you could also avoid chamomile and lavender for the first few months, although in general these are excellent oils for pregnancy.

Because of their potentially toxic nature and strong abortive qualities the following oils should never be used except by a qualified aromatherapist, and must be avoided during pregnancy;

Oreganum • Pennyroyal • St John's Wort • Tansy • Wormwood

for hormonal imbalance.

To ease any perineal pains, a bath with lavender is soothing. Tea tree can also be added, since this is a powerful antiseptic and helps heal internal wounds and stitches.

RECOMMENDED OILS FOR PREGNANCY
Chamomile • Geranium (in low doses) *Lavender • Lemon • Neroli Orange • Rose • Sandalwood*

PREGNANCY MASSAGE

These simple touch massage movements can help to relieve many of the stresses and discomforts of pregnancy, and the back massage is particularly welcome during labour. The basic essential oil massage is modified in various ways to take account of the pregnant condition.

❧ Check the previous page to find which oils are suitable and which are to be avoided.

❧ Use a lower concentration of essential oil to base oil; ½–1 per cent is ideal.

❧ Keep strokes lighter than usual.

❧ In addition to the steps suggested, you can incorporate a facial and gentle breast massage.

❧ It is particularly important to observe the rest period after the massage and to help your partner get up gently.

❧ The positions you work in need to be adapted for a pregnant woman, as she cannot lie out straight on her front or back and needs to be well supported.

THE BACK
After about the fourth month of pregnancy it becomes uncomfortable to lie on the stomach, so work with your partner sitting up with a towel-wrapped pillow or back of a chair to lean over for support.

1 Make sure your partner is comfortable and place your left hand over the forehead and the palm of your right hand across the back of the neck. Hold for a few moments and then release.

2 Apply a little oil to your fingers and using a slight but gentle pressure, softly massage each side of your partner's neck and shoulders, kneading mainly with the thumbs. This will help to relieve the tension often caused by the weight of enlarged breasts.

3 Stroke the oil evenly over the back and begin an *effleurage* movement (a soothing, stroking motion with two hands, moving up the sides of the spine and out over the shoulders). Repeat several times to establish a rhythm and relax your partner.

4 Using the thumbs, work upward on each side of the spinal column from the lower back to the neck to help release congestion along the spinal nerves. Repeat four times. Clear the movement by sweeping up the back using the calming *effleurage* stroke.

5 Starting from the centre of the back, begin working up and outward across the width of the back with superficial *effleurage* movements. Repeat the movements several times until your partner is relaxed. This will help to stimulate the circulation and has a soothing effect on the nerve endings.

6 Using a double handed movement, press down and then gently lift the muscles to the side of the neck, rolling with the thumb, and then release. Work out from the neck across the shoulder, and then repeat across the other shoulder. Performed slowly with rhythmic movements this is very relaxing and will alleviate stiffness.

THE ABDOMEN

For a pregnant woman, the weight of the uterus can constrict important blood vessels if she lies down flat on her back, so provide plenty of pillows, cushions, bolsters or rolled towels to support your partner behind the back, under the neck and knees and anywhere else she needs to feel comfortable.

1 BELOW: It may seem alarming to massage the abdomen during pregnancy but, providing the strokes are light and careful, it is safe and relaxing for mother and baby. Gentle massage all over the abdominal area can be very soothing and is beneficial for relieving the stretched feeling often experienced during pregnancy. Apply oil evenly over the area to help feed the tissues and lessen the possibility of stretch marks.

2 Using the flat of your hands, carefully glide them up from either side of the waist, lifting your hands off as they reach the navel, and then start again. Continue to stroke the area with a light, soft touch, working over the whole of the abdomen to soothe and calm.

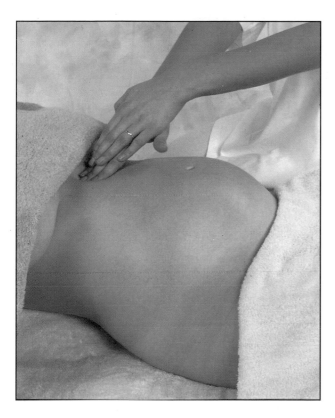

3 After a minute of gentle circular movements, place the fingertips of your left hand on the higher section of the solar plexus region and cover with your right hand. Rest both hands for a moment and then release to help alleviate stress.

LEGS

Make sure your partner is comfortable, with the knees supported by cushions.

Begin gently stroking the leg with an *effleurage* from the ankle to the knee, smoothing up the shin and then glide around the calf.

It can help to relieve the swelling, varicose veins or cramp which afflict many pregnant women. Do not use any heavy movements to the legs and avoid any reflexology movements to the feet, though gentle stroking around the ankles may well be appreciated.

TO FINISH

With both hands positioned at the back of the neck, apply light circular pressures to the cranium (skull) with your fingertips working in an upward direction to help release tension.

End the massage by smoothing the hair away from the neck and forehead, releasing all the negative energy. Allow your partner to rest for 15 minutes and then help her to get up very gently.

BEAUTY BASICS

✦━◉○◉━✦

Looking good starts with great skin, and aromatherapy can help you achieve this in various ways: the remarkable penetrative properties of essential oils make them excellent moisturizers, and the wide range of their properties means there is always the right oil for the right condition. For instance, rosemary stimulates the circulation and thyme helps the cells to regenerate. As well as being stimulating to the lymphatic system, which helps cleanse the tissue that causes sluggish skin, essential oils can be used as part of your daily skin-care routine and to treat specific problems such as acne.

FEED YOUR SKIN

Skin needs to be fed and nourished – inside and out. Healthy diets can keep the body in shape but to keep skin in peak condition it needs to have a ready supply of valuable vitamins and minerals. Many factors can drain the body of this valuable resource – canned and over-processed foods, caffeine, alcohol, nicotine, sunlight, central heating, carbon monoxide and habitual drug taking. The effects of these can build up and attack the skin so from time to time you need to give it a break.

A one-day fruit and vegetable diet is an excellent regime to adopt once a month to cleanse your body and give a boost to your system.

SKIN TYPES

Choose the right oils for your skin type and use them to blend your own cleansers, toners, masks and moisturizing facial oils. Remember that skin types can vary: skin may be drier in winter or more prone to oiliness around the time of your period, and it can change several times between puberty and menopause. So review the oils you use to suit your skin now and vary them to meet your changing complexion.

Few people are blessed with normal skin and even those who are may tend towards dryness or oiliness at times. Letters in parentheses indicate what other skin types an oil is suitable for. D = dry, S = sensitive, O = oily, A = all skin types.

OILS FOR NORMAL SKIN
Chamomile (D, S) • Fennel (O)
Geranium (A) • Lavender (A)
Lemon (O) • Patchouli (D)
Rose (D, S) • Sandalwood (D, S)

OILS FOR DRY SKIN
Chamomile • Geranium • Hyssop
Lavender • Patchouli • Rose
Sandalwood • Ylang-Ylang

OILS FOR SENSITIVE SKIN
Chamomile • Lavender • Neroli
Rose • Sandalwood

OILS FOR OILY SKIN
Bergamot • Cedarwood • Cypress
Frankincense • Geranium • Juniper
Lavender • Lemon • Sage

Combination skin has an oily T-zone panel from the forehead down to the nose and chin area, and may be normal or dry elsewhere. Double up on the treatments, using oils for oily skin on the greasy patches and oils for normal skin on the rest of the face area.

CLEANSERS

Choose the correct essential oils for your skin type and blend them in with an ordinary unperfumed brand of cleanser, liquid soap, or tissue-off lotion/cream, and they will do nature's work of rebalancing the skin.

FACIAL STEAM

Add 5 drops of chamomile for a soothing steam or try lavender, peppermint, thyme or rosemary to stimulate; or use comfrey or fennel for their healing properties.

ABOVE: Cleanse the face, paying particular attention to the oilier areas.

ABOVE RIGHT: For a facial steam, boil the water, cool slightly and add the oils. Steam for 5 minutes.

TONERS

Essential oils are the gentlest way of toning up. Rose water for normal or dry/sensitive skin or witchhazel for oilier skins are ideal bases for fresheners. These can be applied with cotton wool or for a more refreshing tone, sprayed on to the face.

Herbal tea infusions are also ideal toners. Boil a cup of water and infuse chamomile, marigold, rosehip or nettle teas (you can use herbal tea bags if you cannot get hold of the herbs), add 2 drops of orange or lavender oil and leave to cool. Oily skin benefits from juniper or lemongrass whereas drier skins would appreciate rose or sandalwood.

FACIAL OILS

Well-moisturized skin is soft and supple, reflects a healthy glow and ages less quickly. Younger skin only needs light conditioning whereas older skin needs specific nourishing treatments. Most moisturizers soothe and sit on the surface of the skin, but essential oils, with their fine molecular structure, work their way through from the surface to the inner dermis (the skin's deeper regenerating layer). Mixed with the correct amount of base oil, these pure essentials do not clog up pores on lubrication: they are light enough to be absorbed spontaneously by skin.

Use 30 ml (2 tbsp) of base oil and add 6 drops of essential oil (maximum of 3 different oils) to suit individual needs.

MASKS

Both clay and oatmeal are ideal ingredients for any face mask. A natural powdered clay is fuller's earth, which can be mixed into a paste with hot water. Cool and then add yogurt for a smoother consistency. Similarly, finely ground oatmeal can be mixed into a paste and left to cool. Add 15 drops of essential oils to suit your skin type per cupful of paste. Smooth on to your face, leave to dry slightly and then sponge off. For particularly dry/sensitive skins add 15 ml (1 tbsp) evening primrose base oil to give a more moisturizing mask. When applying, avoid the eye area.

EYE TREATS

While relaxing with a face mask on, close the eyes and cover with cotton pads soaked in rose water, or soothe with 2 slices of fresh cucumber.

ACNE

Because of their anti-bacterial, anti-inflammatory and rebalancing properties, essential oils are ideal skin treatments for acne sufferers.

It is often a mistake to scrub oily skin over-zealously: this only activates the sebaceous glands which in turn produce more sebum. If you suffer from pustular acne then avoid excessive facial steams which may spread the condition: use a mask instead. Often it is better to opt for a daily sensitive-skin type cleanser and moisturizer, adding 2 drops of juniper, which is stimulating and antiseptic. Opt for a deeper clay-type mask treatment once a week, adding a couple of drops of juniper, which is healing, soothing and tightening, or eucalyptus which is anti-inflammatory, antiseptic and antibiotic. Increase your intake of Vitamin E, which is a great skin healer.

BROKEN VEINS

These small, red, spider-like thread veins often appear on the surface of the skin around the cheek area. They are broken capillaries and seem to affect those with a delicate or fragile skin type. Hot and cold elements, along with stimulants such as alcohol and caffeine, can often trigger this condition. To treat it at home the secret is to protect the skin from losing excess moisture and to give it extra essential oil treatments using parsley, geranium, chamomile, rosemary or cypress in a heavy base oil.

COLD SORES

Cold sores are small blisters on the lips or surrounding area which are caused by the virus herpes simplex. Any lip sore that persists should be treated medically but for the common cold sore a dab of undiluted tea tree oil will help.

ODD SPOTS

If prone to occasional spots then mix 1 drop each of neroli, lemon and lavender in 5 ml (1 tsp) of base oil and treat just the affected area. For a single spot use a cotton bud and dab on 1 drop of undiluted sandalwood.

FACIAL MASSAGE

Massage helps the skin to absorb oils and creams easily.
Give skin a clear start with our step-by-step facial.

1 Pour a small amount of the blended oil into the palm of your hand and gently apply all over the face, avoiding your eyes.

2 With the backs of your hands, gently tap the skin around the jaw-line and underneath the chin to stimulate the skin cells.

3 Apply small circular movements to the chin area, using your thumbs, this will tone, help circulation and eliminate toxins.

4 Make an "oooh"-shaped mouth. Massage either side easing out fine lines.

5 With your fingertips, press along the top of the cheekbones and massage outward up to the temples to release toxins.

6 With the middle fingers, apply pressure to points above the bridge of the nose and underneath the eyebrows. Hold for 5 seconds and smooth across from the inner to the outer corners of the eyebrows and continue up to the temples.

7 To relieve tension, apply firm pressure at either side of the temples, and rotate backward.

8 Stroke up the forehead to the hairline with the palms of the hands, smoothing out fine lines.

HEALTHY HAIR

✧⟢══◦══⟣✧

Hair can define your image and style but it is also a mirror of your health. Emotional or physical problems can soon result in a lack of bounce or shine. Keeping hair in peak condition is a combination of caring for it on the surface and nurturing it from inside with a well-balanced diet.

SCALP MASSAGE OILS

Dry hair is rough to touch, thick in texture and dries out at the first sign of heated rollers or tongs. Avoid chemical colourants and perms and opt for shampoos and conditioners with jojoba and almond oils. Hot oil treatments allow essential oils to soak in easily and condition the hair. After massaging warm oil into the scalp, wrap the head in a warm towel and leave on for half an hour.

OILS FOR DRY HAIR
Geranium • Lavender
Rose • Sandalwood • Ylang-ylang

Greasy hair tends to look dull, lank, lacks body and will not hold a style. Central heating and environmental elements aggravate the condition but it can stem from a hormonal imbalance. Check your diet and avoid harsh degreasing shampoos. Clean brushes and combs weekly. Plastic brushes are better for brushing through as bristle continually stimulates the scalp. Choose light conditioning rinses to detangle but try a scalp massage to regulate the oil-producing sebaceous glands.

OILS FOR GREASY HAIR
Basil • Cedarwood • Chamomile
Cypress • Eucalyptus • Lemongrass
Rosemary • Sage

Normal hair is glossy with plenty of natural body and bounce. An occasional

hot-oil scalp treatment will keep it looking good and growing healthily.

OILS FOR NORMAL HAIR
Geranium • Lavender
Lemongrass • Rosemary

Combination hair has ends that are dry or normal and the roots are greasy. Avoid using hot appliances near the scalp and keep the ends regularly trimmed and conditioned. Use a scalp treatment with oils for greasy hair but do not comb through to the ends.

HOW TO MIX
Base oils Choose from sweet almond, apricot kernel, avocado, jojoba, evening primrose or sunflower.

Essential oils For one scalp treatment, choose up to 3 oils and use 5 drops of each for 30 ml (2 tbsp) base oil (for very long hair you may need more oil). Warm the blended oils by placing the

container in a bowl of boiling water, and then massage into the scalp. Wrap with a hot towel, leave for 15 minutes and then shampoo.

HAIR PROBLEMS
DANDRUFF
There are two types: dry and the more common oily. It is not catching! It can be caused by factors such as chemical body changes, stress, poor eating habits or wrong application of hair products. Both flaky and dry scalps can be treated with essential oils. Use special dandruff shampoos and conditioning rinses and treat the scalp by gently massaging with oils to suit. Use a base oil formula with patchouli and tea tree. For a dry, itchy scalp try cedarwood and lavender.

GREY HAIR
Grey hair is more porous and needs extra conditioning, particularly if it is chemically treated or coloured. Use a scalp formula for dry hair adding essential oil enhancers like chamomile to lighten or sage to darken any discoloration.

HAIR LOSS
Hair coming out in handfuls is often due to a hormonal imbalance, stress or anxiety, so first, learn to relax. Any unusual thinning patch should be looked at by a trichologist but, as a general remedy, use a scalp massage with lavender and rosemary oils.

SCALP MASSAGE

This is a wonderful way to condition hair, stimulate the scalp and relieve tension. You can use these steps to treat your own hair but it is even more relaxing if you can persuade a friend to help, especially if you have long hair.

1 Shampoo the hair and towel dry to absorb excess water. Comb through with a wide-tooth comb. Tilt your head back and pour some oil on to the hairline, massaging in with thumbs on the temple and fingers spread apart over the centre of the head.

2 Loosely run fingers and oil over the top of the scalp from front to back, lifting hair at the crown. Keep dipping your fingertips in the treatment oil to spread through the hair while massaging.

3 Massage the head by kneading. Grip and push (with fingerpads, rather than fingernails) against the scalp. The scalp should gently rotate against the skull. Concentrate on one area at a time, with the hands positioned on either side of the scalp.

4 Scalp massage works from front to back, from the forehead, frontal hairline, temples and sides, over the crown of the head to the base of the neck, following the natural flow of blood. If the scalp feels particularly tight then concentrate on areas where the scalp does not want to move. At the base of the skull, press firmly and push the whole scalp up toward the crown to release tension.

5 Pull any extra oil through the hair, working out from the roots to the tips. Make sure all the hair is well oiled, and then leave towel-wrapped for at least 15 minutes before shampooing.

THE AROMATIC BATH

The relaxing and remedial properties of water and of massaging oils into the body were recognized in ancient Greek and Roman cultures, when bathing first became a daily ritual. A bath with essential oils is one of the simplest and most effective aromatherapy treatments. It can be stimulating or relaxing, depending on the temperature of the water and whether you choose oils with uplifting or calming properties. An aromatic bath can detoxify the body, help problems like cellulite, joint stiffness, general aches and pains, colds and headaches, tone and condition skin and relieve anxiety and tension.

RUNNING THE BATH

Bath temperature and the time spent in the tub are important. A cooler bath is more stimulating and warmer water relaxes. Very hot water is damaging, however: it causes blood vessels and capillaries to expand and increases the heart beat. You should particularly avoid hot water if you have varicose veins, haemorrhoids, high blood pressure or are pregnant. A 15–20 minute soak is long enough before skin cells over-hydrate and swell with water. Wait until the bath is almost full before adding the oils, as they evaporate so quickly.

OILS FOR THE BATH

Essential oils are the best way of making a bath both aromatic and therapeutic. They sink into the skin easily and at the same time impart their lovely herbal or floral fragrances. You can add drops of oil directly to the bath and they will float on the surface in a fine film and evaporate, giving you the full benefit of their aromas. Or if you want to absorb them more you can disperse them through the water by mixing with a base carrier oil such as sweet almond, apricot kernel, jojoba or evening primrose (these rich base oils all nourish and rejuvenate the skin in their own right).

Mix a bath oil with a combination of up to 3 essential oils, 5 drops of each, in 15 ml (1 tbsp) skin-softening base oil. Choose oils with similar or complementary effects so they do not counter-balance one another.

THE RELAXING BATH

To calm yourself after a fraught day or to prepare yourself for a peaceful night's sleep, turn your bathroom into a private sanctuary. Keep the light soft if possible, or use an eye mask or burn aromatic candles. Support your head with a bath pillow, close your eyes and inhale deeply. Concentrate on your breathing, empty your mind and let the oils soothe away the stresses and strains. After a 15–20 minute soak, get out slowly and wrap yourself in a large, warm towel.

OILS FOR RELAXATION
Basil • Bergamot • Cedarwood Chamomile • Frankincense • Hyssop Juniper • Lavender • Marjoram Melissa • Neroli • Patchouli • Rose Sage • Sandalwood • Ylang-Ylang

Although these oils have a predominantly calming effect some can also be used to stimulate the circulation and lymphatic system, in particular lavender oil and also bergamot.

THE STIMULATING BATH

Best for the morning to get you started or to revive you before an evening out. Keep the water fairly cool and use an invigorating bath mitt to rub down and stimulate the circulation. When you have soaked, rinse yourself with water as cold as you can bear, either by splashing directly from the tap or shower, or by adding more cold water to cool down your bath.

As you get out, either slap yourself dry to make the skin tingle or rub yourself vigorously with a towel.

OILS FOR STIMULATION

Cypress • Eucalyptus • Fennel Geranium • Juniper • Lavender Lemon • Lemongrass • Peppermint Pine • Rosemary • Thyme

THERAPEUTIC BATHS

OILS FOR DERMATITIS

Chamomile • Hyssop • Lavender

OILS FOR ECZEMA

Chamomile • Geranium • Hyssop Juniper • Myrrh • Rosemary

OILS FOR PSORIASIS

Bergamot • Chamomile • Lavender

OILS FOR ARTHRITIS/RHEUMATISM

Chamomile • Eucalyptus • Juniper Lavender • Rosemary • Thyme

SHOWERS AND COLD RINSES

Invigorating jets of water are ideal for getting the blood pumping and there is no need to forgo the benefits of aromatic oils. Skin tends to be sluggish in the cold winter months but sloughing off dead top layers can help regenerate cells and allow moisturizers to be absorbed more easily. An aromatic shower is an excellent way of aiding recovery from a certain illness, lifting the spirits, or promoting relaxation after a busy day. Showers are ideal for smoothing skin with exfoliating rubs using wet salt, a loofah or a mitt to slough off the top surface of dead skin cells. A dry friction glove or loofah is too harsh for most skins so soften first in warm water. Soft bristle brushes can also help to get the circulation going with gentle massage on problem areas like hips and thighs. To keep friction brushes and mitts fresh always rinse them well and hang up to dry.

Essential oils can be used under the shower: try a base oil mixed with invigorating essences and with a clean face-cloth or sponge, pour on the oils and rub all over the body in circular motions whilst showering. To clear the sinuses and help coughs and colds, sponge the chest with a mix of eucalyptus and peppermint oils. A cold-water shower after cleansing improves the circulation and tightens skin pores.

Start off your shower or bath routine by whisking off dead skin cells with a friction mitt. Moisten the palm of the mitt with warm water or softening oils such as sweet almond or evening primrose. Concentrate on outer thighs, working from the knee in upward circular movements across the buttocks.

AFTER-BATH BODY TREATMENTS

Moisturizing oils and lotions applied after the bath or shower help to nourish the skin, keeping it soft and supple. As we get older our skin dehydrates since the oil glands do not produce as much oil as in youth. Apply a body oil all over the body, starting from the feet and working right up to the neck and tips of the ears. Avoid talcum powders which clog the pores and tend to have a drying effect.

BODY-OIL FORMULA

The use of essential oils for skin care combines simple pleasure with health benefits. Essential oils sink beautifully into warm damp skin. For a lasting effect, mix the 3 chosen bath essential oils, 5 drops of each, in 30 ml (2 tbsp) base oil. If you want to make up a larger quantity of body oil, use a concentration of 3 per cent essential oil in base oil.

PROBLEM ZONES

Hands and nails take some rough treatment with everyday chores. The ideal time for a manicure or pedicure is after soaking in a bath when nails and skin are softened, making it easy to clean around the nail bed and to clip uneven nails without snagging.

Fragile or flaky nails benefit from a rich, nourishing treatment: rub them with apricot kernel, wheatgerm or jojoba oil. Restore hands with a soothing, moisturizing mix of 15 ml (1 tbsp) sweet almond oil and 5 drops each of patchouli, lavender and lemon.

Feet are often neglected until they hurt. Polish hard skin around heels and soles with a handful of damp salt or use a pumice stone. While in the bath, bend one knee, grip the toes and then work with the fingers massaging in an upward direction, from the toes to the heels and up the calves in order to stimulate blood flow and relax tired feet. Massage a body oil into the feet after a bath, shower or pedicure.

For a deodorizing and soothing footbath add 3 drops each of cypress and lavender to a basin full of water. Chilblains can be treated with a massage blend of 3 drops of geranium and a drop each of lavender and rosemary in 15 ml (1 tbsp) sweet almond base oil.

ABOVE: Condition hands and nails with a simple finger-pulling exercise. Spread and stretch the fingers straight out; massage each finger with oils, working from the tip of the nails to the cuticles and up to each finger knuckle.

RIGHT: Soften the feet after a bath by massaging between the toes and then working around the tougher skin and heel areas. Finish with sweeping movements all over to stimulate the circulation.

ABOVE: Apply body oil to the arms with smooth upward strokes, concentrating on the elbows and upper arms where the skin is often rougher and drier.

Elbows can soon build up hard protective layers of grey, unsightly skin. A good softener for tough elbows is a sweet almond oil and oatmeal scrub. Mix 45 ml (3 tbsp) of sweet almond oil with 45 ml (3 tbsp) of fine oatmeal and mix to a paste with fresh milk or yoghurt. Smooth and rub over the elbows and any grey, goosey areas of skin around upper arms. Add 6 drops of fennel if arms are flabby. Another great elbow booster is the traditional recipe of cutting a lemon in half, squeezing out the juice and rubbing the elbows in the hollow of the lemon.

LEFT: When it comes to applying body oil, the back, neck and shoulders are often neglected because they are difficult to reach, but these are key areas for releasing tension and the skin needs to be nourished, so smooth as far as possible, or enlist the help of a friend.

IN THE REALM OF THE SENSES

〜〜⚬〜〜

The power of perfume to inspire romance has been known since the Babylonians, and perfume and flow-ers are still today the favourite gifts for lovers. Cleopatra's seduction of Mark Antony was carefully staged with a carpet of rose petals and rare and exotic scents in every conceivable form – even the sails of her barge were drenched in perfume to catch the breeze and announce her arrival.

The sense of smell is fundamental to our sensuality. Pheromones, chemicals secreted in human sweat, act as the most basic trigger to sexual attraction. The smells of flowers and plants are the plant equivalent of pheromones, irresistible to birds and bees and just as attractive to humans. We can use natural aromatic plant oils to relax, heighten our awareness, excite the senses and create a mood for love.

SETTING THE SCENE

Create a calming and sensual atmos-phere with scented candles or a few drops of essential oil evaporated in a fragrancer or light-bulb ring. Dim the lights and turn up the heat.

Scent your lingerie or bedlinen by adding 3 drops of your favourite oil to the final rinse, or store them in drawers with aromatic bags or scented balls. Sprinkle drops of rose or jasmine on the pillows.

PREPARING YOUR BODY

Luxuriate in an aromatic bath or hot tub, or, better still, share it with your partner. After soaking, perfume your whole body with a rich body oil or use a strong concentration to dab pulse points such as wrists, temples and behind the ears and knees, and wait for your partner to discover these secret scented areas.

PARTNER MASSAGE

We are all sensual beings and yet at times we may need help to switch off from everyday concerns and tune in to our senses. The loving touch of partner massage is always enjoyable; it is relax-ing and yet sensually stimulating – a total physical experience.

You can adapt the basic essential massage, using plenty of *effleurage* all over, deeper kneading for tense areas and light feather strokes with the fin-gertips to excite the surface of the skin. Avoid the lymph drainage movements as these are distinctly unerotic! Dis-cover your partner's erogenous zones – explore the ears and feet and the inside of the forearms and thighs. Find some more. Be tender and loving, playful and creative – let your imagination guide you.

OILS FOR SEDUCTION

Most of the aphrodisiac oils combine well with each other, but be careful not to use too many together or they may clash and work against each other.

❧ CLARY SAGE – sweet, sensuous and slightly intoxicating, but be careful as in high doses its sedative effect will inhibit sex drive.

❧ GERANIUM – a strong floral scent that both relaxes and uplifts.

❧ JASMINE – the heady floral fragrance boosts confidence and creates a luxurious atmosphere.

❧ NEROLI – fresh and sweet, its fortifying effect helps overcome shyness and inhibitions.

❧ PATCHOULI – heavy and exotic, it is stimulating in small doses and heightens the senses.

❧ ROSE – the quintessential oil for lovers. Rare and powerful.

❧ SANDALWOOD – woody, sweet and exotic wih spicy undertones.

❧ YLANG-YLANG – the long-lasting floral scent gives a feeling of relaxed well-being, helpful for impotence or frigidity.

You can also try the warm, spicy exotics such as black pepper, ginger, cardamom, cinnamon or cedarwood, but be sparing with these as they can easily overpower.

With a massage oil blended from floral and spicy aphrodisiac essences you can arouse the intimate senses of touch and smell simultaneously as you explore the skin and curves of your partner's body with strong smoothing strokes. Let the heady scents work their spell on the senses and emotions.

AMBIENT AROMAS

A lingering smell, whether pleasant or foul, is usually the first thing we notice when we enter a room, and it can strongly affect the way we feel. Fragrancing the home to cover unpleasant smells and delight the senses is an old tradition. For centuries the Chinese have suspended balls of jasmine flowers over the bed to clear the air and promote pleasant dreams, while posies of jasmine were handed to guests to refresh them on leaving banquets or dances. Lavender sachets placed in drawers and bowls of pot pourri to scent a room were particular favourites of the Victorians.

STUDIES AND OFFICES

Work-places are often stuffy and full of unpleasant smells, but if you work in an open-plan space fragrancing the whole area may not be a viable option. Inhaling a few drops of oil from a hand-kerchief is the most personal way of using a fragrance, or you can spray your immediate environment with a room spray, or add a couple of drops of oil to

a cup of hot water on your desk. Useful oils for the work-place are basil, rosemary, bergamot, lemon and melissa. Bergamot and lemon are particularly antiseptic, and lemon has the added advantage of helping efficiency. Basil stimulates a tired brain and rosemary is a great aid to concentration. Rosemary is also helpful in relieving headaches. If you are feeling overwrought, try clary sage or juniper, but watch the dosage as too much will cause sleepiness.

LIVING ROOMS

The methods for fragrancing a room are many and diverse. Those that involve evaporating the oils, such as fragrancers/diffusers, water bowls, light-bulb rings and room sprays, are best for preventing ill-health, balancing the emotions and disguising unpleasant smells such as cigarette smoke or cooking odours. All these methods disperse the fragrance through a large space extremely quickly and effectively. For more lingering and subtle scents, blend your own pot pourri or, alternatively, use pomanders.

Rose, geranium, orange and lavender are pleasing and uplifting scents for

a room, used individually or blended together. For an exotic, intimate atmosphere use sandalwood or patchouli, or to unwind in the evening try geranium, lavender, sandalwood or ylang-ylang.

PERFUMES FOR PARTIES

Clary sage or jasmine will create a heady, "feel-good" atmosphere for a party, or use orange, lemongrass or neroli for a lighter, fresher touch.

For a festive blend choose from the spicier oils such as frankincense, cedarwood, sandalwood, cinnamon and orange.

BEDROOMS

Whether to ensure a restful night's sleep or to turn your bedroom into a place of passion, fragrancing the bedroom just before retiring will create an appropriate atmosphere. Rose, neroli and lavender are delightful all-purpose oils for the bedroom. Use lavender to freshen a musty spare room to make it welcoming for guests.

INSECT REPELLENT

Use tea tree, eucalyptus, melissa, lemon grass or the closely related citronella in a diffuser to keep insects at bay.

DISINFECTING

Vaporized molecules of any essential oil will neutralize airborne bacteria, but some – such as tea tree, bergamot, lemon, pine and lavender – are particularly antiseptic. Use these in a fragrancer or room spray. Pine, lemon and tea tree can be used on a damp cloth to disinfect surfaces in the kitchen or bathroom. Clear the atmosphere of a sickroom with bergamot, eucalyptus and juniper.

POT POURRI

To make your own pot pourri assemble fully-dried flowers, petals, herbs, leaves and other plant materials. There are no hard and fast rules about quantities and proportions, but an allowance of 30–40g (2–3 tbsp) ground spices, 30g (2 tbsp) orris-root powder, 10g (2 tsp) dried lemon, orange or lime peel, and 6 drops of essential oil to every 4 cups of dried plant material makes a pleasant, balanced mixture.

If your pot pourri loses a little of its aroma over a period of time, it can be revived. Simply stir in another 2 or 3 drops of essential oil. And if the mixture loses its colour sharpness just stir in a few dried flowers such as miniature rosebuds, santolina flowers or tansy clusters.

Cottage Garden Mix

1 cup dried lavender flowers
1 cup dried rose petals
1 cup dried pinks (*Dianthus*)
1 cup dried scented geranium leaves
15g (1 tbsp) ground cinnamon
10g (2 tsp) ground allspice
5g (1 tsp) dried grated lemon peel
30g (2 tbsp) orris-root powder
3 drops rose oil
3 drops geranium oil
Mix ingredients together in a covered container, and set aside for 6 weeks. Stir daily to distribute the fragrances.

Woodland Mix

1 cup lime seedpods, or "keys"
1 cup cedar bark shavings
1 cup sandalwood shavings
1 cup small cones
15g (1 tbsp) whole cloves
15g (1 tbsp) star anise
1 stick cinnamon, crushed
30g (2 tbsp) orris-root powder
4 drops sandalwood oil
2 drops cinnamon oil
Mix ingredients together in a covered container and set aside for 6 weeks. Stir daily.

Ingredients which can be used to make pot pourri. From the left: dried rosemary, lavender, and bay leaves, dried ground orris-root powder, dried rosemary leaves, a selection of essential oils, ground cinnamon, dried chillies and cinnamon sticks, whole cloves, a blend of dried flowers, limes and lemons. The dried peel of citrus fruit is finely grated or chopped for use in the spice mixture.

THE STRESS FACTOR

Pressure can be stimulating, challenging and motivating, but if it builds up we may be left feeling unable to cope. Our response is often to deny the pressure and ignore the physical signs of stress such as fatigue, self-doubt, sleeplessness and headaches. If the symptoms and causes of stress are left untreated they will affect your general health and well-being, and can even lead to serious illness, such as ulcers, heart attacks and clinical depression, so it is important to start tackling problems at an early stage, before they erupt. De-stressing requires a positive tactical plan for learning how to cope and retain a balanced outlook on life. Aromatherapy is a marvellous antidote to many of the problems associated with stress.

ANXIETY

Whether it is a temporary bout of nerves, caused by something like an impending examination or interview, or an ongoing response to a persistent problem, anxiety can be a debilitating response to stress. It prevents you from dealing effectively with a problem and makes you feel tense. Essential oils, when inhaled, stimulate the lymbic portion of the brain which is responsible for all our feelings of well-being and discontent. They can balance the senses before deep depression sets into a more serious state. Temporary anxiety can also trigger skin eruptions so watch your diet and boost levels of Vitamin C and E and B-complex.

Anxiety can be alleviated with a combination of uplifting and calming oils.

Basil (uplifting) • *Bergamot (uplifting)*
Geranium (relaxing) • *Lavender*
(soothing) • *Neroli (sedative)*
Sandalwood (calming)

SOLAR PLEXUS STROKE

A marvellous way of unlocking tension by calming the main nerves that run through this area. Use your left hand (for calming) to stroke the solar plexus (located just below the breast bone) in anti-clockwise circles. Close your eyes as you do this and try to empty your mind. It can help soothe you even if you are clothed, but the effect is enhanced if you use a relaxing oil such as lavender or geranium. Try it while your bath is running, or when lying in bed before you go to sleep.

You can use the oils individually or mix them, using two relaxing oils to one uplifting oil. A good combination is basil, neroli and lavender. Stick to the same blend and proportions for bath and body, mixing 5 drops of each of the three oils in 15 ml (1 tbsp) of base oil for the bath and 30 ml (2 tbsp) for the body. All of the oils can be used individually in light-ring burners or fragrancers.

MILD SHOCK

This is a temporary form of stress, but the impact on the system can nonetheless be very strong, so a fast-acting remedy is needed.

Chamomile (calming) • *Melissa (antidepressant)* • *Neroli (relieves anxiety)*
Peppermint (invigorating pain-reliever)
Rosemary (stimulating)

Use only two essential oils: both camphor and melissa work well individually with neroli, and peppermint has an affinity with melissa. Use a total of 6 drops in 20 ml (1½ tbsp) of base oils, with smaller quantities of rosemary (for example, 4 drops of rosemary to 6 drops of melissa). For fast relief add 4 drops to a handkerchief and inhale.

HEADACHES

Often one of the first signs of stress and a regular affliction for many people. Cold compresses of lavender or geranium across the forehead provide pleasant relief. Add 5 drops of one oil to a small bowl of cool or warm water, soak a cloth in the water, wring out and lay it across the forehead. To help a headache caused by tension in the neck, try a sandalwood compress across the neck. Scalp massage is soothing, or try the shiatsu headache relief steps (see page 318).

DEPRESSION

The blues can hit us all from time to time, as financial, emotional or work problems hang over like a dark cloud. In the long term, if problems are not resolved, depression lowers the immune system, leaving you prone to a spiral of worsening mental and physical health. Essential oils can work wonders in lifting the spirits to prevent this.

UPLIFTING OILS
Bergamot • Cypress • Lemongrass Rosemary • Sage

SOOTHING OILS
Chamomile • Geranium • Jasmine Lavender • Marjoram • Neroli Patchouli • Rose • Sandalwood Ylang-Ylang

Start off with three soothing oils, and then drop one of these in favour of an uplifting oil to give an element of stimulation, and eventually introduce two

stimulating elements. Geranium, lavender and bergamot can make up a good combination. Use your formula for bath and body treatments.

Depression can be difficult to lift and if it persists you should consult a doctor or mental-health professional.

MENTAL FATIGUE

When you feel near to exhaustion or cannot concentrate on one thing at a time because problems seem to be crowding in on you, listen to your body's warning signals. Take time to unwind (try a bath with any of the soothing oils listed for depression), clear your head with a walk or deep-breathing exercises, and then revive yourself with oils such as eucalyptus and peppermint. Rosemary is helpful in concentrating the mind and stimulating the body so that you can continue to work if you feel you really cannot afford to take a break.

INSOMNIA

Sleeplessness is a common response to stress, as your mind and body refuse to let go enough to give you the rest that you need. Learning to relax has to be built into a daily pattern with a healthy diet, regular exercise, and a calming routine to wind down before bedtime. Try a milky drink or herbal tea last thing at night. Have a relaxing bath and massage, drawing on the sedative powers of up to three of the following oils:

Cedarwood • Chamomile Frankincense • Hyssop • Lavender Marjoram • Melissa • Neroli Orange • Patchouli • Rose • Sage Sandalwood • Ylang-Ylang

Breathing aromatic vapours in the bedroom helps to induce sleep:
❧ *Frankincense* is warming and relaxing, and encourages tranquillity. Use in a fragrancer.
❧ *Lavender*'s relaxing quality can be harnessed by dabbing 2 drops on the edge of your pillow.
❧ *Marjoram* has excellent soporific properties. Release in a light-bulb ring or fragrancer.
❧ *Neroli*'s wonderful floral fragrance is also sedative. Disperse unpleasant thoughts with 2 drops on the pillow or in a fragrancer.

HEADACHE RELIEF

Headaches and migraines are common symptoms of stress. Follow these simple shiatsu steps to sweep away the tension, relieve pain and clear the head. The sequence is quick and easy to administer; it can be used anywhere and friends and colleagues will be grateful for the relief of their pain. You can perform some of the steps on yourself, though the healing touch of another's hands is more effective.

1 Establish communication with your partner by placing both hands loosely on either side of the neck. Gently massage the shoulders; this helps to relax the breathing and creates a feeling of well-being.

2 RIGHT: Tilt the head to the side and support with the palm of the hand so that the neck muscles can relax. Place the forearm across the shoulder and apply gentle downward pressure; hold for 5–10 seconds and then repeat with the other side. This movement is particularly good for opening the meridians running along the shoulders and neck.

3 Supporting the head with the left hand, work with thumb and forefinger applying gentle pressure from the base of the neck to the nape. Hold at the nape of the neck for 5 seconds and then release the built-up tension.

4 Tilt the head back slightly, supporting it on your chest. Place your thumbs on the temples with the fingers loosely resting on either side of the face. Gently rotate the thumbs in small forward movements.

5 Find the pressure points just above the inner corner of each eye. Apply gentle pressure with the middle fingers to help disperse the pain. Hold the pressure points for 5 seconds.

6 Position your thumbs on either side of the head just above the hairline – approximately 5 cm (2 in) apart – with palms pressed flat along the sides of the face. Press the thumbs evenly back along the top of the head.

A shiatsu treatment is usually very effective for relieving stress and headaches but if your headache persists, consult a doctor. Avoid the treatment during pregnancy.

LEARNING TO RELAX

Relaxation is a prescription for health. Along with a well-balanced diet, an exercise programme, and a positive attitude towards recognizing and coping with stress, relaxation will help you balance the body and mind, even when you are worried and under pressure.

Exercise combats stress. The physically fitter you are, the better the body and mind can cope. Even burning off steam without losing self-control can be beneficial: a competitive racket sport, thumping the pillow, or going for a long walk can all release built-up tensions. Times of stress and emotional upset can make the body cry out for certain foods. Resist chocolate, cakes, ice cream or addictive stimulants like caffeine. Feed the mind with a high intake of Vitamin C from fresh fruit and vegetables, in particular citrus, berry and tropical fruits, and all the B-complex vitamins.

WHOLE-BODY RELAXATION

Lie down straight with shoulders relaxed and even on the floor. Arms should be straight with elbows alongside the waist, palms turned upward. Relax your head and close the eyes. Breathe in deeply; allow your body to sink into the floor. Breathe out slowly; relax. Focus attention on your breathing; listen as you inhale and exhale and see how quiet the deep breathing can become.

Focus on breathing in and out, slowly and evenly.

Feet slightly apart and allowed to roll out naturally.

Let go any tension in the knees.

Head relaxed and eyes closed.

Shoulders relaxed and even on the floor.

Arms straight with elbows alongside the waist.

Palms of hands relaxed and turned upward.

HEAD ROLL

To help ease tension around the head, neck and shoulders, try a simple head roll to start the relaxation process. Begin with head straight down toward the centre of the chest and roll the head slowly round to the right shoulder and then raise the chin. Lower the head and roll back to the centre and continue round to the left shoulder. Repeat the movement five times.

MASSAGE

❦

Massage techniques are described in other parts of the book but this section presents the system developed by the Swede, Per Henrik Ling, who was inspired by the massage tradition of the Chinese. Using a few simple techniques and strokes, you can learn how to do a whole-body massage, designed especially to be practised at home. Ideas are given for massaging babies, elderly people, even yourself! Learn, too, how massage can be a highly pleasurable and sensual experience.

THE HUMAN TOUCH

The sense of touch is a powerful and highly sensitive form of communication. It is a natural reaction to reach out and touch, whether to feel the shape or texture of something, or to respond to another person, perhaps by comforting them. A mother cuddles her baby, family pets are stroked, sexual partners caress, and if we accidentally knock a limb we instinctively "rub it better".
Fortunately, we are now rediscovering the healing power of massage and other touch therapies which have been understood in other cultures for thousands of years.

THE DEVELOPMENT OF MASSAGE

History shows that although the early Egyptians made references to the benefits of massage, the Chinese were among the first to recognize its healing value at around 3000 BC. Roman and Greek philosophers and physicians prescribed it both for its restorative powers after battle and for general preservation of the body and mind. Although the Romans believed in its curative powers, the art of massage also became part of a daily ritual for relaxation. After bathing, oils would be used to anoint the body from head to toe, followed by a luxurious massage.

Herbalists throughout history have used massage to heal body and soul, both by applying balms and by laying their own hands on the afflicted to expel evil spirits and clear the mind. It was not until the eighteenth and nineteenth centuries, though, that massage became popular throughout Europe, thanks to the work of Per Henrik Ling (1776–1839). Ling was a Swede who travelled to China and returned with a detailed insight into their massage techniques. From these he developed his own system of massage based on a variety of movements, involving pressure, friction, vibration and rotation.

This wealth of practical knowledge soon spread, and medical and non-medical professions worldwide began exploring the benefits of massage. This eventually established the basis of massage today, which in many ways remains much the same now as those early Swedish techniques.

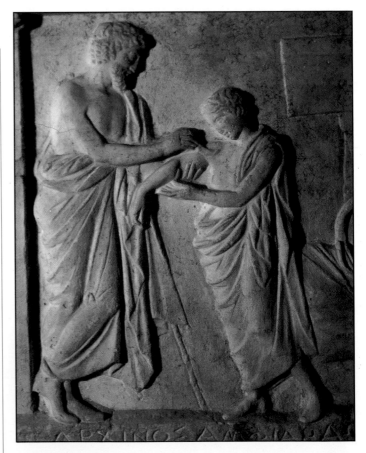

Along with basic massage we are now experiencing a revival of interest in many of the ancient arts which place such great importance on touch. These include aromatherapy, reflexology and shiatsu – all distinctive natural therapies which have a specific role to play in "alternative" health-care and are described in this book.

BELOW LEFT: This Greek stone relief from the fourth century BC shows the physician Aesculapius treating a patient by "rubbing", as recommended by Hippocrates.

RIGHT: As Europe emerged from the Middle Ages, massage once again became part of the bathing ritual, as shown in this sixteenth-century German woodcut of a public bath house.

EFFECTS OF MASSAGE

Massage can stimulate and relax the body and the mind. The skin, blood and lymphatic systems are stimulated, which boosts circulation, aids cellular renewal and removes toxic wastes. As tense muscles relax, stiff joints loosen and nerves are soothed, an all-over feeling of relaxation and well-being comes about.

THE NERVOUS SYSTEM

The nervous system is a highly complex network which relays messages from the brain to the rest of the body. The part of the nervous system which regulates many physiological functions leaves the brain at the base of the skull and runs down the spinal cord, protected by the spine's bony vertebrae. Millions of nerve endings run throughout the body, controlling much of the way it functions. Depending on the depth of the massage movements used, the nerve endings can be stimulated or soothed.

THE SKIN

With massage comes an increase in blood circulation. This helps the exfoliation of superficial dead skin cells, tones the skin and encourages its renewal process. Massage helps maintain the collagen fibres, which give skin its elasticity and strength, and keep wrinkles at bay. The activity of the sweat and sebaceous glands, which lubricate and moisturize the skin, is regulated.

MUSCLES

With the increase in blood flow, the blood's vital nutrients circulate more efficiently. Massage is popular with sportsmen and women because it can improve muscle tone, restore mobility, and ensure the elimination of waste products after exercise. With regular massage, strains and sprains heal more rapidly, while calf cramps and stiff muscles can become a thing of the past. Massage before an exercise session will help loosen and warm up the muscles, or afterwards it will ease sore, aching limbs.

CIRCULATION AND LYMPHATIC SYSTEMS

By dilating the blood vessels, massage increases the blood circulation. A good circulatory system means that an efficient supply of the blood's constituents, including oxygen and nutrients, reaches the billions of individual cells. This is vital for the healthy functioning of the whole body, from the muscles to internal organs such as the kidneys and liver.

At the same time the increase in blood circulation helps accelerate the lymphatic system, which absorbs and eliminates waste substances. Unlike the blood circulation, which has the heart to pump it around, the lymphatic system has no pump of its own and is dependent on muscular action for its efficiency. Massage is an important means of speeding up the flow of the lymph, encouraging a more effective filtering and elimination of waste throughout the body. An efficient lymphatic system provides the body with a strong immune system to fight against infections and disease.

DIGESTION

Massage mobilizes the digestive system so that the processes of assimilation and elimination are improved, helping problems like constipation and flatulence. The digestive system is quick to respond to stress, and the reduction in anxiety and tension which comes with regular massage has a regulating effect on the digestion.

THE BASIC TECHNIQUES

When many people think of massage they picture the vigorous pummelling and slapping often associated with puritanical health spas. In truth, firm massage can be highly beneficial without causing discomfort. You can alternate firm and gentle flowing strokes to create a combination that will alleviate tension and muscular aches and pains whilst energizing and invigorating the body.

In Swedish massage there are four basic types of movement. Familiarize yourself with these different techniques before beginning the step-by-step, whole-body massage.

EFFLEURAGE

Effleurage describes long, soothing, stroking movements using the flat of the hand (or fingers if working on small areas). These are often used to apply oil evenly to the body. You can use one hand on its own or with the other providing support on top of it, both hands simultaneously, or one hand alternating with the other.

Relax the hands and mould them to the contours of the body. Apply slightly more pressure when you take the stroke in the direction of the heart to improve circulation and lymph flow. If you are working away from the heart, keep the pressure firmer on the return stroke. The movements should be fairly slow and continuous.

Effleurage is used to start off a massage, soothing the nerve endings and helping your partner get used to your touch. It is used again at the end of a massage for a relaxing finish. In between, *effleurage* movements provide an important link between other more stimulating strokes and are used to make first contact with a new area of the body. If you feel hesitant about what to do next, you can always insert some *effleurage*, so the continuity is not lost.

You repeat *effleurage* strokes several times. Each time try to start the first complete stroke with fairly light pressure, then apply slightly more pressure with the next complete stroke. Where there are larger muscle areas, such as the thighs and back, you can apply the most pressure for a more stimulating effect.

PETRISSAGE

Petrissage describes a number of movements which involve various ways of kneading, rolling and picking up the skin and muscles. These firm and strengthen the structures by stimulating the deep layers of tissue, and increasing the supply of blood to the area. They also improve the flow of lymph. Generally a single group of muscles, or an individual muscle, is worked on at one time.

For petrissage, start with your fingers pointing away from you, press down with the palm, grasp the flesh between fingers and thumb and push it toward the other hand. As you release the first hand your second hand grasps the flesh and pushes it back toward the first hand. It is a continuous action, alternating the hands to squeeze and release.

With light kneading you are tackling the top muscle layers, whilst firmer kneading works on the deeper muscles, easing taut muscles and breaking down congested tissues to help the elimination of waste products.

FRICTION

Friction, or "connective tissue massage", is a penetrating circular movement which applies deep direct pressure to one particular site of muscular tension, using the thumb, fingertips or knuckles. It is a valuable technique for concentrating on specific areas of tightness and muscle spasm in the back.

As you make the circular rotations you should actually feel the underlying tissues moving; you are not simply sliding over the skin's surface.

A variation on circular friction pressures is static pressure, where you lean gradually into the muscle, slowly deepening the pressure without the rotation action. Press for a few seconds, then gradually release.

Another friction movement is knuckling: use the knuckles in a loosely clenched fist to produce rippling, circular motions. This is used to release tension up the sides of the spine and in other areas. Remember not to work right on top of the spine bone.

TAPOTEMENT

Tapotement, or percussion movements, are fast and stimulating. They include cupping, hacking, pounding (also called pummelling), which all sound like painful practices but when carried out properly should certainly not cause bruising or pain. (Do not use *tapotement* on particularly bony areas or on broken or varicose veins.) For all the movements, remember to keep the hands and wrists relaxed. All the percussion techniques are fast, precision actions, bringing one hand quickly after the other into contact with your partner. It is particularly important at the beginning to ask your partner whether you are applying the right degree of pressure.

These sequences stimulate the blood circulation, tone and help strengthen sagging skin and muscles. In particular, *tapotement* can tighten up soft tissue areas, such as thighs and buttocks, which are prone to cellulite.

For cupping, gently curve the hands to make a loose cupped shape, bending at the knuckles while keeping the fingers straight and firm. Do not bend the fingers too far over. Using the cupped palm, make a bouncy, brisk, cupping action against a fleshy area, alternating the hands quickly. The fast, cupping action creates a suction against the skin. Try this movement on the back, buttocks and thighs.

For pounding (or pummelling), loosely clench your fists, but keep the wrists relaxed. You can use the wrists in two ways: either striking your partner with the outer edges of the loose fist or with the front of the knuckles. Either way, the speed and rhythm of the movement is similar: brisk and firm, alternating the hands, without thumping your partner too enthusiastically. Once again, keep to the fleshier parts of the body, particularly cellulite zones such as hips, buttocks and thighs.

In hacking, the outer edge of the hand is used to stimulate the area by striking it quickly with alternate hands. You need to practise a brisk, bouncing movement, working rhythmically and rapidly over a fleshy area of the body. You need to have very relaxed wrists and fingers, and use the sides of the palm rather than the fingers. Used over the buttocks and thighs, hacking tones up muscles and disperses fluid.

Intersperse these brisk movements with the gentler, *effleurage* strokes, then go back to the pounding or pummelling for as long as you both feel comfortable.

WHOLE-BODY MASSAGE

Our whole-body massage is a comprehensive, top-to-toe sequence based on Swedish massage techniques, specially adapted for home practice. At first, you may find the full sequence too tiring. Until your hands and wrists build up their strength and you get used to positioning your own body comfortably to perform the massage, it is best to work on just a few parts of the body or to perform fewer movements on each part of the body. Always include *effleurage* strokes to begin and end a sequence, and never leave the body unbalanced – if you work on one leg or arm, you should repeat the same movements on the other side of the body.

COMFORT AND CLOTHING

If you are going to massage on the floor, put down a thick layer of blankets or towels, or a futon, to provide your partner with a firm, comfortable cushion. There is nothing more likely to reverse the relaxation process than a hard surface, a cold room and noise. Choose a quiet time, when you will not be disturbed. Your partner may need the room quite a lot warmer than you might expect. Being massaged on the floor might be extremely comfortable for your partner, but it can put a strain on the masseur's back and knees so, if you prefer, set up the same cushioning surface on a large table. It is not a good idea to massage on a bed – the give of a soft mattress can counteract much of your effort.

Have ready several towels, so that you can cover areas of the body which are not being worked on. Often a sense of modesty is crucial to relaxation, and the towels will also keep your partner warm. Move the towels around to cover most of the body, and especially an area you have just finished working on. You will need a cushion or towel to support the head, and it can be helpful to put a roll of towel under the knees when your partner is lying on their back. This relaxes the lower back. When your partner turns over on to the front, a towel under the chest can improve comfort.

Massage in loose-fitting clothes, with soft-soled, flat shoes, or work in bare feet. Take off rings and jewellery, so there is nothing to distract your partner, and make sure your nails are short! The more relaxed you are, as the masseur, the better. If you feel keyed up, try some deep, regular breathing exercises before you start. Take a few stretches, shake your hands to loosen any tension, and you are ready to start.

OILS

There are several oils which are appropriate for body massage. Stick to vegetable oils, rather than mineral oils such as baby oil. Grapeseed, sunflower or almond oil are good, basic vegetable oils, which are light and therefore not too sticky. Jojoba is a good oil for the face, especially if your partner has oily skin. Avoid oils with strong smells, such as olive oil. Also try experimenting by adding a little avocado, apricot or peach kernel oil if you wish, or buy ready-mixed massage oil.

Measure 45–60 ml (3–4 tbsp) oil into a saucer or small container before starting your massage. You will quickly get used to how much oil to apply. The amount varies with the dryness of the skin, and how readily it absorbs the oil, but in general you need enough to facilitate the strokes without applying so much that your hands simply slide over the skin. If you need to apply more oil during a sequence, simply smooth a little oil into the palms of your hands and do some extra *effleurage* strokes.

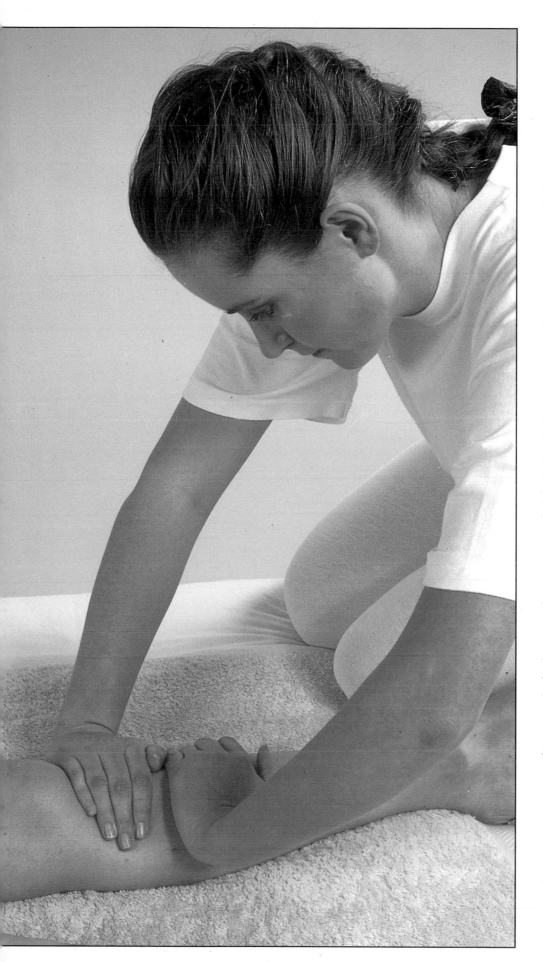

CAUTION

Exchanging a regular basic massage is a luxury for both giver and receiver. However, specific problems should be tackled by a trained practitioner. Never massage right on top of the spine. Working down each side of the bony spinal column is fine, and produces many benefits, but you should avoid working directly on top of the spine.

There are occasions when it is not appropriate to massage. Avoid if there are any of the following conditions:

❦ heart condition
❦ high blood pressure
❦ bacterial or viral infection
❦ nausea or abdominal pain
❦ severe back pain which may be caused by the spine, especially if there are shooting pains in other limbs
❦ temperature or fever
❦ open wound or skin infection
❦ cancer
❦ post-operative recovery

If you are in any doubt, it is always best to check with your doctor first.

THE FULL MASSAGE SEQUENCE

FRONT OF BODY

*1 Legs 2 Feet and ankles
3 Arms and hands • 4 Chest, shoulders and neck • 5 Face
6 Abdomen and waist*

BACK OF BODY

*7 Legs and buttocks
8 Back and shoulders*

FRONT OF BODY

The full massage begins with the front of the body, so your partner should lie face up
with cushions or rolled towels wherever needed for support.

LEGS

Since legs carry the full body weight, the bones and muscles in the legs are the largest and strongest we have. A good leg massage can not only help to relieve strain and tension in the legs, but can benefit the well-being of the whole body. It is not unknown for backache to be traced to problems in the legs, and for a good leg massage to help alleviate the pain.

Leg massage stimulates both the blood circulation and the lymphatic system, and done regularly it helps to prevent varicose veins. Any congestion in the lower legs will be lessened with *effleurage* movements taken up toward the lymph nodes at the back of the knee and in the groin. If legs feel puffy or swollen to the touch, make sure you use the gentlest of pressure. Firm massage on the larger muscles, such as those around the thighs, can dispel tiredness and stimulate a sluggish lymphatic system. Work more lightly over bony areas such as the shins and knees.

VARICOSE VEINS

You need to take certain precautions if your partner has varicose veins. Never knead or put any pressure on varicose veins, and only massage the part of the leg which is higher than the area with veins (that is, only massage closer to the heart); never on or below the vein.

EFFLEURAGE

1 BELOW: Kneel beside your partner's left ankle. With a little oil in the palm of your hands, start with your hands crossed over the ankle, in readiness to begin several long *effleurage* strokes. You will need more oil if the legs are particularly hairy or dry, but do not add too much in the first instance.

2 Keeping your hands crossed over the leg, slide the palms up the front of the leg, over the knee and up to the thigh, in one continuous, sweeping movement to oil the front of the leg evenly.

3 Turn the hands outward around the hip, separate them and bring the hands back down each side of the thigh.

4 Continue to sweep the hands back to the ankle, and then over the foot to the toes. Then place your hands crossed over the ankle again, ready to repeat the entire movement.

Use some more oil if necessary, and this time use slightly firmer pressure on the upward stroke, then lighter again for the return. The stroke is smooth and continuous throughout.

Repeat the sequence over the whole leg once again.

THIGHS

1 Bring both hands up to just above the knee and move them up together, pressing the muscles firmly toward the upper thigh. You should apply enough pressure to see movement in the muscles.

2 At the top of the thigh separate the hands and, using lighter pressure, come down either side of the leg to the knee.

3 Begin kneading the inner thigh with both hands. Squeeze, then release the muscles, picking up and rolling them as you do so. Continue the kneading action over the top and outside thigh.

4 Now use a hacking movement all over the thigh. Briskly strike the area with the outside edge of one hand after another, using short, sharp movements. Keep a fast repetition going.

5 Continue with cupping all over the thigh, working quickly. Expect quite a loud cupping sound, but check with your partner that the strokes are not too powerful.

6 Begin at the knee and do some *effleurage* strokes up to the top of the thigh, sweeping the hands outward and back down to the knee, to soothe the area after the stimulating movements.

KNEES

1 Place both hands just below the knee. Lightly massage around the kneecap, using your fingertips to work gently into the muscles. Repeat three times.

2 Starting with your thumbs above the kneecap, with your hands under the knee for support, slowly draw them lightly around the outside of the kneecap and release. Repeat three times.

3 Support the back of the knee with your hands and use your thumbs to circle gently around the kneecap, working downward. Return to the top of the knee and repeat three times.

4 RIGHT: Raise the height of your hands above the knee. Work around the kneecap with one hand, loosening the muscles with your thumb and fingers. Use gentle, circular rotations to cover the area thoroughly.

You may find it easier to support your wrist with the other hand.

Do some more *effleurage* strokes, sweeping them up from the ankle to just below the kneecap and back down to the ankle. Repeat this several times.

CALVES

1 Knead the calf muscles. Squeeze and release them, working from the ankle up to the knee.

2 Lightly and quickly pinch the fleshy part of the calf with the fingers and thumbs, one hand after the other.

Check with your partner that you are not pinching too hard, although this needs to be felt to be effective.

3 Using the outside edge of both hands, alternately and rhythmically strike the calf muscles, working up and down the entire length, but keeping away from the shin area itself. Keep the hacking action short and brisk.

4 LEFT: Starting at the ankle and crossing your thumbs on top of the shin for support, with loose knuckles make semi-circular kneading movements, working up and down the calf.

Finish the leg with some *effleurage* movements from ankle to thigh.

FEET AND ANKLES

A foot massage is particularly relaxing after the legs have been worked on. It can alleviate anxiety and stress, stimulate the circulation and nervous system, help insomniacs to sleep, and energize anyone feeling tired and lethargic. There are thousands of nerve endings in the foot, particularly on the sole. Try to include the ankles to improve their flexibility.

Change the pressure of the strokes to suit your partner, remembering that deeper pressure tends to revitalize whereas gentle strokes increase relaxation throughout the entire person. When working on the feet it is best to use only a very little oil, otherwise your hands will slide around and tickle. If your partner's feet are hot, use talcum powder instead.

Before starting, you may wish to raise your partner's knees slightly with a rolled towel under them, to relax the muscles around the knees and in the lower back.

1 Kneel at your partner's feet. Starting with the hands at the ankle, gently slide your hands toward the tips of the toes and then release them. Repeat several times. If you are using oil, apply it with this stroke.

2 With the heels of your hands, give a good stretch to the top of the foot. Draw the heel toward the sides of the foot to give the stretch. Repeat a few times, working slightly further down the foot too.

3 Supporting the foot in both hands, find the furrow between each tendon and, using small, circular movements, work both thumbs up the tendons toward the ankle. Repeat three times on each tendon.

4 Resting the thumbs across the top of the ankle, work the fingers right around the ankle bone using light, circular movements.

5 Lightly tap the toes with your fingers to build up some gentle friction.

6 Now knead the foot firmly, working particularly well into the arch. You will need to use different parts of the hand, such as the heel, knuckle and thumbs.

7, 8 Supporting the lower leg with your left hand, gently rotate the ankle three times in each direction, without forcing.

9 RIGHT: Give the foot a gentle stretch backward and forward, to relax and flex the tendons. Supporting the back of the lower leg, use your other hand at the toes to push the foot gently away from you. To reverse the stretch take the hand over the top of the foot, and press the foot down, still supporting the lower leg with the other hand.

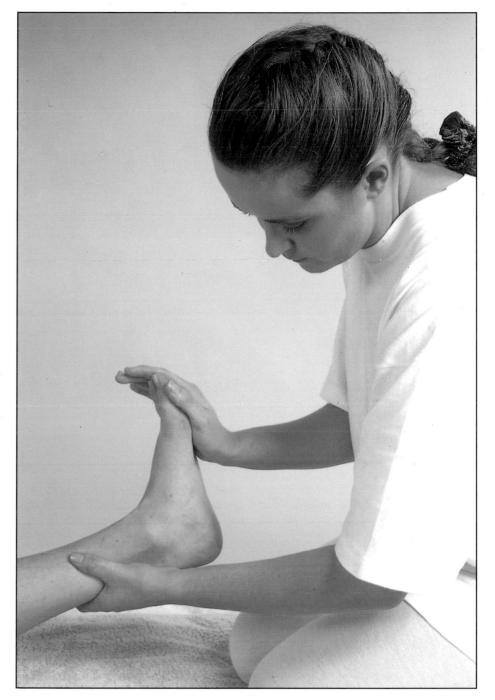

10 Finish the foot and ankle sequence with some long sweeping, *effleurage* strokes from the top of the foot up the lower leg and back down to the foot, to help reintegrate the foot and the leg. Repeat several times, varying the pressure.

Move around your partner to kneel on the other side.
Repeat the entire sequence on the front of the other leg and the other foot.

ARMS AND HANDS

Arms and hands can hide the most powerful emotions. Tight, clenched arms and hands often reflect insecurity, self-protection and unresolved anger. Tension in the arms can cause headaches, neck pain, and aching shoulders. Do not be put off if your partner's arms are slim and bony, there are still important muscle areas there.

A hand massage feels surprisingly good, almost on a par with having the feet massaged. A lot of tension creeps into the hands: a massage is a reminder of how it feels to relax them. Massaging the arms and hands can liberate and relax not only the muscles but also the pent-up emotions, as your partner starts to feel the wonderful sensation of letting go.

ARMS

1 Kneel halfway along your partner's right side. Holding the wrist with your left hand, lightly oil the arm using *effleurage* strokes, starting from the wrist and sweeping your hand up around the shoulder and down again. Repeat three times.

2 Changing hands, so that your partner's wrist is supported in your right hand, use the left hand to stroke gently from the wrist to the shoulder, and back down again. Repeat several times.

3 Lift the arm and rest the hand on your right shoulder ready to start kneading. Support your partner's wrist with your left hand and use your right to knead lightly the muscles of the upper arm, working from elbow to shoulder.

4 Keeping your partner's hand supported by your shoulder, use the fingers of both hands to continue the kneading.

5 Still holding the arm across the front of your chest with your right hand, do some *effleurage* strokes from the elbow up to the shoulder and back down again. Repeat three times.

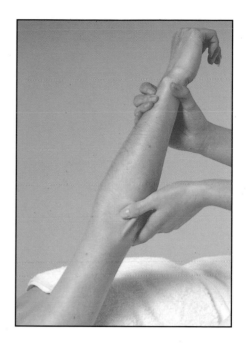

6 Bend your partner's arm and rest the right hand on the left shoulder. Using the outside edge of your hands, do some short, brisk hacking on the outer and under sides of the arm.

7 With your partner's arm still bent, firmly knead the muscles of the upper arm with your right hand, using the left hand to keep your partner's arm stable.

8 Holding the wrist for support with your right hand, work around the outside of the elbow with your fingers and thumb, using smooth circular movements and covering the area thoroughly. As the elbows can get dry you may need some more oil.

9 To encourage further relaxation, hold the wrist with the left hand and do some *effleurage* strokes up and down the top of the forearm. Keep the pressure fairly firm.

10 Repeat these *effleurage* strokes on the inside of the forearm.

11 Rest your partner's elbow back on the towel. Supporting the weight of the lower arm in your left hand, use your right hand to knead the inside of the forearm, starting from the wrist. When you reach the elbow glide back to the wrist to begin again. Repeat three times.

Finish the arm with a few *effleurage* strokes and then massage the hand and wrist (see the following pages) before moving on to the other arm.

HANDS AND WRISTS

1 Support your partner's hand in both hands and gently use the thumbs to knead the palm. This should be a continuous, circular action, with the thumbs alternately applying pressure.

2 Rest your hands under your partner's wrist and use the thumbs to stroke outward around the wrist. Then work with the thumbs up the inner forearm toward the elbow, using circular movements.

3 Turn the hand over, supporting the wrist. Massage gently over the back of the wrist with your thumbs.

4 Stroke up in between the tendons on the back of the hand with your thumbs, from knuckles to wrist, using circles. Repeat twice between each tendon.

5 Sweep the hands alternately up from the wrist toward the elbow, applying a fairly firm pressure with the inside edge of the hands. Repeat several times.

6 Come back down to the hand and stretch the back of the hand, drawing your hands out toward the sides.

7 With one hand make circular pressure movements around each of the three joints on each finger, starting at the tip. When you have worked around all three joints, gently rotate the finger twice. Then gently stretch each finger to release the joints.

8 Raising your partner's lower arm and supporting it with your left hand, clasp your partner's hand with your right hand, and gently rotate it in a half circle, three times in each direction.

9 Still supporting the lower arm, thread your fingers between your partner's and gently bend the wrist backward and forward three times, making sure that the wrist joint is not forced.

10 ABOVE: Finish the arm and hand sequence by stroking the entire length of the arm and hand with some soothing *effleurage* from palm to shoulder.

11 BELOW: Hold your partner's hand between both of your palms for several seconds then release, lowering the arm gently.

Move around your partner to kneel on the other side. Repeat the arm and hand massage on the left side.

CHEST, SHOULDERS AND NECK

Ideally, a chest massage should follow an arm massage and precede a facial massage. It is not only the hours spent sitting hunched over a desk that tighten and contract the chest muscles – clutching a car steering wheel, carrying heavy shopping, and poor posture all have a cumulative effect. Tension in the chest can also exacerbate inflexibility and stiffness in the neck and the shoulders. This sequence includes work to help these problems.

First, check if your partner would be more comfortable with a small cushion or a folded towel under the head. They may or may not, but it is important that the neck should be comfortable. Kneel behind your partner's head to start the sequence.

CHEST

1 Lightly oil the palm of your right hand, and with the flat of the hands placed on the chest, fingers pointing toward your partner's feet, place the left hand on top of the right. You will be doing reinforced *effleurage* on the right side of the chest first.

2 Sweep your hands over the chest, toward and around the right shoulder, keeping the left hand over the right. The movement should be a continuous *effleurage* stroke. You should apply enough pressure to press the chest and shoulder toward the floor, so that they release as you lift off after the stroke. Repeat three times.

3 Continue the *effleurage* stroke, sweeping both hands around and up the right side of the neck.

Repeat the sequence twice more, starting from the centre of the chest.

4 Repeat the sequence once again, but this time finish by bringing both hands up to the jawline with the fingers resting lightly under the centre of the jaw.

5 With both hands, knead the fleshy area in front of the armpit. Pick up and release the muscles, squeezing them from one hand to the other.

6 On the same fleshy area, lightly pinch the surface muscles between the thumb and first finger. Alternate the hands swiftly in a rhythmical action, checking with your partner that there is no discomfort.

Repeat the *effleurage* strokes from the centre of the chest and over the right side of the neck in one continuous movement, to soothe the area you have worked on.

Then repeat the entire sequence on the left side of the chest and neck, lightly oiling the palm of your left hand before you begin.

SHOULDERS AND NECK

1 Place both hands fairly firmly, side by side, over the front of the chest.

2 Sweep them out toward each shoulder with firm *effleurage* strokes, taking them over the shoulders, around under the upper back and up the back of the neck.

3 When you take the movement around the back and the neck gently lift the weight of your partner to give the muscles a gentle stretch.

4 LEFT: With the fingertips, work with circular pressures up the back of the neck to the base of the skull. These should be small, firm rotations which you can feel easing taut muscles. You should spend some time on this area, which is often extremely tense.

5 With loose fists, use the knuckle area to ripple your fingers in semi-circular frictions all over the upper chest. Keep the half circles fairly small and apply quite firm pressure on the fleshier area, but avoid working directly on the collarbone.

6 Bring your loose fists under the upper back and continue to knead behind the shoulders and around the base of the neck.

7 BELOW: Finish with several *effleurage* strokes, starting at the front of the chest and stroking the hands over each shoulder, and up behind the neck.

FACE

The face constantly mirrors our health and emotions. Stress and tension are reflected in a furrowed brow, and lines around the eyes, mouth and jawline. A face massage can soothe away headaches, anxiety and exhaustion and replace them with a feeling of serenity. It improves the circulation, giving the skin a healthy glow.

If your partner wears contact lenses make sure they are removed before you start a face massage. Use a little, light facial oil, and do not let the oil get too near or in the eyes. Keep the hands relaxed. You may be surprised to find that the face is less fragile than it looks and you can apply quite deep pressure without discomfort.

Your partner will probably still prefer to have a small cushion or towel under the head.
Use a towelling hairband to keep the hair off the face.

1 Kneel at the top of your partner's head and lightly oil your palms. With your hands placed over the collarbone, pointing away from you, get ready to begin some gentle *effleurage* strokes.

2 Sweep your hands out across the shoulders, keeping the pressure light.

3 In a continuous movement, bring your hands up around the back of the neck to the nape, pause for a moment, increasing the pressure slightly with the fingertips, then release and lift your hands away.

Repeat the *effleurage* sequence a minimum of three times.

4 Bring your right arm across the front of your partner so the hand supports the left shoulder. Using light, upward strokes, sweep your left hand up from the top of the shoulder, up the side of the neck to the edge of the jaw. Repeat three times.

5 Now repeat this movement on the other side of the neck.

6 Starting with both hands over the front of the chest, fingers pointing toward each other, lightly sweep the flat of one hand up the front of the neck to the jaw, flicking the hand away when you get there. As you flick the first hand away, bring the second up, so you stroke up with alternate hands. Repeat several times.

7 Bring both hands up to the front of the jaw. Alternately sweep one hand and then the other up along the jawline toward the ear. Repeat several times.

8 Briskly tap the length of the jawline using the middle and ring fingers, starting from the centre front and working toward the ears. This should be a stimulating movement, so keep the patting quick and fairly firm.

9 Afterwards, soothe the area by cradling the face gently with both hands. Pause for several moments, then release the hands.

10 Bring your hands up to the forehead. Loosely interlock your fingers, and, using the palms, apply gentle pressure over the forehead. Slowly unlock the fingers to release. Repeat three times.

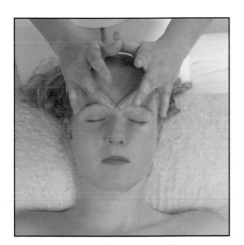

11 Left: Starting with the third finger of each hand placed on the bridge of the nose, stroke out over the brows toward the temples at each side of the forehead. Come up the forehead a little and, starting again with both fingers at the centre front, repeat the strokes out toward the hairline.

Repeat a couple of times more, bringing the fingers higher up the forehead each time, until the whole forehead is covered.

12 To finish, place your hands on each side of your partner's head, and pause for a few seconds before lifting them away.

ABDOMEN AND WAIST

Many people feel exposed and vulnerable when baring their abdomen so you will need to be particularly sensitive to your partner when it comes to this part of the massage. Start with very gentle strokes, but try to be confident, as a gentle touch which is also tentative can feel unnerving for your partner.

Massage of the abdomen calms the nerves and can soothe stomach aches if they are caused by tension, poor digestion or period pains. It also stimulates the digestive organs. You should wait for at least an hour after your partner's meal before giving an abdominal massage.

Kneel beside your partner to do the massage. With a little practice you will find it is possible to tackle both sides from the same position. It helps to start and finish the massage by focusing on your partner's breathing so that your strokes coincide with the intake and exhalation. To begin with, try slowly stroking your hands up from the lower abdomen to the chest on inhalation and down the sides on exhalation.

ABDOMEN

1 Kneel beside your partner, level with the hips. Lightly oil the palms of the hands, and make contact by gently placing your hands together in a diamond shape over the lower abdomen, pointing toward the head. Keep the fingers together and the hands relaxed. Encourage your partner to breathe into the abdomen so you can feel it expand and contract. Work with the breath.

2 Slowly slide your hands up the centre of the abdomen until you reach the ribs, making sure the pressure is even and not too firm.

3 Continue the movement by sweeping the hands out and around the sides of the waist. As you take them out from the ribs toward the sides you can apply a little more pressure, so that you feel the muscles being drawn outward.

4 Return to the starting position with both hands placed on the lower abdomen and repeat this continuous movement several times. Apply more oil as necessary.

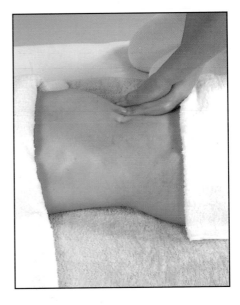

5 Place both hands on your partner's lower abdomen at the right side, ready to circle the navel. Your left hand rests over the right for support.

6 Stroke upward, keeping the left hand over the right, until you reach the ribs. The pressure can be quite firm to stimulate the digestive system. Keep the stroke smooth and continuous.

7 Continue the stroke by bringing your hands across under the ribs, and down the left side of your partner's abdomen. It is important that the direction you work in is up your partner's right side, across and down the left side.

Repeat the navel-circling movement three times, each time returning to the centre of the lower abdomen.

WAIST

1 Begin kneading around the waist area by squeezing and releasing the flesh from one hand to the other. These movements are firm and stimulating.

2, 3 RIGHT AND BELOW RIGHT: Cross your hands over your partner's waist so the palms are grasping the sides of the midriff. Briskly draw them up the side of the waist, uncrossing the hands over the top of the abdomen and turning the palms as they travel down the other side. Draw up again and recross the arms to the original starting position. Keep the speed of this fairly quick and apply firm pressure to draw the flesh up the sides, then lighten your touch across the top of the abdomen. Repeat four times.

4 Starting at the far side of the waist, lightly pinch the flesh between fingers and thumbs with brisk, short stimulating movements. Repeat on the other side of the waist.

5 With loosely cupped hands, lightly cup the side of the waist, keeping the pace fast and stimulating, but at the same time checking that it is not causing discomfort. The action should be enough to increase the flow of blood to the area without hurting.

6 Working on the top of the hip area, squeeze and release the flesh in a kneading movement, using deep and stimulating pressure.

7 LEFT: Finish the massage of the abdomen by repeating the soothing *effleurage* strokes from the beginning of the sequence. End with both hands placed over the centre of the abdomen, fingers pointing toward the head. Hold for a few seconds before lifting off.

BACK OF BODY

Ask your partner to turn over on to their front, ready for you to start work on the back of the legs and buttocks. Rest their head to one side.

LEGS AND BUTTOCKS

The backs of the legs and buttocks offer plenty of scope for massage techniques. Most people can take plenty of firm massage on the larger muscles in the thighs and buttocks. The fleshy parts are ideal for kneading and squeezing and the firmer pressure can feel wonderfully satisfying.

In contrast though, the most gentle *effleurage* can still stimulate other body functions, and poor circulation and a sluggish lymphatic system can be considerably improved with a good leg massage. Tiredness and heaviness in the legs is alleviated and your partner should have renewed energy afterwards.

EFFLEURAGE

1 LEFT: Start by kneeling on one side of your partner's ankles. You should be able to work on both legs from the same side. Begin by working on the leg furthest away from you.

Lightly oil your hands and place them crossed over the back of the left ankle.

2 In a smooth and continuous movement, *effleurage* up the leg, with right hand leading the left. When you get to the back of the knee pause for two seconds.

3 Carry the stroke up the leg and at the top of the thigh cross the hands, keeping the pressure even and light.

4 Bring your hands back down the sides of the leg until you reach the back of the ankle again.

Repeat the sequence three times, each time increasing the pressure slightly on the upward stroke toward the heart.

UPPER LEGS AND BUTTOCKS

1 Move to a kneeling position beside your partner's upper leg. Using a firm kneading movement, squeeze and release the back of the thigh muscles, working up to the buttocks. You should be able to pick up quite a large area of muscle between the hands.

2 With the outside edge of the hands, do some short, sharp hacking movements. Alternate the hands in a quick, repetitive action. Continue the hacking all over the back of the upper leg and the buttocks.

3 Continue working on the upper leg and buttocks, with some cupping. The cupping action should be short and fast to stimulate the whole area.

4 With loose fists, briskly pound the top and outside of the thigh. You can use the backs of your fingers or the outside edge of the fists. Use a firmer knuckling action over the buttock area.

5 Follow this sequence of friction movements with soothing *effleurage* strokes from the back of the knee to the top of the thigh, sweeping out and back down the leg to the knee.

CALVES

1 Move back down to kneel beside your partner's ankles. Lightly oil your hands again if necessary. Start with both hands on the back of your partner's ankle. Smooth your right hand up toward the knee, keeping your left hand on the ankle for support.

2 Continue to stroke the right hand toward the thigh, keeping the pressure light as you reach the back of the knee.

3 As you continue the stroke, taking your right hand up toward the top of the thigh, simultaneously slide your left hand up the lower leg to the back of the knee. Try to make this a flowing movement.

4 Without pausing, bring your right hand in a continuous stroke back down the leg. When you reach the knee you will need to slide the left hand off the knee, so the right hand can continue right down to the ankle again.

5 Start kneading the calf with both hands, working from the ankle up to the knee. Do not knead the back of the knee. Squeeze and release the calf muscle as you go. If your partner's calf muscles are particularly tight this kneading action may feel uncomfortable, so ask your partner if the pressure is right.

Repeat three times, or until you feel confident with the movement.

7 LEFT: Lifting and supporting your partner's leg in the left hand, slide your right hand up from the back of the ankle to the knee. Keep the pressure as firm as is comfortable. Repeat three times. Gently return the leg to rest on the floor.

6 Do some short, sharp pinching movements all over the calf muscle, again checking that you are not hurting your partner.

8 With your thumbs together start at the back of the ankle, and work up the back of the calf to the knee, applying pressure firm enough to release tightness in these muscles. When you reach the back of the knee, lighten the pressure and sweep your hands back down the sides of the leg to the ankle. Repeat three times.

9 To complete the back of the leg massage, repeat the *effleurage* strokes from the beginning of the sequence, stroking the leg from ankle to thigh and back down to the ankle again. Repeat three times to soothe the leg.

Repeat the entire back of leg massage on your partner's other leg, covering the leg you have worked on with a towel to keep the muscles warm.

BACK AND SHOULDERS

The back is an area of great strength and mobility, and it is the main supportive structure of the body. It therefore warrants more attention than most other areas. By working on the back you can reach nerves affecting every part of the body.

Full back massage, with emphasis on the spine and lower back, greatly alleviates effects of stress throughout the body, enhancing physical and psychological well-being. Smooth, flowing strokes stretch the muscles and tissues around contours of the back, and help restore flexibility for health and mobility, whilst stronger strokes along the spinal muscles and over the lower back bring deeper relief to aching or knotted muscles.

You should never massage directly on the spine itself, although working down each side is highly beneficial. Avoid using percussion strokes such as hacking and cupping on the kidneys, which are level with the waistline in the centre of the back.

First, make sure your partner is comfortable, lying face down with arms resting beside the face. Support the forehead with a rolled towel and, if helpful, use a pillow, cushion or rolled towel under the chest. It helps to have hair clear from the back of the neck.

EFFLEURAGE

Kneel beside your partner's right hip and oil your hands. With your first long *effleurage* strokes try to concentrate on finding areas of particular tension and tightness.

1 Starting at the lower back, begin the *effleurage* strokes. With thumbs crossed to connect the hands together, move slowly up the centre of the back, putting firm pressure on the fingertips.

2 Take the stroke up to the top of the back in a continuous movement.

3 Without a pause, separate the hands at the top of the back, sweeping them out and around the shoulders.

4 Continue the stroke, bringing both hands down the sides of the back to the lower back, ready to begin again.

Repeat this *effleurage* sequence three times, oiling your hands each time.

SHOULDERS

1 Using your thumbs each side of the spine, start level with the shoulder blades and make circling pressure movements, working quite firmly into the muscles.

2 Continue working up each side of the spine until you reach the nape of the neck.

3 Carefully bring your partner's arm across the hollow of the back and clasp their right hand with your left to support the arm. The shoulder blade should now stick out slightly. With your right thumb make circular pressure movements over the shoulder area. Strong muscles support the shoulder blade and you can work firmly under the bone itself to release tightness in this area.

4 With your left hand resting over your right to increase the pressure, work in small, circular movements from the base of the neck out over the shoulder.

5 Continue round to the shoulder blade, using firm pressure to release tension in the muscle.

Move to the other side of your partner and repeat these steps on the other shoulder.

BACK

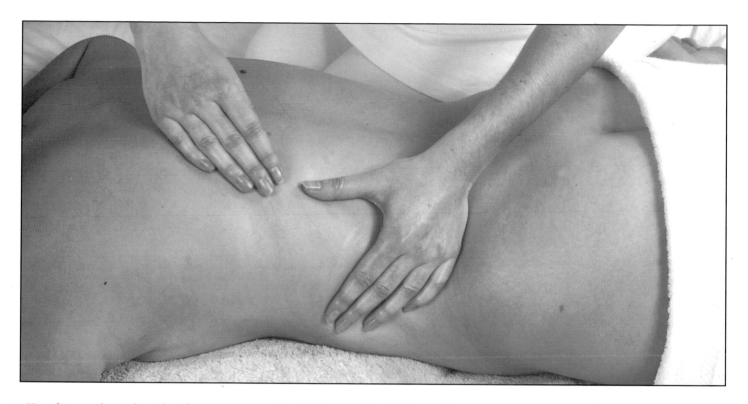

1 Kneeling to the right side of your partner, start to knead the far side of the back firmly with both hands, beginning at the outer sides of the waist. Pick up, roll and release the muscles, alternately pressing one hand toward another. Continue kneading up the back until you reach the shoulders.

Start again at the waist but this time come closer to the spine and repeat the line of kneading up the back.

Repeat the kneading on the near side of the back. You should be able to do this without moving your kneeling position.

2 Using the outer edge of the hands, briskly and rhythmically hack from the lower back up to the shoulders, but avoid the bony shoulder blade. Try to visualize each side of the back divided into three sections, so you cover the whole back thoroughly.

3 Start cupping from the lower back up the back and across the shoulders. The action should be quick, with alternate hands striking the back briskly.

4 Repeat the *effleurage* strokes from the beginning of the sequence to soothe the back. Repeat several times.

SPINE

1 LEFT: With loose fists, and thumbs crossed for support, push the top of the hands up each side of the spine to the napc of the neck.

2 RIGHT: Uncurl the fingers when you get to the nape and sweep them back down the sides of the back. Repeat three times.

3 Starting at the lower back, place the thumbs on either side of the spine, resting your hands either side of the back. Rotate the thumbs in small circles, travelling up the sides of the spine until you reach the hairline. Use firm pressure. Reverse the movement, circling your thumbs back down each side of the spine.

4 Starting at the lower back, use loose knuckles, crossing your thumbs over each other for support, to work up either side of the spine and back down again. Repeat twice.

5 Using the backs of your hands and starting at the lower back, push up either side of the spine to just above the waistline. Then sweep your hands outward and back down around the hips. Repeat three times.

6 To finish the massage, repeat the *effleurage* strokes from the beginning of the sequence, starting at the lower back, up the back, around the shoulders and down again to the lower back, in a continuous sweeping movement.

SELF MASSAGE

✦◦✦

A simple, effective self massage can do wonders to ease away tension and restore energy after a stressful, tiring day. After a shower or bath, massaging the body with lotions and oils is very relaxing and helps keep the skin in glowing condition. You can use self massage to target particular aches and pains or areas of tension, for relief just where you need it. The beauty of self massage is you can do it to suit your needs and moods at any time – to unwind in the evening or to energize yourself in the morning.

SHOULDERS

1 Sitting upright, start from the base of the neck and press down with your fingers along the top of the shoulders. As you reach the bony part of the shoulder, slide your hand back to the base of the neck, and repeat the pressing at least three times. Finish by stroking firmly from neck to shoulder and then repeat on the other side of the neck.

2 Use the fingertips of both hands to make small, circular movements, working up the back of the neck. Gentle circular movements, where you can feel yourself easing muscular tightness, are better than direct, static pressures on this area. Continue up and around the base of the skull.

3 Knead each shoulder with a firm, squeezing action, rolling the flesh between your fingers and the ball of the hand. Repeat several times on each side.

4 With your hand in a loose fist, pummel your shoulder lightly, keeping the wrist and elbow relaxed. Use light, springy movements to stimulate the area. Repeat on the other shoulder.

ARMS

1 Stroke firmly up the arm from the wrist to the shoulder, returning with a lighter touch. Repeat the stroke several times on different parts of the arm.

2 Pressing your fingers toward the palm of the hand, knead up the arm from the elbow to the shoulder. Cover the area thoroughly, working right around the arm.

3 Starting from the wrist, knead up the forearm toward the elbow, this time using your thumb to make circular movements.

4 With thumb and fingers, make circular pressures around the elbow. First, work around the far side of the elbow with your working arm coming over the top of the arm you are massaging, then bend that arm up and work from the inside of your elbow. You may need more oil for dry elbows.

5 RIGHT: Gently but briskly pat your upper arm, or use some gentle cupping. Follow with some *effleurage* stroking up and down the whole arm again to finish. Work on the hand before massaging the other arm.

HANDS

1 Squeeze the hand firmly, spreading the palm laterally. Cover the whole of the hand, fingers and wrist.

2 Using circular pressure, squeeze each finger joint between your finger and thumb. Then hold the base of each finger and pull the finger gently to stretch it, sliding your grip up to the top of the finger in a continuous movement.

3 With circular thumb pressures, work up each of the furrows between the bones in the hand, from the knuckle to the wrist. When you have covered each furrow, smooth the hand by stroking.

4 Turn the hand over to work on the palm. Cover the area with circular thumb pressures, paying particular attention to the heel of the hand and the wrist. Follow this with some deeper, static pressures all over the palm.

5 Finish by stroking the palm of one hand with the other. This can be quite a firm stroke, working from the tips of the fingers to the wrist, leading with the pressure from the heel of the hand.

Stroke back to the fingers and repeat twice more, each time using slightly less pressure. Finally, stroke the inside of the wrist.

Repeat the whole of the arm and hand massage sequences on the other side.

BACK AND ABDOMEN

1 Lie on your back, clasp your knees and gently rock backward and forward to massage the lower back, buttocks and hip joints and gently stretch out the vertebrae.

2 LEFT: Bend your knees up and use some gentle *petrissage* to knead the whole of the abdominal area. When you have finished kneading, place both hands flat on the centre of the abdomen, fingers pointing slightly together, and pause for a few moments. Then smooth your hands outward over the hips and thighs in a long, slow, moulding movement.

BUTTOCKS, HIPS
AND THIGHS

1 Kneel up and pummel your hips and buttocks, using a clenched fist and keeping your wrists flexible.

2 With the thumb and fingers, squeeze and release the muscles firmly and slowly, working from the top of the thigh over the buttock. Repeat on the left side.

3 Use both hands to squeeze and release the muscles on the front and side of the thigh, kneading the entire upper leg. Repeat on the other side.

4 Starting at the knee, stroke up the thigh with both hands to soothe the leg.

LEGS

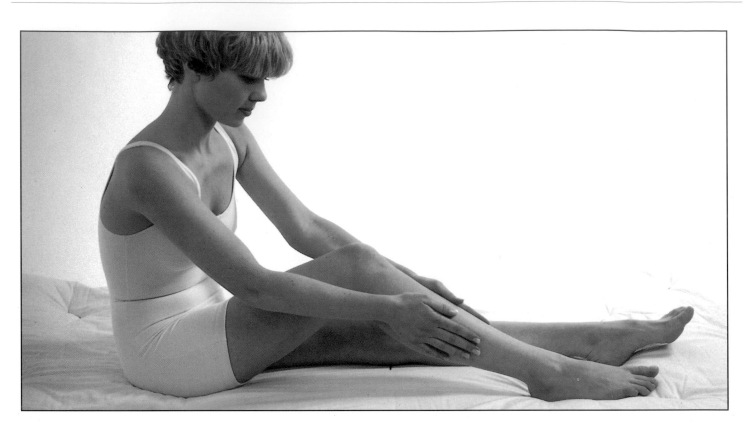

1 Sitting down, with one leg raised slightly, stroke the leg with both hands from ankle to thigh. Begin the stroke as close to the ankle as you can reach.

Repeat several times, moving around the leg slightly each time to stroke a different part.

2 Massage the knee, stroking around the outside of the kneecap to begin with, then using circular pressure with the fingertips to work around the kneecap more firmly.

3 Knead the calf muscle with both hands, using a firm *petrissage* to loosen any tension in the muscle.

4 Continue the kneading on the thigh, working over the top and outside areas with alternate hands. Whilst the leg is still raised, do some soothing *effleurage* strokes up the back of the leg from ankle to hip.

Continue with the foot massage (opposite) before repeating all the steps on the other leg.

FEET

1 Sitting down and leaning back, raise a leg, supporting the weight with your hands. Rotate the right ankle five times in each direction.

2 Gently bring your foot over the other leg. With one hand on top of the foot and one underneath, stroke up the foot from toes to ankle. Repeat three times.

3 With the thumbs, apply circular pressure over the ball of the foot. Work in lines from the inside of the foot to the outer edge. Repeat three times.

4 Supporting the foot with one hand, continue the circular pressures over the raised instep, working from the inner to the outer edge. Repeat three times.

5 Still holding the foot with one hand, make a loose fist with the other and firmly rotate your fist over the instep. Work thoroughly into the arch.

6 Massage each toe individually. Slowly stretch the toe between the thumb and finger, and pull gently, moving your fingers up the toe each time, until you reach the tip.

7 Repeat the *effleurage* strokes of the foot, with one hand over and one under the foot, working from toes to ankle, several times.

Repeat the leg and foot massage sequence on the other side.

MASSAGE AND EXERCISE

Professional sports people value massage very highly, not least because it works on several levels. Used before exercise it can prepare the body for the increase in activity, not only by warming and loosening the muscles and joints (increasing their flexibility and helping to prevent cramp and injuries), but also by stimulating the system, both physically and mentally. This is the key to improved performance. After an exercise session, massage speeds up the elimination of waste products (in particular lactic acid) by stimulating the lymphatic system. The accumulation of these waste products during exercise is the cause of much of the stiffness and pain experienced afterwards.

STRAINS AND SPRAINS

A burning sensation under the skin is likely to indicate that muscles, fibres or ligaments have been strained – stretched beyond their natural limits. This is often the result of exercising without an adequate warm-up routine or over-exertion. A routine of pre-exercise massage and limbering will help to prevent strains. Gently massaging the affected area will also help to speed recovery.

Sprains are more serious and are caused by violent wrenching of a joint, most commonly the ankle, wrist or knee. The surrounding muscles, ligaments and tendons may also be damaged and the affected area may be extremely painful and swollen. Apply an ice-pack or cold compress for 15–20 minutes to reduce the swelling. When it is removed you can start to massage the area gently (as shown opposite), taking care not to work directly on the swelling. Rest the ankle as much as possible and use a support bandage.

A serious sprain should always be checked by a doctor in case a bone has been fractured, and a sprained knee always requires medical attention.

CRAMP

You do not have to be a fitness fanatic to suffer from cramp. On the contrary, it is usually under-used or ill-prepared muscles which go into cramp. It does not even take movement to set it off: the searing pain of cramp can occur in the middle of the night, when the reduced circulation has caused muscles to contract. Frequent cramps may indicate generally poor circulation or a deficiency of calcium or salt. Massage will increase the blood circulation to alleviate the pain. You should also try to stretch out the affected muscle.

BACKACHE

Back strain is the most common source of debilitating pain. Most sports put increased strain on the legs, buttocks and back. Previous injuries can make the back prone to recurrent pain. Awkward, inappropriate or excessive exercise can also cause trouble. You should never subject the back to unnecessary strain. With regular and thorough back massage (particularly before exercise) the likelihood of injury is reduced. If, however, you want a quick warm-up for the back, or an after-exercise sequence, follow the instant back and shoulder massage. Always consult a doctor, osteopath or chiropractor if in any doubt about the seriousness of a back problem.

WITH OR WITHOUT OILS

You do not always have oil at hand, and it certainly is not crucial for massaging unexpected strains, sprains and cramps. If you do have some light vegetable oil nearby, all the better, but do not worry if you have not.

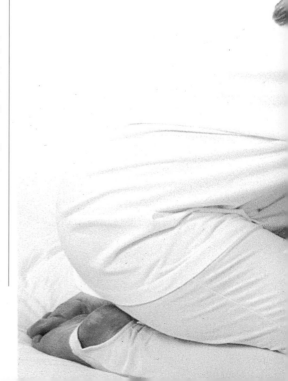

ANKLE STRAIN OR SPRAIN

1 ABOVE and BELOW: Avoid working directly on the swollen area. Start with gentle *effleurage* strokes working from the knee toward the thigh. Massaging in the direction of the lymph nodes in the groin will help drain away the fluids that have accumulated around the joint. Lightly stroke back to the knee. Repeat several times.

2 Help your partner to bend the affected leg. Continue the *effleurage* strokes on the lower leg, this time working from the ankle to the knee, alternating your hands. Repeat several times, then gently squeeze the calves with one hand, with the other supporting the foot.

3 Concentrating on the ankle area, stroke extremely gently all around the ankle with short, upward movements. Check that this is not causing discomfort.

CALF CRAMP

1 With your partner lying face down and the foot supported across your leg or a small pillow, gradually apply direct thumb pressure into the belly of the cramped calf muscle for 8–10 seconds.

2 Do some *effleurage* strokes, working from ankle to thigh and back down again.

SELF-HELP STRETCH

A good way of dealing with calf cramp is to sit down with the affected leg straight and stretch the toes toward you. Hold this position for 8 seconds and then release. Repeat a few times, until the spasm seems to be lessening. Then knead your calf muscle using firm pressure. When the muscle feels more relaxed switch to *effleurage* strokes, working up the leg.

HAMSTRING CRAMP

1 With your partner lying face down and the ankles raised on a small pillow or cushion, begin massaging up the back of the thigh using alternate hands in slow, rhythmical stroking movements.

Then apply static pressure to the middle of the thigh with the thumbs, holding for 8–10 seconds.

2 Firmly knead the calf muscle. Squeeze, press and release the muscle using one hand after the other. Finally, do some soothing *effleurage* strokes up from ankle to thigh and back down again.

HAMSTRING SELF-HELP STRETCH

Lie down flat, with the affected leg raised and the other knee bent. Stretch the muscle by pulling the thigh gently toward the chest.

Then firmly stroke up the back of your thigh for 8–10 seconds. Start to knead the back of the thigh until you feel the muscles begin to relax. Finally, stroke over the area to soothe it.

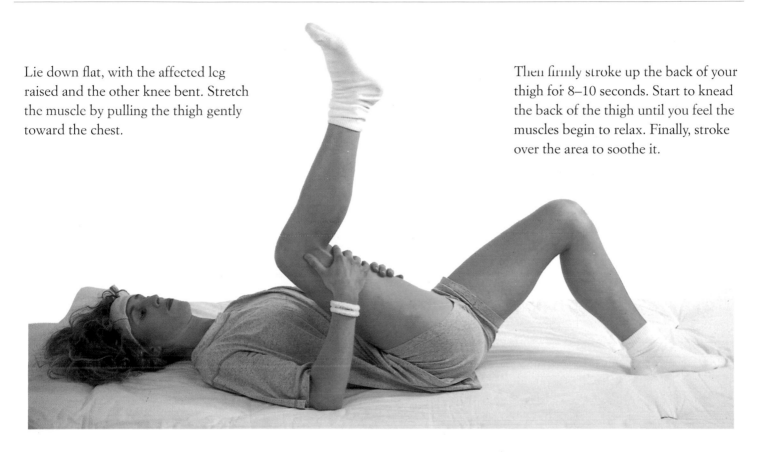

TENNIS OR GOLFER'S ELBOW

1 Support your partner's wrist in one hand and use soothing *effleurage* strokes along both sides of the arm, stroking from the wrist to the elbow and back again. Repeat several times.

2 Rest your partner's hand against your side. Continue working up from the wrist to the elbow and back, making small, circular movements with both thumbs, paying particular attention to the muscles in the forearm.

3, 4 Secure your partner's hand in yours, and with the other hand supporting the elbow, flex the elbow forward, bringing the hand back to give the tendons that attach to the bones a good stretch.

BABY MASSAGE

A newborn baby instinctively responds to touch, and massage between mother and baby is a marvellous way of enhancing the natural bonding. All babies have this powerful sensitivity to being caressed and cuddled. Watch how a baby tightly curls its hands or toes as soon as something touches them. There is no fixed sequence for massaging a baby. Keep the movements gentle and flowing. The simple action of gently stroking a baby will strengthen the natural bonding, and soothe and reassure the baby too. Massage has been shown to help calm difficult or colicky babies, and alleviate wind and other digestive problems. It may also build resistance to coughs and colds. Use a little light vegetable oil which is easily absorbed, such as sweet almond or sunflower, taking care to avoid the eyes.

GETTING COMFORTABLE

Lay the baby gently on the back on a warm, soft towel between your legs, or on your lap, whichever is most comfortable. Pour about 5 ml (1 tsp) sweet almond oil into a small dish. Make sure your hands are warm and that the room is quiet, very warm and there are no draughts. After a baby's bathtime is ideal.

WORKING ON BABY'S FRONT

1 Slowly and gently, smooth a little of the oil all over the front of the baby's body, shoulders to feet, avoiding the face. Lightly stroke down the chest and abdomen, with the tips of your fingers. This is a delightful stroke which can be used to calm a baby at anytime.

2 Keeping the pressure very light, smooth both hands over the abdomen in continuous, circular strokes, working up the baby's right side, across and down the baby's left side. Keep the movement continuous by lifting your left hand when your arms cross. Repeat these circular strokes several times.

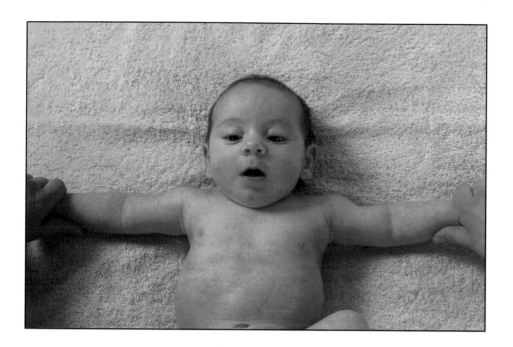

3 LEFT: Gently stretch out both arms to the side, spreading the hands and fingers if the baby will let you. Gently squeeze out along the arms, then massage the wrist and palms with light, circular thumb movements. Finish by stretching out each finger with a slight pull.

4 Move on to the legs and feet, working on one leg at a time. Support the leg with both hands and gently squeeze and release the fleshy part of the thigh. Then, supporting the leg with one hand, stroke the leg from the knee to the thigh and back down again.

5 RIGHT: Move your supporting hand down to behind the ankle. Gently smooth the palm of your other hand over the top of the foot from toe to ankle and back again. When you get to the toes, very gently stretch each one in turn.

Repeat steps 4 and 5 on the baby's other leg.

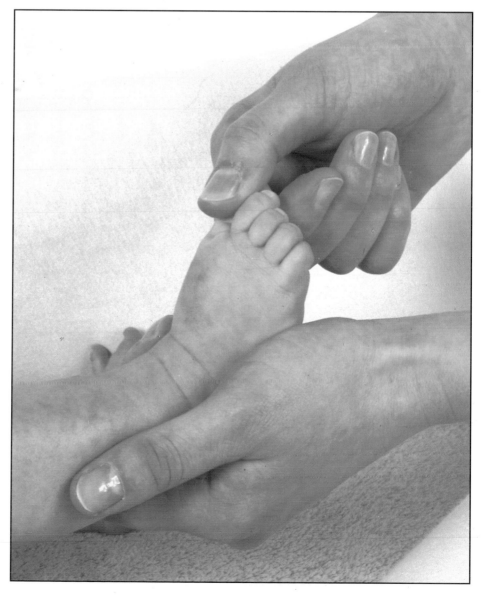

WORKING ON BABY'S BACK

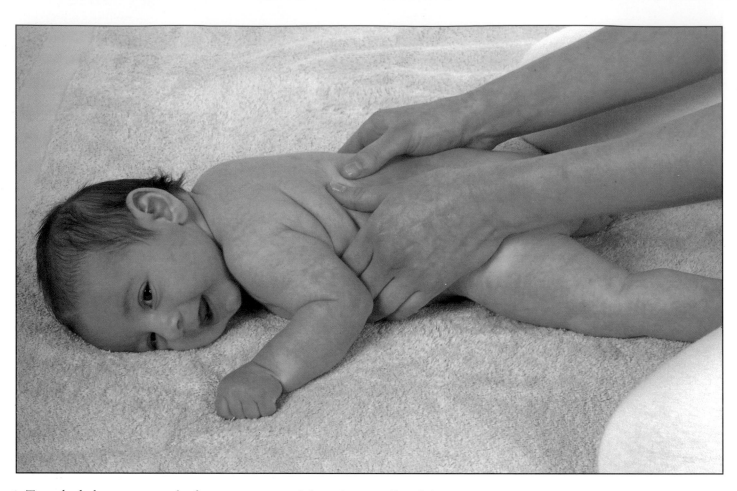

1 Turn the baby over on to the front. Begin by stroking up the whole back to distribute a little oil. Take your strokes around the sides as well and then up the legs, back and out over the arms. Gentle massage on the back like this is particularly soothing because of its calming effect on the spinal nerves.

2 Gently knead and squeeze the buttocks to stimulate the circulation. Make a loose fist and rotate over the buttocks, in circular movements.

3 Alternating your hands, one over the other, gently stroke up one side of the back to the shoulders and down again. Repeat on the other side of the back.

4 Bring both hands around the sides of the upper body, and use your thumbs to massage gently up the back to the base of the neck, and down again. Include some gentle massage with the thumbs on the shoulders.

5 To finish, repeat the feather strokes used at the beginning of the massage, working all over the back from neck to buttocks.

MASSAGE FOR OLDER PEOPLE

As we get older, painful, stiff joints, rheumatism and other signs of wear and tear become all too common. There are many ways to minimize the discomfort that the aging process brings. Good nutrition and remaining as active as possible are as crucial as ever, and massage can help in reducing pain, alleviating stiffness and retaining mobility. It is not necessary to lie down – sitting on a chair is fine for massage of the neck and shoulders, and you can raise the leg on a stool for a leg, foot and ankle massage.

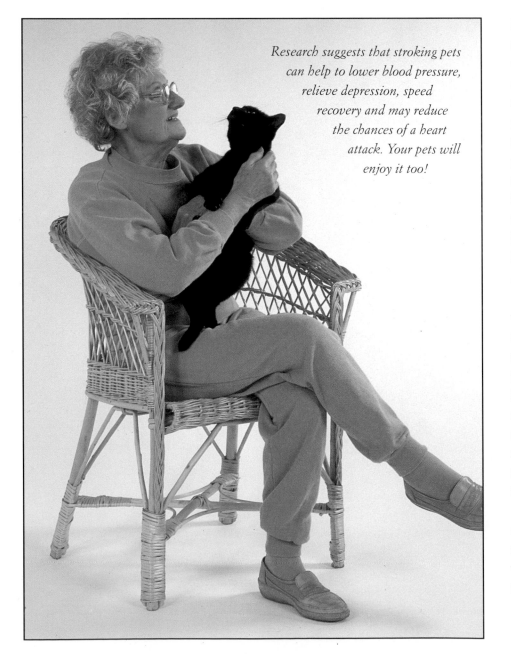

Research suggests that stroking pets can help to lower blood pressure, relieve depression, speed recovery and may reduce the chances of a heart attack. Your pets will enjoy it too!

Many older people suffer from aches and pains brought on by cold damp weather. A warm bath using aromatic essential oils such as lavender or sandalwood can comfort, soothe and relax you. Follow the bath with a gentle massage, and you will make headway in practising self-help. Massage stiff joints such as at wrists, knees, ankles and the hip. If the joint is affected by rheumatoid arthritis, massaging above and below the swollen area can relieve pain by relaxing the surrounding muscles. Avoid any swollen or inflamed areas.

The general wear and tear of joints which comes with aging is called osteoarthritis, and usually affects hips and knees in particular. Because the pain is often caused by the surrounding muscles, rather than the joint itself, massage can help to soothe the spasm and relieve pain. So long as the area is not swollen or inflamed you can massage the joint itself, working gently into the area which hurts most.

Massage can help to fulfil the deepseated need for touch and communication, bringing psychological as well as physiological benefits, and contributing to a well-balanced lifestyle.

1 Start by gently resting your thumbs on the base of your partner's skull, just under the bony part. Relax your hands around each side of the head. Slowly and without too much pressure, slide your thumbs up through the hair, until you get halfway up the back of the head. Repeat three times, from the base of the skull to halfway up the head, to stimulate the nervous system.

2 Place the thumbs on the back of the neck and press gently, starting at the base of the skull and working down in a straight line toward the shoulders. This will loosen stiffness and relieve tension in the area. Repeat three times, down the centre each time.

3 With your hand on either side of the neck, gently knead the tops of the shoulders, squeezing and releasing the muscles between your thumbs and fingers. Repeat three times, the full length of the shoulder.

4 Bring your hands lower down the back near each shoulder blade, and use thumbs and fingers to massage upward over the shoulder blades, right up to the top of the shoulders. Slightly push into the back and release. Repeat from start to finish three times. You can vary the movement slightly by rotating the fingers as you work up.

5 Use any of the massage or self-massage techniques for the hands or feet, but avoid working directly on any joints inflamed with arthritis. Work above and below a swelling and then stroke up the limb toward the nearest lymph node. This stimulates the elimination of waste products and reduces inflammation.

6 If there are no signs of inflammation, you can use circular thumb movements all over the palm, then turn the hand over and work along each finger to the tip. Gently stretch each joint as far as it will go without causing pain, and then soothe the whole hand with firm strokes toward the wrist.

THE SENSUAL TOUCH

In the right circumstances, with a softly lit room, relaxing music, and using some of the more aphrodisiac essential oils such as rose, patchouli, neroli or sandalwood, a massage can be a highly pleasurable and sensual experience, relaxing the body and arousing the senses. Intuition will play a larger part in a sensual massage, as you discover which areas have the strongest impact on your partner's senses.

1 With your partner lying on their front, start by resting your hands gently on the back of their shoulder blades. Fan the palms out across the back, sweeping your hands out and around over the shoulders.

2 Knead firmly along the top of the shoulders, squeezing and releasing the muscles each side of the neck and shoulders. As the shoulders start to relax, work more deeply into the muscles.

BELOW: The back can be extremely sensitive to touch of many different kinds. Try sitting back to back and moving gently together, feeling the contours of your partner's back against yours. Press against each other so that you can feel the pelvis, the spine and the shoulders. Rest your head back on your partner's shoulder, and enjoy the feeling of your backs exchanging warmth and energy. Hold for a count of 10 and repeat on the other side.

3 Check that your partner's head is still comfortable then, beginning at the nape of the neck, let your thumbs gently stroke down each side of the spine. When you get to the lower back return up each side of the spine, this time working with slightly more pressure and rotating the thumbs to release muscular tension. Work up and down the spine two or three times.

4 Move round so your partner can rest their head on your thighs, and with long, *effleurage* strokes, massage the length of the back from the neck right down to the buttocks and back up the sides of the trunk. Repeat three times.

5 Starting at the lower back, gently stroke up either side of the spine, making light feathery strokes with your fingertips. Repeat three times, making the strokes lighter each time, until they can barely be felt.

6 LEFT: Massage the lower back with some kneading. Using the flat, and in particular the heel, of the hand, knead the buttocks, then come back to the start and work over a different area. The nerves that cross this area relate to the man's groin, and the woman's uterus. The buttocks themselves are highly erogenous areas.

7 Curling your third and fourth fingers under, place your hands toward the top of the upper legs and circle your first and second fingers outward, one hand alternating with the other. This should be a slow, leisurely stroke with varying pressure.

  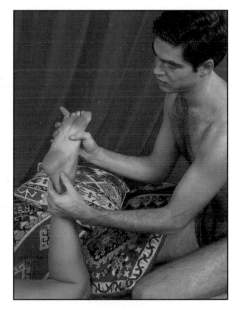

8 Support your partner's leg across your thigh and circle your thumbs over the calf, alternating the thumbs and applying firm pressure.

9 Raise your partner's foot, supporting its weight in your hands. Knead the instep firmly, using the thumbs to apply the pressure. Work all over the ball of the foot up toward the big toe.

10 Support your partner's foot in one hand, and place the thumb of that hand firmly over the centre of the instep. This has a wonderful, calming effect. With the thumb and first finger of the other hand, stroke around the ankle using circular movements.

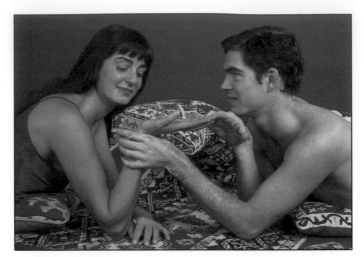

11 At this stage, lie down facing each other, making sure you are both comfortable and well supported with plenty of cushions. Gently caress your partner's hands.

12 Gently stretch and release your partner's wrists, by flexing the hand backward and forwards. Softly stroke the inside of the palm with your fingers. Repeat on the other hand.

13 Gently massage each finger, beginning with the thumb or little finger and working from the base joint to the tip. Try squeezing, rubbing and circular movements, and gentle pulling.

14 Supporting your partner's elbow in one hand, use the other to caress and stroke the inside of the wrist just below the thumb, which is a particularly sensitive area. Continue working over the whole of the wrist area, using gentle, circular thumb movements. Repeat on the other wrist.

15 LEFT: With feather strokes, use your fingers to stroke up the soft inner arm. This is a highly sensitive area when lightly touched and the effect is both stimulating and relaxing. Repeat on the other arm.

16 LEFT: Use long *effleurage* strokes up and down the inner thigh area. Then massage closer to the highly erogenous region of the groin.

17 With a feathery touch, stroke across the shoulders and up the neck, covering the sides, front and back. You can run your fingers up through the hair as well.

Spend more time caressing the base of the neck, which arouses strong, sexual responses.

18 RIGHT: Finally, trace around the ear with your fingers, starting at the outside and circling toward the centre. Continue with soft, pinching movements around the outside edge and on the lobe, where you will be triggering sexual responses from the adrenal gland and sexual organs.

INSTANT MASSAGE

Sometimes, the idea of having tension in your shoulders and neck massaged away, without stopping to find the right place and the time to undress, is a particularly tempting one. There is increasing interest in learning how to do a shoulder massage with the minimum of disruption, especially in offices. Even at home, there are times when nothing is better than someone giving you a ten-minute shoulder and neck massage.

1 Ask your partner to sit astride a chair facing the back. You can offer a folded towel or cushion for comfort. Standing behind your partner, begin by leaning on your forearms so that your weight presses down gently on to the fleshy part of the shoulders.

2 With your partner leaning forward, use *effleurage* strokes from the bottom of the shoulder blades, up the back and out over the top of the shoulders to finish at the top of the arms. Repeat four times.

3 With a firm *petrissage*, use both hands to knead out along the shoulders from the sides of the neck to the upper arms.

4 Starting as far down the lower back as you can, work up the spine with small, circular frictions. Continue up the sides of the neck to the base of the skull, then glide back down and work up again, this time moving out over the shoulders as you reach the top.

5 Moving around to the side of the chair, tilt your partner's head forward and support it with one hand. With the thumb and finger of the other hand, grasp the neck firmly and massage with circular movements, working up the neck and into the base of the skull.

6 Working from behind your partner again, massage the back of the head with both hands coming over the forehead and down to the temples with small, circular pressures, moving the scalp against the skull. Lighten your touch at the temples.

7 First on one side and then the other, do some hacking across the fleshy parts of the shoulders and upper back, using the outer side of your hands to make short, brisk movements. Keep the wrists and hands very relaxed.

 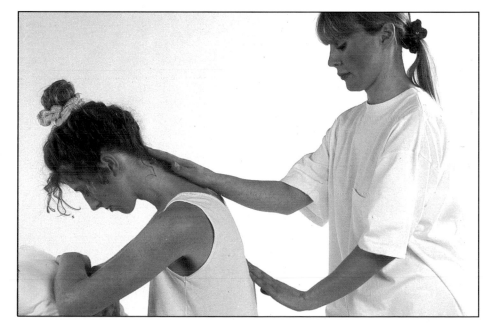

8 Continue with a brisk cupping action across each shoulder, working on one side at a time.

9 RIGHT: Finish the sequence by gently stroking down the entire back with one hand following the other. Repeat five times with each stroke getting lighter.

REFLEXOLOGY

ost people enjoy massage to the feet – one of the most sensitive parts of the body. All foot massage is beneficial and relaxing, but reflexology provides a more specific method of working to diagnose problems and stimulate health in the whole body. It is based on the principle that the body can be divided into ten vertical zones, each corresponding to an area of the foot, so that the feet are, in effect, a map of the body. Reflexology can be an effective way of relieving pain and helping to restore the body's natural well-being.

FOOT CHARTS

The foot charts are only guidelines for interpretation. When you find a tender or congested part of the foot you may look for that part on the charts and see approximately which reflex the tenderness lies on. This is only a rough guide because every pair of feet are different and will not be the same shape as your chart. Also, the charts are two-dimensional and your body is three-dimensional and therefore the reflexes on your feet reflect this. In reality your organs overlap each other, whereas the charts are much simplified for clarity, to give an idea of where things are.

CROWN

CERVICAL

SPINE

THORACIC

LUMBAR

SACRUM

COCCYX

SPINAL REFLEX

SCIATIC/LOWER BACK

LOWER LYMPH & FALLOPIAN TUBES OR VAS DEFERENS

CHEST/BREAST

OVARIES OR TESTES

ARMS   HIP/KNEE

LEGS

PELVIS

OUTER FOOT

LOWER LYMPH & FALLOPIAN TUBES OR VAS DEFERENS

CHEST/BREAST

UPPER LYMPH

TOP OF FOOT

SCIATIC/LOWER BACK/RECTUM

LOWER LYMPH & FALLOPIAN TUBES OR VAS DEFERENS

CHEST/BREAST

UTERUS OR PROSTATE

PELVIC FLOOR

BLADDER

PELVIS

INNER FOOT

THE BACKGROUND

The concept of using the body's reflexes for therapeutic purposes is not new – the early Chinese developed the technique of acupressure thousands of years ago. This provided the basis of knowledge about reflex zones and points and connections between different parts of the body. We know that the early Chinese, Japanese, Indians and Egyptians worked on the feet to promote good health, and many of the long-established principles developed by these civilizations are used today.

Reflexology as it is known today is based largely on the work of Dr William Fitzgerald and Eunice Ingham. Dr Fitzgerald devised his own system of acupressure points which produced an analgesic effect when stimulated. He found that the body could be divided into ten zones running from the top of the head to the tips of the toes, and that everything occurring in a specific zone of the body could affect the organs and other parts of the body in that zone.

The theory was refined in the 1930s by a young physiotherapist called Eunice Ingham, who introduced a special grip technique and the action of the thumb on the foot and developed a more intricate zone system. The system has been further refined into the internationally recognized method now practised.

Modern reflexology offers tremendous health benefits: it reduces stress, improves circulation, cleanses the body of impurities and toxins, and can revitalize energy levels.

RIGHT FOOT

LEFT FOOT

KEY

Ag Adrenal glands
e Ears
Et Eustachian tubes
Ee Eye/Ear helper
E Eyes
Gb Gall bladder
H Heart
K Kidneys
Lg Lachrymal glands
Lv Liver
L Lungs
M Mouth
N Neck
n Nose
Ps Pancreas
Pt Para-thyroid
Pg Pituitary glands
SN Side of neck
Sp Spleen
S Stomach
Tb Trachea bronchi oesophagus
th Thymus
T Thyroid

BASIC REFLEXOLOGY TECHNIQUES

THE TREATMENT

Advanced diagnosis is a trained professional skill but some basic techniques can easily be used in a foot massage. You can also use them to work on your own feet, sitting with one ankle supported on the opposite thigh.

The following points will ensure a relaxing session:

❧ Work with your partner's foot in your lap or supported at the right height with cushions or bolsters.

❧ Your partner can sit in a comfortable chair with a footstool or small table to raise the feet.

❧ Ensure the back, neck and knees are supported, so your partner can relax.

❧ The massage is given without oil. Dust the feet with talcum powder or work directly on the skin, if you prefer.

❧ Make sure your nails are short and well filed.

The following sequence of movements offers an introduction to reflexology. It is necessary to hold the foot correctly so that all points can be reached and stimulated with ease. The hands will swap their holding and working roles according to the part of the foot to be reached, so practise with both hands.

Apart from proper holding, the main principle to observe is leverage. Use the rest of the fingers in opposition to the working thumb to obtain more effective contact with the foot, or the thumb in opposition to the working finger in finger walking.

GREETING THE FEET

BELOW: The initial contact with the feet sets the tone for the whole treatment. Gently holding both feet relaxes them, allows you to learn about your partner and establishes a relationship.

ANKLE ROTATION

Begin with some relaxing movements. Stabilize the ankle by holding the right foot in the left hand, supporting the heel.

Gently wrap the fingers of the working hand below the base of the toes. Rotate the foot several times in each direction.

ANKLE STRETCH

Using the same hold as for the ankle rotation, stretch the foot back and forth slowly to release tension in the Achilles tendon, taking care not to force the ankle joint. Then work all around the ankle, applying pressure. This area corresponds to the reproductive organs, legs and lower back.

SOLAR PLEXUS RELAXATION

Place both thumbs on the solar plexus point located in the centre of the ball of the foot where there is a little indentation. This is a good relaxation exercise, particularly if your partner is very tense or nervous. You can also work on both feet simultaneously.

THUMB HOOKING

Place the outer corner of the thumb on a reflex point, with the thumb flat. Bend the thumb at the first joint to apply pressure, and pull back across the point. Use the other fingers for counter-pressure and raise the wrist to increase the pressure. Hooking is used to stimulate points that are too small for the walking technique (see right), such as the pituitary point, the solar plexus and lymph drainage points, and any point of soreness.

THUMB WALKING

This is the principal technique for covering large areas. Thumb walking starts in the same way as the thumb hook and then the outside corner of the flexed thumb is rocked slightly forward. Maintain steady pressure as the thumb walks, avoiding an "on-off" movement. Press along the diaphragm line under the ball of the foot, then stimulate the spinal area along the main arch of the foot from the heel to the big toe.

FINGER WALKING

1, 2 This technique is used to work on the top of the feet. The principle is the same as for thumb walking: flexing the first finger joint and rocking forward. With the holding hand, support and spread the toes, and push on the ball of the foot with the thumb of the working hand to provide leverage. Finger walk from the base of the little toe up to the ankle. Begin again, walking between the troughs of the next toes, toward the inside of the foot.

This helps to relieve tension in the chest and lung area, and the areas for lymph drainage and vocal chords which are located between the big toe and second toe at the top of the foot.

STROKING THE FEET

LEFT: Using alternate hands, stroke the foot softly from the ankles to the toes to smooth and relax the whole area of each foot.

DESSERT STROKE

RIGHT: Take the foot in both hands and slide the hands gently up and down. Dessert strokes are enjoyable and can be used throughout the treatment to soothe and relax your partner after a sensitive reflex has been worked on. Always end the session with dessert strokes to rebalance the whole foot.

FOR AN EFFECTIVE TREATMENT:

❧ Explore the foot with the outside edge of the thumb, by the nail, but be careful not to dig with your nail.
❧ Make regular eye contact with your partner to check responses to specific pressures and to detect painful or sensitive areas.

❧ Pay extra attention to sensitive areas, which may feel granular, as these are usually due to calcification or deposits of lymph fluid. Work on them thoroughly to disperse the blockages and release energy in the zone.
❧ Work on each area of the foot several times and make sure that no area is left out.

❧ Work through each foot once to find sensitive areas and then a second time to reintegrate the foot and body.
❧ Join the movements and areas of the foot with dessert strokes.
❧ Always keep contact with at least one hand.
❧ Knuckling can be used to cover large areas of the foot.

alexander technique

alexander technique
alexander techn

People tend to associate the Alexander technique with relaxation, alternative medicine, body massage and with "posture". Yet it is actually much more than that.

One way towards a clearer understanding of the technique is to begin by stating what it is not. The Alexander technique does not train its teachers to make a medical diagnosis of their students, nor does it focus on any division between the mind and body. The technique believes in the indivisibility of the two and in their psycho-physical unity. Above all, the technique's main objective is to encourage people to use themselves, their bodies and minds more effectively in their day-to-day lives.

The technique's preventive role is an efficient tool which maintains tone and general well-being. It also helps to improve posture and relieve related pain. In fact it can assist people with stress-related illnesses such as respiratory and gastro-intestinal problems, as well as psychosomatic conditions. It can help those who suffer from psychological distress, such as depression, as well as facilitating recovery from accidents and injuries. The technique can even assist people with mechanical problems, such as frozen shoulder, tennis elbow and arthritis. Above all, it helps promote muscle tone and general well-being while encouraging poise and flexibility. The technique aids the well in addition to those with ailments.

the alexander technique principles

Once you start studying the technique, it quickly becomes clear that it helps you in all kinds of ways that other alternative remedies do not. That is not because it is superior, but because of its key agenda. As shown here, it helps us focus on our minds and bodies in new ways, and on aspects of our being that we might take for granted. The technique gets us back to basics.

Primary Control

"Misuse" occurs by contracting the muscles of the neck and pulling the head back and down into the shoulders. This has the twin effect of actually compressing the spine and narrowing and shortening the stature, creating tensions throughout the body. It is definitely something to be avoided.

Frederick Matthias Alexander discovered that the relationship between the head, the neck and the back, or "primary control", mechanically controlled movement and co-ordination in the whole body. To make ourselves aware of this consciously in our daily activities is the basis of good use.

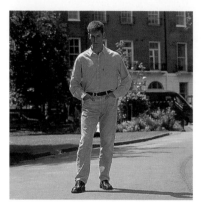

See how this model is misusing himself. He is leaning over to the right, shortening and creating an imbalance in his body.

Inhibition

In its psychological-physiological sense, inhibition means a fast-moving yet natural control of your reactions, suppressing and smothering any possible spontaneity.

However, Alexander discovered that if he managed to stop himself from behaving in his habitual way, he could choose how he wished to respond to a stimulus. If someone rings the doorbell, your immediate response may be to go straight to the door. In doing so, you will be responding habitually. If you stop yourself from responding automatically, you then choose exactly how you will approach the door with the minimum effort.

Concepts

The concept of end-gaining is extremely important in the work of Alexander technique teachers. Alexander realized that the habits he was encountering were far more deep-rooted and powerful than he had at first thought. The most serious of these was the tendency to try to react impulsively – end-gaining. End-gaining means reacting immediately and too quickly to a stimulus, without thinking. You respond by wanting something to happen, and become interested in the end result instead of being in the present. A typical example is if you are going to be late for an appointment and start to worry about the consequences. You get worked up during this process, forgetting that you might be sitting on a train, and that things are happening around you. In effect you are letting your thoughts take the situation into the future, instead of being in the "here and now", in the present.

Cutting yourself off from your environment has inevitable consequences for body positioning. It tends to lead to a pulling back of the head, a rounding of the back, a tightening of the legs and a loss of connection between the arms and the back. The gaze becomes fixed, the breath held. Essentially, the whole person is affected, both in mind and in body.

Alexander suggests you should use your "means-whereby". To put Alexander's conclusion into context, if we accept that we cannot change circumstances, we can change our approach to our bodies and allow ourselves to experience the new. It is then possible to learn to be in the moment rather than the past or the future, and to maintain a sense of inner balance and unity.

Direction

Directions are signals given by the brain to parts of the body prior to or during physical action. It is possible to alter these signals to promote a positive change. You will find that the combination of direction and inhibition enables one to transform habitual ways of moving and eliminate old patterns of misuse.

Note how this model is walking. Her head, neck and back are all correctly aligned. Her arms are free to move in a relaxed way.

Natural Poise

Nothing is more elegant and enviable than someone with perfect poise. It is something most of us have when young, but sadly it can be quickly lost to laziness and bad postural habits. In fact, it is quite easy to be totally unaware just how bad our posture is. At various times during the day it is worth freezing your movements, and taking a good look at yourself. You will be surprised at how often you fall well short of the ideal. Sitting at work is probably the one situation when your back is almost always wrongly positioned, becoming increasingly hunched, tense and stiff. Once you have ascertained exactly when and how you are going wrong, you can start putting matters right. If in any doubt, just look at young children. They instinctively know how to move gracefully and effortlessly without strain. That is something we should all try to emulate.

This child carries his toy close to his body., allowing it to lengthen and relax. This ensures good nervous energy and blood flow and allows full expansion of the lungs for breathing.

Primary Directions

• Think of freeing the neck.
• Let the head go forward and up.
• Let the back lengthen and widen.

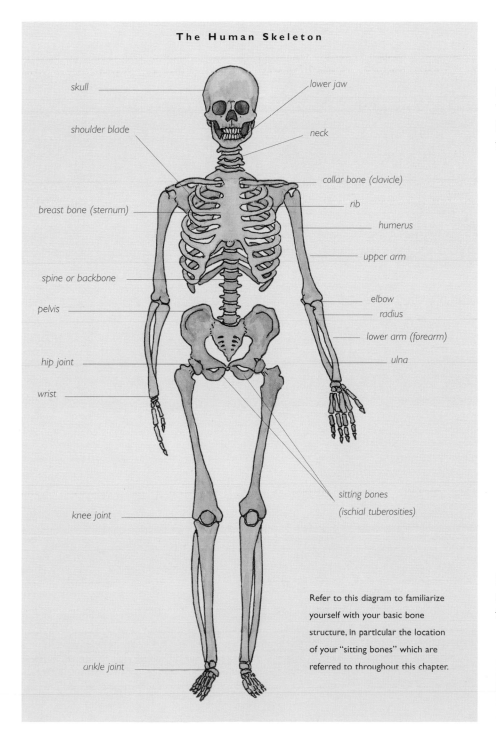

The Human Skeleton

skull — lower jaw

shoulder blade — neck

collar bone (clavicle)

rib

breast bone (sternum) — humerus

upper arm

spine or backbone

elbow

pelvis — radius

lower arm (forearm)

hip joint — ulna

wrist

knee joint — sitting bones (ischial tuberosities)

ankle joint

Refer to this diagram to familiarize yourself with your basic bone structure, in particular the location of your "sitting bones" which are referred to throughout this chapter.

Note how this child is using his joints to squat, and how he simultaneously holds the plastic bag quite effortlessly.

"Possession of property ... a means to happiness not an end."
Thomas Jefferson

putting the alexander technique into practice
putting the alexander technique

putting the alexander technique into practice

A certain, rightful degree of commitment is paramount during a course of lessons because the older and more set in your ways you are, the longer it can take to change, to release unnecessary muscular tension, and to re-educate the system. Success, however, is not hard to achieve but note that it will not happen overnight, and that some slight pitfalls are always going to be inevitable, so do not be put off.

For example, you may well find yourself trying to do the directions as a routine mechanical exercise when in reality success lies in the power of the body and mind uniting as one, and in the power to think about what you are doing. Do not imagine there are any short cuts, there are not. There is also the distinct possibility that you might be tempted to give up out of sheer frustration because your time scale is too unrealistically short and limiting, and you have not allowed sufficient time for a significant, quantifiable improvement. Do not be hard on yourself, and do not imagine that you can become an expert in a ridiculously short space of time. The technique deserves more respect.

What therefore follows is the identification of the main procedures that we use most often in daily life, the areas that most concern us. In fact, the use of the word "procedure" is quite deliberate because it totally avoids the suggestion of a mind-body split and maintains a sense of psycho-physical unity. The emphasis throughout is on the means of achieving these procedures, but with the minimum of muscular tension and effort. Many students have said that a course of lessons in the technique could be compared to learning to drive or learning a new language. Dedication and determination are a sure basis for total success.

use of the eyes
If you want to know something about someone, just look straight into their eyes. They reveal an amazing amount about their current frame of mind. You can easily spot the depressed, dull and lifeless by their deadpan, almost one-dimensional eyes; the totally alert looking for a lively reply; the sad; the plaintive; the cheeky; and the happy. The technique reminds you how to stay lively and alert, and in touch with the rest of the world.

STAYING ALERT

If you observe people when they are either standing or walking, they often seem to be completely locked in a private world of their own, totally unaware of their own surroundings. They have stopped communicating with that is out there. When the gaze is fixed, the breathing also tends to suffer. It becomes rather restricted and there is less freedom in the body. The gaze should therefore be directed towards the outside world, taking in information so that you are not exclusively concentrating on what is happening within.

One of the strongest habits that a teacher perceives is the tendency of certain pupils to look down, not with their eyes, but by a general collapsing motion from the neck. This is the result of a fundamental misunderstanding of the alignment of the head, the neck and the back, and the position of the joints in the body.

Note how the models in this sequence of photographs (*below*) are using their eyes. Which do you think is the correct position? Can there be any doubt?.

"It's no good shutting your eyes if you're crossing a busy road."
F. M. Alexander

Here children are using their eyes to look at their toys. They have not disturbed the alignment between their heads, their necks and their backs, thus maintaining their good use.

In this position, the model is breaking the alignment between her head, her neck and her back as she looks down, thus using her neck inappropriately.

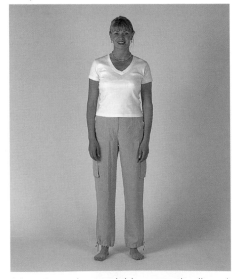

Note how the model is correctly aligned. She is maintaining her length and her width. Her eyes are alert and taking in her surroundings.

Here the model is breaking at the neckline and pulling her head back to look up, disturbing the alignment between her head, neck and back.

the semi-supine position

Standing for long periods easily compresses the spine. Lying down in a semi-supine position is a way of alleviating unnecessary tensions in the muscles and joints, and should be practised every day for at least 20 minutes. It encourages a better awareness of the head-neck-back relationship. This position does not necessarily need monitoring by a teacher, and it also gives you much needed time for yourself.

THE POSITION

Try to keep your eyes alert and open. It is preferable to avoid closing them because you will probably find it quite difficult not to fall asleep, which is definitely not the point of the exercise!

During your daily 20-minute session try and give yourself the time to practise some sharp, well directed thoughts to avoid your mind from wandering and spreading out, covering other possible important issues. This session can also encourage you to put into practice your excellent skills of observation. A good practice is to go over the primary directions, and to notice if you are aware of any tension in your body and to address it without trying to correct it. That is the secret of success.

Books are used to support the head. If you have too many, however, your chin will drop and you will feel pressure on your throat.

Correspondingly, if you do not have enough books your head will tilt back and will not be properly supported.

MOVING INTO THE SEMI-SUPINE

It is preferable to lie down on a hard, carpeted surface or alternatively on a rug on the floor. Avoid beds as they will not offer you adequate support. The number of books you need will depend on their thickness, and will also vary from person to person.

To lie down on the floor, place the books far enough behind you to give enough space for the whole of your torso and your bottom. When sitting, you can place your hands palms down on the floor behind you to help you lower your back. Take care not to stiffen the arms or to hold your breath in the process. To get up, it is preferable to roll over to one side, leading with your eyes rather than your head, and following with your torso and legs. Then place the free hand flat on the floor and go on to all fours. Be careful to maintain the alignment between your head, your neck and your back and not to hold your breath. Walk your hands back so that you move your bottom back towards your heels.

Make sure that your legs are about hip-width apart and that your knees are directed towards the ceiling.

If your knees are falling out, you will probably lose the contact between the inner side of your foot and the floor.

sitting and standing

Correct posture is as much about what is right as what is wrong. It is vital that you know what to do, and what not to do. It is easy to start out with correct posture, but fall into bad habits. You must know when to correct yourself. Remember to keep a straight alignment between head, neck and back, and to keep your legs hip-width apart with knees pointing forward, in the same direction as your feet.

SITTING

Correct: think of the shoulders going away from each other.

Incorrect: rounded shoulders and feet wrapped around chair legs.

Incorrect: arching the back, folding legs and leaning to one side.

FROM SITTING TO STANDING

It is well worth practising this basic technique several times to perfect it. You will be surprised how ingrained bad habits are. Start by placing your legs about hip-width apart. Avoid pushing firmly up with them; that is not the object. Also, make sure that your feet are flat and are not placed so far forwards that coming up to stand is in any way difficult. Finally, remember to lead with the head; that is the key to getting this technique right.

I Here the model is relaxed, feet apart, hands resting comfortably, ready to go into the standing position.

2 As she stands she has managed to keep the correct alignment between her head, neck and back.

3 Having hinged from the hip, sending her knees forwards and away over her feet, she is now properly upright.

reaching and handling

It is impossible to avoid two basic movements, reaching and handling. Yet how many of us know how to do them properly, according to the Alexander technique? Reaching means keeping the alignment between the head, neck and back, whether you are low down or standing up. If you are indeed squatting, it is important that you allow your hand to lead your movement. Let everything else follow behind.

HANDLING

See how the model's weight is balanced over the feet, and how she is allowing her hand to lead her wrist and arm.

Here, the legs are straight and the head is pulled back, causing a lot of strain on the neck, and the shoulders are tense.

See how the arms remain well connected to the shoulder blades and back. Also, there is no tension in the arms and wrists.

GOING UP ON TIPTOES

When going on tiptoes correctly, the weight that is placed on the middle of the feet when standing is placed on the balls of the feet, as the head leads the body forwards and upwards. It is important to maintain the alignment between the head, the neck and the back. The breath is not held, and the eyes are alert.

Look at how this model is going on tiptoes to enable her hand to lead her arm to close the window.

Note how the model is well poised and correctly aligned. There is no undue stress on the body.

Here the head contraction is severe. The model is holding his breath, causing unnecessary tension in the body.

"monkey" or bending

The position known as the "monkey" enables us to move with more flexibility in our daily activities. It is a useful means of moving from standing to sitting or squatting, as well as helping with lifting, picking things up, working at a desk, washing, ironing, and participating in sports such as skiing and golf. The "monkey" respects the relationship between the head, neck and back.

THE POSITION

The "monkey" position might sound tricky, but it really is not. Try it slowly, see how it works, then try it again at a more natural speed. It basically involves the head moving forwards and up, and then the knees moving forwards and away over the feet to counterbalance the bottom going back over the heels, enabling the arms to move freely. It is also important to remember that when you go into "monkey" you must review your primary directions. What is more, stay alert at all times, and avoid fixing your gaze or holding your breath. Such moves will quickly undermine the marvellous effects of the "monkey".

To be more precise then, stand with your legs hip-width apart, with the feet slightly turned outwards. Your weight should be evenly distributed, neither too far forwards nor too far back on your feet. To start going into the "monkey", allow the knees to bend slightly over your feet as you tilt forwards from your hip joints, making sure your head, your neck and your back are aligned. Avoid collapsing over yourself!

One final point is to make sure you think of widening and lengthening your back as you widen across the shoulder girdle, to allow free movement and your arms to hang freely. This extra tip will ensure you enjoy the full effect of "the monkey".

This model is in the correct "monkey" position. Her head, her neck and her back are aligned. Her knees are bent forward and away from her hips.

When going into the "monkey" avoid retracting the head back and down into the spine. Note how the model has rounded her shoulders and pulled in her knees.

Here the model is not bending her knees as she bends forwards. Her back is collapsed over her body, and her legs are straight and braced.

everyday situations

In everyday situations it is important to pause before reacting, to make sure you are so positioned that you do not misuse yourself. The more aware you are, the more likely you will encourage muscular release through your whole system. Equally, the more at peace you are, the easier it is to apply the principles of the Alexander technique. The following excellent examples show how the "monkey" can keep you healthy.

Note how the model's back is correctly aligned, keeping to the head-neck-back principle. See how she is using her joints and allowing her widening arms to handle the dish.

How things can go wrong. Here the model has started pulling her head back. Also, her back is rounded, her legs are braced and her arms have become much too tense.

In this highly incorrect stance, the man is collapsing from his waist down as he begins works in the garden. His shoulders are far too rounded, and his head is being pulled back.

In this correct procedure, the model is neatly poised and balanced, and she is well aligned to begin her ironing. Her hand, wrist and arm are also free as she holds the iron. The other crucial point to note is how she is widening across her upper arms. It is clear that she looks balanced and feels alert.

See how the model is using the whole of his back quite correctly. He is sensibly allowing his weight to come back on to his heels, and his knees go forwards and away over his feet.

An example of how not to do it. Here he is completely out of alignment. You can sense it is not right, but why? He is actually pulling his head back, rounding the back, and holding in the arms. This position is entirely the result of bad habits. Without the Alexander technique, he would never know how to right this.

"lunge monkey"

The "lunge monkey" is similar to the "monkey" because the knees go forwards and away, and the torso tilts slightly forwards from the hip joints. Also, one foot is placed behind the other, and the legs are placed hip-width apart, enabling you to balance the upper part of your body on to the forward or the back leg whenever the need arises. In this way, your weight is placed forwards or backwards according to your activity.

BENDING

The "lunge monkey" is extremely useful when you need to lift something heavy from the floor; when you need to move an object from one side of a surface to another, for example during cooking; or when you need to push or pull something rather heavy into place.

When you adapt the "lunge monkey" it is important to remember to keep your head, your neck and your back correctly aligned. The legs must be hip-width apart, with the arms hanging freely on either side of your torso.

Also, allow your weight to move to the right on to the right foot (or to the left, as the situation demands). If moving to the left, reverse the instructions.

See how the model has collapsed badly from the waist down. Her shoulders are rounded, the legs are straight and the knees are braced, causing tension.

Observe how the model has gone into the "lunge monkey". Her head, neck and back are neatly aligned, and her knees are going forward away from her hips.

Note how the model has completely lost the correct alignment with her back as she squats. Her head has dropped, and her shoulders are hunched and rounded. Furthermore, she looks ill at ease and uncomfortable. There is no poise or grace. This position is definitely one to avoid.

In this correct procedure, observe how the model's head, neck and back are correctly aligned. Her shoulders are widening across her upper arms. She looks well balanced, and fully in control of her movements. Also note how her heels are tucked in under the bottom. The position is also easy to get into.

SQUATTING

In Western societies most people find it difficult to squat in their everyday lives. Young children have very little difficulty in doing so, but as we grow older we lose the necessary flexibility to squat as our joints become less mobile.

A low "monkey" or semi-squat is the best way that an Alexander teacher can re-introduce a student to squatting over a series of lessons. To squat, follow the same guidelines as for the "monkey", but with a wider stance. Remember to maintain the alignment between the head, the neck and the back, and to allow the joints in the hips, the knees and the ankles to be free. As you go into a deeper squat you might find that your heels come off the ground. This does not present a problem as far as the technique is concerned, so long as you keep your balance. As a general rule, go only as far as you feel comfortable.

the technique in the home

The key point to note about the Alexander technique is that it is not an abstract theory that you can apply when the mood takes you. It is a specific, practical everyday guide that will help you enormously whether you are bending, squatting, lifting or carrying. It gives you terrific control whatever you are doing, injecting extra confidence that will keep you alert and relaxed.

BENDING

Note how the model is tilted forwards to get a greater range of movement. His arms are free, supported by his back.

Now he is incorrectly bending forwards from the waist. His legs are braced, and his head is pulled back.

Here the model has aligned herself nicely to make the bed. Her legs are bent, creating a greater range of movement.

SQUATTING

This model is lunge squatting to brush up dirt from the floor. She has maintained her good use, giving herself a maximum range of movement. She looks good and feels good.

Here, in an incorrect example of how you should sweep the floor, the model is badly restricting his range of movement. He is quite clearly unbalanced, and feels totally uncomfortable.

Note how this man is squatting sensibly to plant a rose bush in his garden. By placing himself at the same level as the rose, he is allowing himself a greater range of movement.

lifting and carrying

A lot of back pain is the result of lifting heavy weights. To avoid back strain, stand near to the load by placing your feet either side of it, and maintain the alignment between head, neck and back. Go into the "monkey" or "lunge monkey" and squat. Then bend your arms so that your elbows are close to your body. Make sure that you widen out across the upper arms, and avoid tension in the arms and wrists.

LIFTING

1 Once you are holding the load as closely to your body as you can, come out of a squat or lunge squat into a "monkey" before standing.

2 Lift the weight in a flowing action, that does not jar or suddenly pull against the back. If the weight proves too heavy, it is easy to bend and put it down.

3 To place the load back on the ground, reverse the process and apply the same principles, making sure that your head, neck and back are aligned.

CARRYING

Here the model is carrying all her shopping bags in one hand, creating an imbalance as she is pulled down to the left. She is raising her right shoulder in an attempt to support her handbag.

This model is carrying her shopping bags sensibly and correctly so that they are evenly distributed on both sides. She is well balanced and able to walk freely. She looks content.

Look at the excellent way this mother is carrying her child. Her weight is evenly distributed and she is holding the child close to her body, firmly supporting his upper and lower body.

daily routines

The most surprising point about the Alexander technique is that it is not just for big, set piece movements such as lifting heavy weights, when doing it incorrectly can obviously lead to back problems. The technique even extends to the minutiae of life, routines that we completely take for granted, such as eating, drinking, and driving. If you had always wondered how they should be done, read on. These tips will make all the difference.

EATING AND DRINKING

If you are standing upright while you are drinking remember that you still need to be fully alert at all times. Therefore, make sure that you do not fix your gaze rigidly and thereby lose all communication and contact with the outside world. You also need to ensure that your head leads you away from your heels (see the section on Standing for further guidance). You will find that your shoulder girdle brings mobility to your arms, and that the pelvis provides stability which simultaneously facilitates mobility in your legs.

The very same principles also apply to eating. Whether you are going to eat something from your hand or use a fork, it is all too easy to forget your posture completely. Remember that you should not totally focus on the matter in hand, but that you must also consider your stance, alertness and poise.

Avoid gripping or clutching your glass. Be aware of the connection with your arm, which links to your back and then into your heels. As you raise the cup to your lips, bring your weight back on to the heels, so as not to pull in your lower back. Also, bring the glass to the lips, rather than leaning down into it.

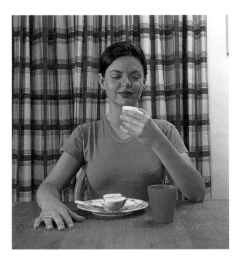

Take some time to consider how you are seated at the table and then bring the food up to your mouth, rather than the reverse. Your feet should be correctly positioned on the floor. You should also be aware of both your sitting bones, and how your back should be lengthening and widening. This position also aids digestion.

DRIVING

Most of the problems experienced by drivers are due to fixed postures, long journeys and poor seating support.

Too many people who spend huge amounts of time driving find themselves constricted by the position of the steering wheel and the pedals. Such a cramped environment is bound to lead to stress and strain on the back, and equally on the arms and legs.

When choosing a car take time to see whether the seat is firm and supportive. If you already own a car and it does not have a lumbar support adjustment, you can use a wedge-shaped cushion to give you adequate support in the lumbar area and the pelvis. It makes a vital difference.

You should be able to reach the pedals quite easily. A wedge-shaped cushion is extremely useful to avoid a poor, slumping position.

See how the model is badly collapsing forward, how the neck is being strained and the arms are rigidly tense. Such a position will cause lots of discomfort.

office work

Before reading it is important to spend some time considering exactly how you are going to sit in order to avoid badly slumping, which is very easy to do, especially in a big old comfortable armchair. Once you get drawn into what you are reading it is virtually certain that you will completely forget about your posture. It is vitally important that you do not end up creating all kinds of stresses and strains in your body.

READING AND WRITING

When you are sitting at your desk or at a table, it is important that you adjust your chair in such a way that your lower arms and hands can be placed on the surface of your table or desk at a right angle. If your chair is too close you are likely to end up lifting your shoulders to adjust your arms. If your chair is too high, you will probably find that you start slumping. You must also avoid crossing your legs, and do make sure that your feet remain comfortably flat on the floor.

A useful trick when reading is to use a sloping board to avoid slumping over your desk or table.

Note how the model is holding her body badly with her arm, and how her legs are folded, offering no support.

Keep the alignment between your head, your neck and your back.

This model is firmly gripping the pen, causing tension in her wrist and hand.

Here the model is tensing her wrist, hand and arm, restricting her movement.

DESKWORK

An increasing number of people are complaining of neck and shoulder tension, wrist problems and back pain resulting from their working environment. Some cases are directly linked to badly designed furniture, awkward or unfavourable sitting positions and immobility. In other instances, although chairs and work surfaces are good, the posture is poor. You must therefore remember your primary directions: the head, neck and back should be aligned, and the head should be lengthening away from the sitting bones.

How not to do it. See how the model is slumping badly, causing unnecessary tension in the spine, so weakening the muscles surrounding the torso.

Here the spine is correctly aligned, and the head is poised gracefully above the neck. The feet are well placed on the floor, nicely apart.

office equipment

The office is not what it used to be. It now offers amazing improvements in high-tech equipment, but also plenty of opportunities for repetitive strain injury, aching backs and tense necks. The temptation is to spend far too long in one awkward position. So always be aware of what you are doing, how long it will take, and the best position you need to adopt. Such awareness makes all the difference between a good and bad day.

MOBILE PHONE USE

Observe Yourself When the Telephone Rings

Do you snatch and grab it? Or do you try to give yourself some time before you pick up the receiver? Next time the telephone rings, stop and go over your primary directions. Make sure that you bring the receiver up to your ear rather than suddenly leaning down towards it, thus compromising your position.

Here the model is pulling her head down wrongly towards her mobile phone to talk, and slouching.

In this example the model has maintained her balance throughout her body. She looks poised and relaxed.

WORKING AT A COMPUTER

If you are working at a computer or portable computer, use your eyes to look down towards it. Avoid lurching at the neck as you will lose the correct alignment with your back.

Here the model badly collapses over her computer. She has lost the correct alignment between her hands, her wrists and her lower arms. Her shoulders are far too hunched.

Here the model is incorrectly holding in her wrist, arms and shoulders, causing unnecessary strain and discomfort. She will soon feel very uncomfortable, and have to adopt a new position.

t'ai chi

t'ai chi t'ai chi

T'ai chi ch'uan is an ancient form of slow, graceful and rhythmic exercise which originated in China, where it is still extremely popular, often being performed in public parks in the fresh morning air. It has its roots in Taoist philosophy. The movements of the t'ai chi form gently tone and strengthen the organs and muscles, improve circulation and posture, and relax both mind and body. Its name translates as "supreme ultimate fist", but this is not its true meaning. "Strength within softness", "poetry in motion" and "moving harmony" all come closer to expressing the spirit of t'ai chi.

T'ai chi has been variously described as a system of health, medicine, physical co-ordination, relaxation, self-defence and consciousness raising, as well as a means of exercise and self-development. It is all these things. The style shown here is the Yang-style short form, as developed by Professor Cheng Man-Ch'ing, which is the one most practised in the West.

Unlike the "hard" martial arts which rely on force and speed, t'ai chi is "soft" or "internal". Its emphasis lies in the yielding aspect of nature when overcoming the hard – like the waterfall which eventually wears away the rock beneath. It teaches patience and relaxation, and fosters an understanding of the co-ordination of mind, body and spirit. It is the perfect antidote to the stresses and strains of today's modern lifestyles.

t'ai chi for health or self defence If you

simply want to go out and strike a pose, jumping about like Bruce Lee, t'ai chi is not for you. It is a very serious, highly regarded ancient technique that has two major qualities. It improves your health, and teaches you how to overcome stronger hostile forces when you are under attack. The most amazing part of t'ai chi is the way its movements are almost balletic.

The Benefits of T'ai Chi

Although t'ai chi can eventually be used in self-defence, and most classes do incorporate some of its practical applications, it is initially practised mainly for its health-giving benefits. It is particularly useful for increasing alertness and body awareness, and for developing concentration and sensitivity. It helps with balance and posture, and enhances a sense of "groundedness". However, all the postures can also be used when defending yourself against an attack by an opponent. Its gentleness and subtlety do not preclude its use as a very effective form of self-defence.

It is not easy to separate the physical and mental aspects of t'ai chi, as they are closely interrelated. In Chinese medicine, the interdependence of mind, body and spirit is seen as integral to well-being.

The ancient art of t'ai chi instills enormous grace and confidence.

The Theory of T'ai Chi

Like music, t'ai chi cannot be appreciated purely on an intellectual level. It also has an enormous spiritual side, and when you watch any highly experienced t'ai chi practitioners you will see how they are almost in a kind of trance, in a separate world where they cannot be touched. Correctly done, it is quite hypnotic.

For now, we must look at some of the concepts that are fundamental to the martial arts, as well as to medicine and philosophy. Although these disciplines are all treated quite separately by those in the West, they are all inseparable in the Eastern view. From thousands of years of close observation of patterns of energy, the Chinese successfully evolved a way of life that actually ropes all three ingredients together.

Chi

Chi is the prime driving force of human life, the spark behind thought, creativity and growth which maintains and nurtures us. It can be felt as movement of energy in the body, like the ceaseless flow of an electrical current. Chi flows through the body along channels called meridians.

The Tan Tien

The Chi is stored in the Tan Tien. This is an area about the size of a golf ball, located four finger-widths below the navel, and about one-third of the way from the front to the back of the body. It is the centre of gravity of the body, and in t'ai chi all movement emanates from it. Try to let the breath and the mind sink to the Tan Tien.

Yin and Yang

Yin and Yang describe the complementary yet opposing forces of nature. Their relationship has a harmony and balance: both Yin and Yang are necessary, are constantly moving and balancing each other, and this interaction creates Chi. The Chinese observed that when the balance of Yin and Yang is disrupted so too will be the body's Chi, leading to ill health.

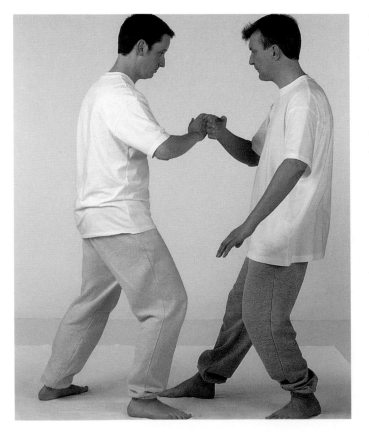

One of the key requirements for t'ai chi is excellent balance.

warm-up exercises

Perform these exercises slowly and gently, with the mind and the breath focused in the Tan Tien. Notice any differences between the right and left sides of your body, and between the upper and lower parts. The object is gradually to enter the world of t'ai chi, and to warm up all your muscles so that you do not get any strains. The more you warm up, the better your technique will be. The movements will flow like a stream.

CIRCLING HANDS

1 Inhale and allow both hands to float upwards a comfortable distance in front of your body, palms facing downwards.

2 As your hands rise above your head, relax the wrists and begin to open the palms outwards. Begin to exhale.

3 Open out your arms to your sides. Draw your hands inwards at the bottom of the circle and smoothly begin again.

4 Inhale as your palms, facing upwards, float in front of your body. Exhale and push your right hand down by your hip and your left hand up by your temple.

5 Breathe in again, relax your palms which now turn to face each other and begin moving them towards each other in front of your body.

6 Repeat step 4 in reverse as you exhale. Breathe in again and bring your hands in front of your body in a mirror image of Step 5.

SHAKING OUT SHOULDERS, ARMS AND HANDS

I Gently shake out any tension in your wrists and hands. Gradually work up to include your shoulders. This exercise is especially useful before, during and after long periods at a keyboard, or repetitive work with the hands.

LOOSENING SHOULDERS

I Make increasing circles with one shoulder. Change direction and decrease the size of the circles. Repeat for the other shoulder. Rotate your shoulders alternately.

ROTATING WAIST

I Place both hands lightly on your hips. Keeping your head up, begin by spiralling your hips slowly outwards, feeling for any restriction, tightness or lack of ease. Change direction and spiral back in slowly.

KNEE ROTATIONS

I Bring your feet together and place your palms lightly on your upper kneecaps. Feel the Chi from your palms radiating deep into your knee joints. Circle your knees clockwise several times, then change direction.

2 Keep your legs and hands in the same position. Rotate your knees in opposite directions – one circles clockwise while the other circles anti-clockwise (counterclockwise). Change the direction of each knee and repeat the rotations.

CALF STRETCH

I Step forward with your right foot. Keeping the heel on the floor, pull up your toes towards the knee. Drop your body forward, keeping your right leg straight. Hold for a few breaths and release. Repeat for the other leg.

FOUR-DIRECTIONAL BREATHING

1 As you inhale, bring your hands up to chest height, palms facing upwards.

2 As you exhale, turn the palms to face away and extend your arms as if pushing something away. On the next inhalation, turn your palms back to face your body, softening your arms and drawing them back in towards your chest.

3 Exhale again, turn the palms out and extend your arms out to your sides.

4 Relax and bring your arms in towards your chest as you inhale.

5 On the next exhalation turn your palms upwards and extend your arms towards the sky.

6 Inhale and let your arms descend, palms facing downwards. As your arms pass the solar plexus, exhale and push down towards the earth. Repeat this sequence several times.

ROTATING FROM THE WAIST WITH FEET FORWARD

1 Imagine a central axis from the crown of your head, dropping down through your body to a point between your feet. Rotate your body around this axis, keeping your arms relaxed.

2 As your waist turns to the left, your weight shifts on to your left leg. As it turns right, move your weight across on to your right leg. Let your arms swing naturally,

3 Repeat the sequence for about 1 minute. As you do it, try to keep each knee over its respective big toe to avoid any strain on the muscles and ligaments.

ROTATING FROM THE WAIST TURNING ON THE BALL OF THE FOOT

1 The arms follow the same movement as above, but each foot pivots in turn on the ball. Keeping your weight in your left leg, turn your waist to the right. Lift your right heel and swivel the right foot 90°.

2 As your waist returns to the centre, straighten your right foot until your feet are parallel and shoulder-width apart. Transfer your weight on to your right foot.

3 Turn your waist to the left, lift your left heel and pivot on the ball of your left foot. Repeat the sequence for about 1 minute, keeping your head up, back straight and arms and shoulders relaxed.

OPENING AND CLOSING THE CIRCLE

1 Place your hands in front of your face, palms facing away. Turn your waist slowly to the right.

2 Drop almost all your weight into your right leg and continue turning your waist, bending forwards which in turn brings your hands around in a large circular movement.

3 As your hands cross the bottom of the circle, shift your weight into your left leg. Continue to turn your waist slowly, bringing your hands up to complete the circle.

4 When your hands reach their starting-point in front of your face, repeat the sequence and continue for several more rotations.

5 Change direction gently at the bottom of the circle to repeat the sequence. This time, join your palms together lightly at the top of each circle.

6 Keep the palms together as you turn, allowing your hands to separate at the bottom. Finish the exercise by keeping your palms connected and spiralling your hands to end in front of your chest.

SHIFTING WEIGHT

ROTATING WHOLE BODY

1 Place your left foot at 45° and your right foot forward, heels shoulder-width apart. Shift your weight from one leg to the other – do not tip your pelvis forwards or backwards.

2 Let your arms swing naturally. Continue for about 1 minute, then change legs and repeat the sequence again. Feel a strong root developing through your feet into the centre of the earth.

1 Hold both arms in front of the chest, palms facing inwards, fingertips almost touching. Turn your waist and arms and shift your weight to the right. Repeat to the left.

WAVING HANDS IN CLOUDS

1 Begin with your right hand facing the Tan Tien, your left hand directly above it, facing your chest. Turn your waist to the left, shifting your weight into your left leg. Turn your palms towards each other.

2 Bring your waist back to the front. As you do so, lower your left hand until it is opposite the Tan Tien and raise your right hand to the level of your chest, with your palms facing your body.

3 Now turn your waist to the right, shift the weight across to your right leg, and turn your palms towards each other in a mirror image of Step 1. Repeat the entire sequence several times.

PUSH TO CENTRE, PUSH TO CORNER

1 Place your right foot at 45° and step forward with your left foot. Begin with all your weight on your right leg, right hand resting palm upwards on your right hip, left fingertips in line with your mouth, palm facing diagonally forwards and to the centre.

2 Bring your weight forward on to your left leg. Your right hand turns diagonally forwards as it comes to push towards the centre of your body; your left hand turns palm upwards as it draws back to rest on your left hip.

3 Shift your weight back on to your right foot, turning your waist 45° to the right. At the same time draw your right hand back to your right hip and push your left hand towards the corner until it is in line with the centre of your body, fingertips opposite your mouth. Repeat steps 1, 2 and 3 for about 1 minute.

4 Repeat the sequence in mirror image as it is shown above. Make sure that all your movements are smooth and flowing and that the weight is gently shifted between your feet.

5 Bring your weight on to your right leg. Your left hand turns diagonally forwards as it comes towards the centre of the body, your right palm turns upwards as it draws back to rest on the right hip.

6 Shift your weight to your left foot, turning your waist 45° to the left. At the same time, draw your left hand to your left hip and push your right hand to the corner. Repeat the cycle in Steps 5 and 6.

NECK ROTATIONS

I Keep the palms of your hands in front of your chest, fingertips almost touching. Relax your shoulders and elbows. Turn your head to look over one shoulder, then the other. Repeat several times, keeping the neck movements fluid.

HIP ROTATIONS

I Turn out your left foot and sink all your weight on to it. Draw a smooth circle with your right knee, keeping the hip movement as fluid as possible. Repeat the same rotation on the other hip.

ANKLE ROTATIONS

I Place your left foot at 45°, bend your left knee and sink all your weight into your left leg. Lift your right foot and slowly rotate the ankle, describing a circle with your big toe. Repeat the exercise for the left ankle.

RETURN TO CENTRE

I As you breathe in, take your hands out to the sides in front of your body, and raise them slowly in a large circle, palms facing upwards.

2 As you exhale, lower your hands in front of the centre of your body, palms facing downwards.

3 At the bottom of the circle, turn your hands outwards again to begin a new circle with the new breath.

KIDNEY MASSAGE

I The kidneys are the most important organs, according to Chinese medicine, as they store the Chi. This massage provides gentle stimulation and helps to break down crystals of uric acid found in kidney stones. Bring your heels together at right angles, and massage around your kidneys with loose fists.

ABDOMINAL MASSAGE

I With your heels together, massage your abdomen in a circular motion with the palms of your hands to assist and bring blood to the digestive area.

STIMULATING THE BACK OF THE NECK

I Lift your hands to the back of your head. Flick your index and middle fingers over each other to tap the base of the occipital ridge at the back of the skull, releasing Chi up to the top of your head. Flick the back of your head about 20 times.

FEELING THE AIR

I With your heels together and feet at right angles, inhale and let both hands float up towards your shoulders, palms facing upwards. Feel the resistance of the air on your palms.

2 As you exhale, let both hands float back down. Try to feel resistance on the backs of your hands, and the air rushing softly between your fingers.

STILLNESS WITHIN MOVEMENT

I Bring your heels together at right angles to each other. Try to feel where your body weight naturally lies. After a few quiet moments of standing still, you can begin some t'ai chi walking, or start the form. Notice the feelings you have, especially in the Tan Tien, and carry these feelings with you into the form.

yang-style short form
yang-style short form

yang-style short form

After completing all the warm-up exercises, and having a moment or so quietly standing to see if you can find a point of equilibrium, a few minutes of t'ai chi walking may now follow. This is known as walking with an "empty step", rather in the manner of a cat tentatively putting out its paw before committing its full weight on to the front leg.

In fact, it is well worth studying an adult cat that is gracefully walking, or gliding forwards when it has spotted its prey. Its whole movement is one of ceaseless flow, of elegant, unforced movement when every part of its body seems to be an extension of another part, and nothing is hurried or rushed.

As you progress through the form, use the following pages as an aide-mémoire for your practice, especially for the transitions from one posture to the next. Remember to keep your movements slow and smooth, like clouds drifting gently by on a summer's day, and relax. If you worry about this new exercise, you will not succeed.

In many ways that is the key problem for the new Western practitioner. Doing these exercises initially means that you will be highly self-conscious because there is nothing like it in our culture. Yet gradually, after a few lessons, and above all after watching expert t'ai chi practitioners, it becomes clear that this is something which you can do successfully, and without having to worry about what you look like.

Once you launch into the first few movements, the rest follow, and you find that an awkward state of self-consciousness is quickly replaced by an inner calm as you become less aware of the outside world, and more aware of inner ones. The key to t'ai chi is being able to make seamless flowing moves, with the emphasis not so much on specific poses as on the linking means of getting there. Ultimately, you too may be able to go into a park in the early morning, as they do in the East, and carry out t'ai chi utterly unself-consciously, gaining spiritual refreshment.

ATTENTION, PREPARATION AND BEGINNING

1 Stand in a relaxed and upright posture, feet pointing diagonally outwards, making a right angle. Distribute your weight evenly through your body.

2 Bend your right knee and sink all your weight down through your right leg into the foot, without leaning across. Then move the "empty" left leg a shoulder-width away, with the toes pointing straight ahead.

3 Transfer 70% of your weight to your left leg, simultaneously turning your waist and therefore your whole body diagonally to the right.

4 Keeping 70% of your weight in your left leg, turn your whole body back to face the front. Bring your right foot around to the front as your waist moves. Your feet should be shoulder-width apart and parallel. Your hands also move with your body, the palms facing the ground as if resting on a cushion of air.

5 Relax your wrists and let your arms float up and away from your body. When your hands reach shoulder height, gently extend the fingertips.

6 Draw your hands back in towards your body by dropping the elbows. This penultimate posture is one of relaxed, graceful ease.

WARD OFF LEFT

7 In the final position, relax your wrists and let your hands float down the front of your body, just in front of and below the waist. The bulk of your weight is in your left leg.

1 Sink all your weight on to your left leg, and turn your body to the right, pivoting on your right heel. Imagine you are holding a large ball, with the right hand in front of the chest.

2 Sink all your weight on to your right leg, as if carrying the ball forward. Pick up your "empty" (weightless) left leg and step forwards, toes pointing to the front.

WARD OFF RIGHT

3 Turn the waist to the left, facing the front. Your left hand comes up, palm facing the chest, and the right floats down with 70% of your weight now on your left leg, as your right moves around.

1 Sink all your weight into your left leg. Turn to the right: the left palm turns face down, the right palm turns up as if both hands are again holding the large ball. The heels should be slightly apart.

2 Turn your waist to face the right-hand side and shift 70% of your weight on to your right foot, and turn your left foot to 45°. Raise your right arm so that the palm faces your chest.

ROLL BACK, PRESS AND PUSH

This posture, together with the one that follows it, "Single Whip", is also known as "Grasping the Sparrow's Tail".

1 Turn your body to the right. Point the fingertips of your right hand to the sky in a relaxed way. Your left arm moves horizontally with the fingertips almost touching the right elbow, palm facing the body. Your weight remains 70% on the right leg, 30% on the left.

2 As you turn your waist to the left, begin to shift weight to your left leg. Follow the movement of the body with your arms until your right hand is horizontal. Your left hand begins to flow down with the movement of your waist. Your weight settles on your left leg.

3 Turn your waist back to the right and let your left arm follow this movement. All your weight remains in the left leg. Bring your palm gradually across to rest against your right wrist, opposite the centre of your chest.

4 Press forward, keeping the hands in full contact. Shift 70% of your weight into your front (right) leg. Ensure that your heels are still shoulder-width apart, and that the right foot is pointing forward, and the left foot at 45°.

5 Separate your hands and sink all your weight back into your left foot. Your fingertips are now shoulder-width apart at shoulder height.

6 Move your weight forward 70% into your right leg. Your arms and hands keep the same position.

SINGLE WHIP

1 As your weight shifts back into the left leg, leave your fingers where they are in space, effectively straightening – but not locking – your arms. The palms now face down towards the ground.

2 Turn your whole body to the left and shift all your weight into your left leg. Your right heel remains on the ground while your toes turn through 120°, following the body round.

3 Sink your weight back into your right leg. Bring your left hand under the right to hold the imaginary ball in front of your body. Then form a "hook" with the fingers and thumb of your right hand.

LIFTING HANDS

4 Ensure all your weight is in your right leg. Bend the right knee and turn your body to the left, sending out the hook in line with, and at the same height as, your shoulder. Take an "empty" (weightless) shoulder-width step with your left foot.

5 Shift 70% of your weight on to your left leg, adjusting your right foot to 45°. Ensure that your heels are shoulder-width apart, your left hand in line with your left shoulder and your right hand hook at 90° to the rest of your body.

1 Place your weight on the left leg, open your hands and palms inwards, the left palm facing the right elbow. Pick up your empty right foot and place down the heel without weight, directly in front of the left heel.

WHITE CRANE SPREADS WINGS AND PUSH

2 Turn your waist to the left, your hands following the movement of your waist. Bring your right toe by your left heel, touching the ground but weightless.

3 Take an "empty" step to the right, and transfer 70% of the weight to the right foot. The left palm ends up opposite your inner right elbow. Your right arm is curved, guarding the groin, and your feet are at right angles to each other.

1 Drop all your weight into your right leg. Turn your waist to the left. As your right hand begins to rise, your left hand sweeps down in front of your left thigh.

2 Pick up your "empty" left leg and touch the toe on the ground but without shifting your weight. Bring your right hand up to guard your temple, turning to face diagonally outwards as it moves up. Your left hand floats down.

3 As you turn your waist to the left, your right hand follows and sweeps down; your left palm opens outwards.

4 As you turn your waist to the right, your right hand continues in a circle. Your left hand follows the move of your waist and faces down in front of your chest. As your waist returns to the centre, the right hand is level with the shoulder.

PLAY GUITAR. BRUSH LEFT KNEE AND PUSH
This posture is also known as "Strumming the Lute".

5 Take a shoulder-width step with your left foot, heel first. Move 70% of your weight into your left leg as your left hand brushes down across it. Meanwhile, your right hand follows a concave curve into the centre to finish by the mouth.

I As all your weight sinks into your left leg, adjust the "empty" right foot by drawing it slightly nearer the left foot, toe first. Bring your weight into the right foot. Your left leg and arm float up simultaneously – imagine a thread connecting them.

2 Turn to the right, dropping your right hand down while your left hand follows the movement of your waist to the centre of your chest, palm facing down. As your waist returns to the front, your right hand comes to shoulder height.

STEP FORWARD, DEFLECT, INTERCEPT AND PUNCH

3 Take a shoulder-width step with your left foot, heel first. Move 70% of your weight into your left leg as your left hand brushes down across it. Your right hand follows a curve ending by your mouth.

I Turn your waist 45° to the left and sink all your weight into your right foot. As the weight shifts back, lift the toes of your left foot and pivot 45° on the heel. Bring your hands down by your left leg.

2 Shift all your weight into your left leg. Form a loose fist with your right hand, but check that the fingers are not wrapped around the thumb. The right toes are behind the left heel.

3 Arc both of your hands and your right foot simultaneously towards the centre line, as your waist turns around to the right. The right foot now lands "empty", in line with the left instep. Check that your position is correct. Note that your left thumb should roughly be in line with your left eye.

4 Continue to turn your waist to the right, bringing the right fist palm upwards to rest on the right hip. You should now commence transferring all your weight on to your right foot. Your eyes should skim across the tops of your left fingers.

5 Place your left foot a shoulder width from the right foot. Shift 70% of your weight to your left leg and bring your right fist forward as if to punch, rotating it through a quarter turn in a corkscrew motion. Then bring your left arm across your body, with the palm facing your inner right elbow.

WITHDRAW AND PUSH. CROSSING HANDS

1 As you turn your waist to the left, your right arm follows your body to an angle of 45° and the fist opens up. Meanwhile, cup your left hand gracefully a couple of inches under your right elbow, as if supporting it.

2 Draw your right arm across your left palm as your weight sinks into your right foot, and your waist turns to the right.

3 Bring your waist back to the centre and turn both palms to face the front.

4 Move your weight forward 70% on to your left leg. Your hands remain at shoulder width and shoulder height.

5 Turn your waist to the right and simultaneously sink all your weight into your left leg. Draw your hands in towards your chest in a softly inverted "V" shape, as if holding the top of a ball.

6 As your whole weight shifts into your right leg, turn your waist to the right. Your left toes turn with your waist and your right hand travels out both diagonally and upwards.

EMBRACE TIGER, RETURN TO MOUNTAIN

7 Sink all your weight back into your left leg. Your left hand now travels out diagonally. Though the position might seem slightly awkward and lopsided, it actually flows naturally into the final step.

8 Finally, bring your right foot shoulder-width away from and parallel to the left, but maintain your weight 70% in the left leg. Both hands circle down and up, stopping opposite your chest, palms facing the body. The wrists are touching, with the right wrist outside the left one. Hold this stance for a few seconds.

I Keeping all your weight in your left leg, turn your waist to the right. Open your hands outwards. Step diagonally back with your right foot. Move your weight 70% on to your right foot. As your waist completes its turn, move your left hand so that the fingertips are in line with your left shoulder, palm facing forward.

ROLL BACK, PRESS AND PUSH: SINGLE WHIP

PUNCH UNDER ELBOW

2 As you turn your waist slightly to the right, allow your left hand to come across so that the fingertips point to your right elbow. Meanwhile, your right hand travels upwards so that the fingertips point heavenward.

I Now repeat the sequence in "Roll Back, Press and Push". This time, perform this section from one diagonal corner to the other rather than from one side to the other. This picture shows your position at the end of the sequence.

I Sink all your weight back on to your right foot. Turn your waist 45° to the left, lifting the left toes and letting your left foot and both arms pivot 45° to the left.

2 Lower your left foot, gradually shifting your weight forward into it. When all your weight is on your left foot, step forward with your right foot so that the heel is in line with your left instep.

3 Rotate your upper body 90° to the left. Your arms follow this waist movement, so that the hook (your right hand) is now out in front level with your right shoulder, and your left hand is level with your face at 90° to the front. Your weight is in your left leg.

4 Transfer all your weight to your right leg, turning your waist to the right and letting your left hand move down, then up, until the fingers are in line with your left shoulder. Your left arm and leg move around simultaneously. Rest your left heel on the ground without any weight.

STEP BACK TO REPULSE THE MONKEY

1 As you turn your waist further to the right, your right hand opens and moves down by your hip, then floats up to shoulder height. The palm of your left hand turns over to face down.

2 Step back with your left foot as your waist turns to the left. Your right hand travels forward, palm facing down, while your left hand travels down towards the left hip with the palm facing up.

3 The right toes also straighten as the waist turns. As you continue to turn to the left, your left hand floats up to shoulder height, while your right hand comes forward, palm facing down.

STEP BACK TO REPULSE THE MONKEY (RIGHT). DIAGONAL FLYING

1 Turn your waist to the right, step back with your right foot and let your left hand travel forward, palm down. Your right hand moves down to rest on your hip, palm up. Your left foot turns to face the front as the waist moves. Your right hand now comes up to shoulder height.

2 With your weight on your left foot, turn your waist to the left. Turn your right hand palm upwards as it travels round in front of your waist, while your left hand, palm downwards, comes in front of your chest. Your hands are now holding an imaginary ball in front of you.

3 Turn your waist 90° to the right, maintaining the position of your arms and hands in front of your chest, as if carrying the ball.

WAVING HANDS IN CLOUDS (RIGHT, LEFT, RIGHT)

4 Stepping with your right foot, turn a further 135° to the right, and then transfer 70% of your weight into the right foot. Your waist also turns to the right and your right hand moves with it, travelling to shoulder height, arm extended and facing diagonally upwards. Your left hand moves simultaneously to just outside your left thigh, palm facing down.

I Bring all your weight on to your right foot. Turn your waist to the right and move your left hand across near your right hip. At the same time, your right hand turns palm downwards at shoulder height. Raise your left foot and move it forward until the left heel is now level and in line with the right.

2 As your waist turns to the front, move your right hand to face it and your left hand to face your chest. The right toes swivel round to face forwards so that your feet are now shoulder-width apart.

3 As your waist turns to the left, turn your palms towards each other, as if holding a large ball to the left of your body. All your weight is in your left leg and your right foot steps in to about half shoulder width.

4 Turn your waist back to the centre. Your hands again change position, the left hand descending to be opposite and facing your waist, and the right hand opposite and facing your chest.

5 Turn your waist to the right, your hands holding the imaginary ball, with the right hand uppermost, palm facing down, and the left hand below it, palm facing up. When all your weight is on your right foot, step back to shoulder-width apart.

WAVING HANDS IN CLOUDS (LEFT, RIGHT, LEFT). THE WHIP

1 Turn your waist back to the centre, bringing your right hand down to face your waist and your left hand up to face your chest. Repeat Steps 3, 4 and 5, then Steps 2 and 3 from "Waving Hands in Clouds, Right, Left, Right".

2 Turn your waist back to the centre and form a hook with your right hand, as it moves in level with your chest, directly above your left hand. It is located in front of your waist, palm upwards.

3 Step forward with your right foot. Turn your waist to the right, then to the left as you transfer your weight to your right foot, sending out the hook at 90° to the front of your body.

GOLDEN ROOSTER STANDS ON ONE LEG (LEFT). SQUATTING SINGLE WHIP

4 Continue turning your waist around towards the left, and then step with your left foot to about shoulder-width apart, with your left palm now facing your left shoulder.

5 Shift your weight 70% on to your left foot, turning away your left palm at shoulder height, and turning the right toes to 45°.

1 Sink all your weight into your left leg, turning your left hand over so that the palm faces upwards. Simultaneously turn out the right toes. This is a nicely balanced, elegant position.

2 Move your weight across into your right leg, bringing your left palm in towards your chest. The left toes turn 45° to the right.

3 Sink down into your right leg, keeping your back straight. Move your waist to the left, brush open your left knee with your left arm and turn your left toes out 90° to the left.

4 Transfer all your weight into your left leg. Open the right hand hook, lower the hand then bring it up in front of your chest. Raise your right leg as your weight shifts forward into your left leg, so that your right thigh becomes parallel with the ground. Bend your left knee.

GOLDEN ROOSTER STANDS ON ONE LEG (RIGHT). SEPARATE RIGHT FOOT

1 Place your right foot down and move all your weight on to it. As your weight sinks into your right leg, your right hand descends to rest on a cushion of air by your right thigh. Your left arm and left leg simultaneously move up to form a mirror image of the previous posture.

2 Step out with your "empty" left foot diagonally to the left, and form a ward-off position with your left arm horizontally positioned across your body, opposite your chest.

3 Shift all your weight into your left leg, bringing your right arm up to cross in front of your left arm, with the wrists touching. Bring your right toe to your left heel. Turn your wrists, maintaining skin contact as you do so, so that your left arm now crosses your right.

4 Then turn your hands away from your body, and open them out in a fan like action. Your eyes should be level with the tips of your fingers.

5 Keep your left hand level with your left ear, palm facing away. Open out your right hand to the corner, below shoulder height, and simultaneously kick gently with your right leg, to knee height. You should be so balanced that you do not fall over.

1 Keeping all your weight in your left leg, turn to the left-hand corner, forming a ward-off position with your right arm.

2 Turn your waist to the right and step to the right with your right leg. As you transfer weight into it, bring your left hand up outside the right so that the wrists meet. The left toes come up to meet the right heel.

3 Open out your hands, the right hand this time remaining level with the head and the left hand travelling to below shoulder height. The left foot follows, kicking gently to the corner.

4 Turn your waist and left knee to the front again. Take a shoulder-width "empty" step with your left leg, toes pointing in the forward direction.

NEEDLES AT SEA BOTTOM

5 Brush your left hand across and above the front of your left leg, to just outside your left thigh. Your right hand curves in, fingertips forward, to finish with the fingers in line with your mouth.

1 Move all your weight into your left leg. Pick up your empty right foot and make a small adjustment step forward.

2 Place your right toes down, then bring your left hand across your body so that the left palm rests above your right wrist. At the same time, pick up your left leg and place the toes down.

IRON FAN PENETRATES BACK. TURN BODY, CHOP AND PUSH

3 Move your right arm forwards and diagonally downwards with your body, then vertically downwards. The arm remains in line with your right leg, and all your weight remains in your right leg.

1 Your weight remains in your right leg and both hands assume a ward-off position. Take a shoulder-width step with the left foot. Shift your weight 70% into your left leg and turn your hands outwards, the left hand by your chest, the right guarding your temple.

2 Turn your waist to the right and sink all your weight back into your right leg, bringing your left toes round. Bring your left hand up, turning the palm diagonally outwards to guard the temple. At the same time, form a loose fist with your right hand, palm facing downwards.

3 Sink all your weight back on to your left leg. As you transfer the weight back, the fist descends in front of your groin.

4 Step to shoulder width with your right foot. Your right arm pivots at the elbow and your left arm folds across so that the left hand faces the right inner elbow. All your weight remains on your left leg. You are nicely balanced as shown above.

5 Transfer your weight forward 70% into your right leg. Your left arm pushes forward, fingertips in line with your left shoulder, and your right fist descends to your right hip, palm upwards. The left toes are at 45°.

STEP FORWARD, DEFLECT DOWNWARDS, INTERCEPT AND PUNCH, KICK WITH HEEL

1 Sink all your weight into the left leg as your waist turns to the left. Bring the right toe to the left heel. The right hand comes across the body, and the palm faces down by the left hip. The left hand is below the right hand, palm up. Go to "Step Forward, Deflect, Intercept and Punch" and repeat Steps 3, 4 and 5.

2 Sink your weight into your left leg, turning your waist to the right. Cross your wrists, the right outside the left. Sink the weight back into your right leg. Your waist turns left and your left foot pivots on the heel 45° to the left. Shift all your weight forward into your left leg, turning your hands palms outwards.

3 Open your hands out gracefully like a fan, the right hand to below shoulder height, the left hand at head height, palms facing away. Your right foot now comes up from the ground, and the heel kicks diagonally away.

BRUSH RIGHT KNEE AND PUSH. BRUSH LEFT KNEE AND PUNCH DOWN

1 Place your "empty" right foot on the ground, toes forward. Your right hand curves down to rest on a cushion of air outside your right thigh. Your left hand curves forward to push to the centre, fingertips in line with your mouth.

2 Sink back into your left leg, turning your waist to the right, with the palm of your left hand facing towards your body in the Yang-style ward-off position.

3 Transfer your weight forward into your right foot, with your left palm turning so that it faces downwards.

WARD OFF RIGHT. ROLL BACK, PRESS AND PUSH. WHIP

4 Take a shoulder-width step with your left foot and bring 70% of your weight onto it. Your right hand forms a loose fist, which comes over your hip and punches down the centre. Your left hand brushes your left leg and rests by the left knee.

1 Sink back into your right leg. Your left hand now assumes a ward-off position, the fingertips of your right hand pointing towards the centre of the left palm. Your right palm faces downwards. Gaze steadily and confidently forwards.

2 Turn your body 45° to the left, pivoting neatly on the left heel. Shift all your weight forward into your left leg. Your left arm should remain in this position, while your right hand now presses smartly down.

FAIR LADY WEAVES SHUTTLES (RIGHT AND LEFT)

3 Step through at shoulder width with your "empty" right foot. As you transfer 70% of your weight into it, your right hand comes up into a ward-off position opposite your chest, with the left fingertips now pointing towards the right palm, left palm downwards. Repeat "Roll Back, Press and Push" and "Single Whip".

1 Transfer your weight to your right leg as you turn your waist to the right, and turn the "empty" left toes through 90°. Bring your left hand across your body and under your elbow. Open the hook of your right hand and lower the right arm, palm turning to face upwards.

2 Sink your weight back into your left leg, turn your waist further to the right and turn out your right foot so the heel is in line with the left instep.

3 Sink your weight into your right leg, drawing your left arm across your right palm, and step at shoulder width to the left corner with your left foot. As you shift your weight forward into your left leg, turn both palms outwards.

4 Transfer your weight into your right foot and turn your waist and left foot to the right as far as possible (135°). Turn your palms to face your body, the right palm by the left elbow.

5 Sink your weight back into your left leg and draw your left arm across your right palm.

FAIR LADY WEAVES SHUTTLES (RIGHT AND LEFT)

6 Turn a further 135° right, to the corner. Step to shoulder width with your right foot, and shift 70% of your weight into it, pushing towards the centre of your mouth with your left hand. Bring the right hand up to guard your forehead, palm facing diagonally.

1 Turn to the left, sinking all your weight into your left leg. Pick up your right foot and draw it in. Transfer all your weight to your right foot, then step to the left (45°) with your left foot. Turn your palms in and draw your right arm across the left palm, left arm in a ward-off position.

2 Your left hand then moves up and turns outwards by your head, while the fingers of your right hand come into the centre in line with your mouth. Now repeat the postures described in Steps 4, 5 and 6 of the previous exercise.

WARD OFF LEFT. WARD OFF RIGHT. ROLL BACK, PRESS AND PUSH. SINGLE WHIP

1 Sink your weight into your left leg as your waist turns to the left. Both arms come round with the movement of your waist, the left hand lower than the right. The right toes come round to the front.

2 Sink your weight into your right leg as your left hand presses down, palm facing downwards. Take a shoulder-width step with your left foot.

3 Transfer your weight 70% into your left foot. Your left hand comes up in front of your chest. Your right hand floats outside your right thigh. Repeat previous step.

SQUATTING SINGLE WHIP. STEP FORWARD FOR SEVEN STARS RIDE TIGER

1 Repeat the postures described in Steps 1, 2 and 3 of "Golden Rooster Stands on One Leg (Left). Squatting Single Whip", ending by brushing open the left knee.

2 Transfer all your weight into your left leg. The right hand hook opens and the hand descends, then comes up in front of your neck, where it forms a loose fist. At the same time, your left hand rises up to form a loose fist, and connects at the wrist inside your right hand. Move your right toes forward to touch the ground without any weight whatsoever.

1 Keep your weight in your left leg and step back with your right foot, toes touching the ground first. Sink your weight into it and turn your waist to the right. The fists open and then move down by your right hip, with the wrists still connected.

2 Pick up your left leg as your waist turns right, then place your toes down as your waist turns back to the left. Your right hand comes round to the front, fingertips level with your right ear, and your left hand rests by your left thigh.

3 Pick up your left toes, turn your waist to the left corner and place the toes down empty of any weight. Your right palm faces your inner left elbow. Your left hand is at the height of your left shoulder, elbow relaxed.

4 Lift your left toes and swing your waist clockwise, pivoting on the ball of your right foot. Your arms swing to the right with the movement of your waist.

5 Drop your left foot and transfer all your weight into it straight away. Look closely at the photograph above to check how you should be standing.

6 When your arms and waist reach the front (the arms at shoulder height and shoulder width with the palms facing downwards), your right foot lifts up and circles clockwise.

7 After circling, your right leg comes to rest with the upper leg parallel to the ground and the foot comfortably relaxed. Your left leg is bent while the arms are still pointing ahead.

BEND BOW TO SHOOT TIGER. STEP FORWARD, DEFLECT DOWN, INTERCEPT AND PUNCH

1 Turn your waist to the right. Your arms follow your waist, dropping down parallel, and your right foot is placed facing the right corner.

2 As your waist turns to the right, shift the weight into your right leg and circle your arms round to the right. As your waist turns back to the left, raise your arms and circle round with the waist. Form loose fists. Bring the right hand up to the right of your forehead, knuckles facing the right eyebrow. The left hand is at shoulder height.

3 Sink your weight into your left leg and pick up your right foot, placing the toes by your left heel. Open the left fist as your arms move across your body following the waist movement.

WITHDRAW AND PUSH. CROSSING HANDS. CONCLUSION.

4 Both hands and your right foot simultaneously arc in towards the centre line, as your waist turns to the right. The right foot lands "empty", completely in line with the left instep.

5 Continue to turn your waist, bringing the right fist palm upwards to rest on your right hip and shifting your weight to the right foot. Step through at shoulder width with your left foot. Shift 70% of your weight to the left and bring your right fist forward to punch in a corkscrew. Your left arm comes across your body.

1 Repeat the postures described in "Withdraw and Push. Crossing Hands". Ensure your weight is 70% in your left leg when crossing hands.

2 From crossing the hands, turn both palms down to face the ground as your body now rises up.

3 Bring all your weight into your left leg, turn your waist to the right and pivot on your left heel, turning the foot out to an angle of 45°.

4 Move all your weight into your right leg. Step in with your left foot so that the feet make a right angle. Bring half your weight to the left foot. Rest your arms and hands by your side with shoulders relaxed. You may now begin again.

yoga stretches
yoga stretches

yoga stretches

Have you ever watched a cat waking up? More often than not, it will give an exaggerated yawn, then arch its back until stretched to its limit, before loosely letting go and gracefully moving off on its way. Have you ever stopped to wonder why it makes these movements? The cat knows instinctively the value of stretching in maintaining flexibility and improving circulation to the muscles; you too can become stronger and more flexible with regular stretching exercises.

Most of us tend to hold in patterns of tension arising from everyday cares and worries, bad posture, lack of exercise and so on. These patterns make us feel stiff and unbending, and directly interfere with our movements. Inflexibility within our bodies can in turn affect mental flexibility, and we can become stuck in thought as well as in action. Regular stretching exercises not only free our bodies, allowing us to move easily, but can also help us to think and act without being so restricted. They are excellent improvers. In fact, by stretching muscles, ligaments and tendons, we make them much more efficient and stronger. The lengthening actions also help us to stand and walk taller, and even with added grace. The joints are better supported and are more able to go through their full range of movements, while the muscles are better nourished from the increased blood supply. The stretches give you that extra edge.

warm-up exercises

As any athlete will tell you, before starting to do any serious stretching or exercise, such as tennis, it is important that you first do some gentle warm-up exercises. They ensure that your muscles are nicely warmed and loosened, and will help to prevent any sudden strain or injury. The best thing is they only take a few minutes, and they can also be practised at any time if you are feeling stiff and need to loosen up.

SHRUGGING SHOULDERS

1 Stand upright with your feet slightly apart and your shoulders relaxed.

2 Lift your shoulders up as high as they will go, then let them fall down again. Stay relaxed and repeat a few times.

ARM CIRCLING

1 Wheel your arms around from the shoulders in slow, large circles.

2 Do this a few times going backwards, then repeat circling your arms forwards.

SQUATS

1 Stand with your feet slightly apart, hands on hips. Go slowly into a squat.

2 Slowly return to a standing position, then repeat. Your back should be upright.

LOOSE TWISTS

▮ In a standing position with feet comfortably apart and knees relaxed, swing your arms loosely backwards and forwards around your body. Keep your head and body facing forward all the time, and keep your feet and pelvis still. Repeat a few times to loosen your arms and shoulders.

ARM STRETCHING

▮ Stand with your arms straight out in front of you, at chest height. Take in a deep breath and exhale.

SIDEWAYS BEND

▮ Stand with your feet at least shoulder-width apart and your arms hanging down at your sides. Bend down to one side, trying not to twist. Slowly return to the upright and then bend to the other side. Straighten up and now repeat.

SHAKE

▮ Try to relax and let your whole body go completely floppy. Shake your limbs to release any tension. Continue for as long as you feel comfortable. If you prefer, shake each limb in sequence, starting with your right arm.

CAT STRETCH

▮ Kneel on all fours, with your hands and knees shoulder-width apart. As you start to inhale, bring your head forward and slightly hollow your back.

2 Now breathe out and, as you do so, arch the back upwards like a cat, allowing your head to drop down. Repeat a few times.

therapeutic movements
therapeutic movements

therapeutic movements

One of the best things about stretches is that you can do some simple, straightforward exercises anywhere, at any time: at home, in the office, standing in a queue or even sitting in the car; there are no restrictions. However, in order to get the most benefit from regular stretching, and particularly from doing yoga practice, it is important to create a quiet, comfortable space and to give yourself plenty of time to do the movements without any pressure or interruptions from the telephone or colleagues. In fact, making this space is in itself a relaxing, unwinding step, and will enhance the effectiveness of the actual exercises.

Ideally, make an area that feels quiet and calming to you, perhaps with softer lighting if it is needed, maybe with a thick, soft mat for the floor-based stretches. If you have any back discomfort, or just need extra support when lying down, then a couple of cushions may be extremely useful. It is helpful to wear loose fitting, airy clothing so that you can move freely and easily. If the weather permits try to let in some fresh air, but do not risk getting cold. These exercises are not intended to work up a good sweat or strain the heart, but to make you feel altogether less stiff and tense, and generally much more flexible. They are great for loosening you up, releasing tensions, improving circulation, toning the body, and generally making you feel much freer and more confident with your own body. They can really perk you up. After each exercise you will also need time to relax quietly, before you plunge back into everyday life.

If you find them an enormous benefit and become inspired, and want to try out more exercises, then do find a good, local class. Yoga exercises are generally best learnt in such a class, with a skilled, experienced teacher for maximum benefit. Alternatively you could create your own class at home, inviting a yoga teacher, friends and family on a regular basis.

tension and backache relievers

In the great majority of cases back trouble is the result of chronic tensions which can build up around the spine. Tired, tight muscles are also much more prone to strain or injury. The stretches that are shown here are intended to aid flexibility of the spine, and to make you feel much more supple, but if you already suffer from back pain or an injury then you must seek professional advice.

COBRA

1 Lie on your front, with your arms bent and your hands under your shoulders.

2 Slowly lift your head and push down on your arms to help raise your trunk.

3 If you can, tilt your head backwards and stretch up and back, then relax.

SIMPLE TWIST

1 Sit on the floor with your legs stetched straight out in front of you.

2 Bend one leg and place the foot on the floor across the other knee.

3 Place your opposite arm in front of your bent leg and twist to look over your shoulder.

FULL TWIST

1 Bend one leg so that the foot rests on the inner thigh of the other leg.

2 Bring this leg over the first one, then grasp your foot with the other arm.

3 Twist as far around as you can, hold, then relax. Swap over your legs. Repeat.

TRIANGLE

1 Stand with your feet shoulder-width apart and your arms straight out to the sides. This should be a well-balanced, easily held position. Your head should feel like a ball balancing on your neck. Stare straight ahead.

2 Bend down to one side without twisting your body, letting the opposite arm rise in the air. If you find this awkward or uncomfortable, do not strain yourself. The object is to loosen the body, not injure it.

3 Stretch the raised arm, look up and hold. Slowly straighten and repeat on the other side. If you can, repeat several times, but be careful to move slowly into position to avoid a strain.

BENDING TWIST   SLOUCH STRESS

1 Stand with your feet shoulder-width apart and your arms straight out to the sides. Bending forward, try to touch your foot, or the floor in front of it if you can, with your opposite hand. Slowly uncurl and return to the starting position. Repeat on the other side.

1 Sit on a tall stool so that your feet are just off the floor. With your hands behind your back, slouch so that your back is rounded, with your head now lowered down towards your chest.

2 Flex one foot, and lift the leg to straighten it if possible. Release the leg, relax, then repeat a few times. Repeat with the other leg. Note that the object is to build up a slow pace, not to go fast.

soothing and removing tension

Many of us suffer at some time from tension headaches and know that they begin with a gradual feeling of pressure in the head or neck, or a taut sensation in the facial muscles. Once you are aware of such tension, tackle it immediately. A few simple stretches can help to relieve these muscular spasms and prevent them leading to a severe headache. They can be done almost anywhere.

SIDEWAYS NECK STRETCH

1 Slowly stretch your head down to one side, feeling the pull in the neck muscles. Return the head to the upright position and repeat on the other side.

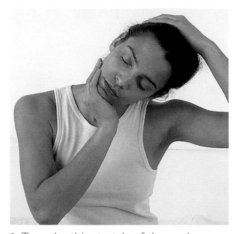

2 To make this stretch of the neck muscles more effective, use your hands to give extra leverage. Place one hand under your chin and the other on top of your head; repeat the other side.

HEAD TO CHEST

1 Lower your head towards your chest, feeling the pull on the back of the neck. Hold at your furthest stretch before slowly raising the head again. Repeat two or three times.

LION POSTURE

1 To stretch the facial muscles and release tension, open your mouth as wide as possible and push out your tongue. At the same time, open your eyes into as wide a stare as you can manage. Repeat a couple of times.

SEMICIRCLE ROTATION

1 Turn the head to one side, then steadily rotate it in a semicircular movement, letting the chin drop down across the chest.

2 Dropping the head backwards compresses the neck, so it is best not to make this a full circle rotation. Repeat, going back in the opposite direction.

posture enhancers
One of the great benefits of an exercise system such as yoga is the fact that it gradually and increasingly gives you considerable grace and poise. In addition it will make a huge difference to your overall posture. If it was previously a bit lax, and you ended up slouching, you will really notice the difference. In fact, learning to hold yourself properly can help you to look and feel much younger, and reduce muscle strain.

1 Stand with feet slightly apart and arms raised in front. Slowly twist to one side. Repeat on the other side.

2 Stand with your feet apart, and hold your arms out. Bend over, sliding one hand down the inside of the same leg.

3 Reach as far as is comfortable, then slowly return to the upright and repeat on the other side.

4 For the tree routine, stand on one leg and bend the other knee, as shown.

5 Either place your palms together above your head, or raise the hands.

6 For the arm and leg stance, stand on one leg and hold the other foot behind.

tired and aching leg revivers
Most of us spend too long each day with our legs stuck in fixed positions, and stiffness of the lower limbs from inactivity or tension can make you feel quite tired. Legs benefit from being stretched, keeping them toned and supple. These exercises prevent the legs, thighs and lower back from getting too tense. Since some of these positions are quite difficult, do beware of straining yourself.

ALTERNATE LEG PULLS

1 Sit on the floor, with one leg out straight and the other bent so that the foot rests on the inner thigh of your extended leg. Do it with care.

2 Lean forward and clasp the straight leg as far down as is comfortable; pull your chest down a little further and hold for a moment. Change legs and repeat.

FULL LEG PULLS

1 The previous stretch can be extended by starting with both legs straight out in front of you. Repeat as described.

SIDE LEG RAISE

2 Lean forward and hold the legs with both hands; pull yourself down a little further and hold for a moment. If this is difficult, bend the legs slightly.

1 Lie on your side with your legs and body in a straight line. Support your head with one hand and place your free hand on the floor for balance.

2 Without twisting your hips, steadily raise the upper leg as far as is comfortable. Hold, then lower slowly. Repeat with the other leg.

CAT STRETCH

1 Kneel on all fours with your hands and knees shoulder-width apart. Raise your head and look straight ahead.

2 Breathe in, and as you exhale lift and arch your back. Hold for a moment before relaxing back into the original position. Inhale, then repeat.

BACK PUSH-UP

1 Lie on your back with your knees bent and your feet on the floor, hip-width apart. Now place your hands on the floor by your shoulders.

SIT UP/LIE DOWN

2 Push up with your hands and feet, arching your back at the same time. Hold for a moment, then lower your body back to the floor. Do not strain yourself with this movement – it works on lots of muscles at the same time.

1 Sit on the floor with both legs straight out in front of you. Your torso should be at right angles to your legs, with your eyes looking forward.

2 Slowly lower your back to the floor, then start to bend the legs and raise them off the floor.

3 As you raise the legs, slowly start to straighten them until they are as close to the vertical as you can manage. Again, take care not to strain yourself.

4 Keeping the legs straight, slowly lower them to the floor.

5 Continue the movement by sitting up and clasping your legs with your hands to bend forwards. Slowly return to the original sitting position.

abdominal tension relievers
We tend to hold and lock up too much tension in our abdomen, especially if we are the kind of people who always bottle up our feelings. Even simple muscular tension can leave us feeling stiff and rather uncomfortable, and much less flexible around the waist. Consequently exercises aimed at reducing stiffness and increasing flexibility in the abdominal region are extremely useful.

LOTUS

1 For the full lotus, the first leg should be bent with the foot on top of the other thigh, and the second leg bent so that the foot goes over the other leg on to the opposite thigh. Hold if possible.

2 For an easier version bend one leg and rest the foot on the inner thigh of the other leg. Bend the second leg and place the foot on top of the opposite thigh. Keep the spine upright.

ABDOMINAL MOVEMENTS

1 Either sit cross-legged or kneel, and place your hands on your waist or thighs. Breathe out completely.

LEG OVER

2 Without inhaling, pull in your abdomen as far as you can, then "snap" it in and out up to five times before taking a breath. Relax for a few moments, breathing freely, before repeating.

1 Lie on your back, with your legs out straight. Raise one leg as close to the vertical as is comfortable, then move it across the body, keeping your hips in contact with the floor.

2 Push the leg as far over as possible, then slowly return to the original position. Repeat with the other leg.

LYING TWISTS

1 Lie on your back, hands behind your head and legs together, knees bent.

2 Twist the legs from side to side, keeping the back and hips on the floor.

SIDE BENDS

1 Stand with feet apart and hands on hips. Bend down to one side.

ROLL TWIST

2 Slowly return to the upright position and bend to the other side. Repeat.

1 Keeping the legs and hips still, roll your upper body around in a clockwise circle.

2 Move slowly and carefully, and bend only as far as is comfortable.

SIT UP/LIE DOWN

1 Sit on the floor with both legs straight out in front of you.

2 Slowly lie back, then start to bend the legs and raise them off the floor.

3 Sit up, bend forwards, clasp your legs and slowly return to the sitting position.

office tensions and stiff muscles For people

who spend their working day sitting at a desk it is very easy to get stiff, aching muscles. Badly designed chairs do not help, and as you get tired, so posture suffers and you can end up getting round-shouldered. It is therefore absolutely essential that every now and again you get up and walk around, relax your body, and try some of these excellent loosening-up exercises.

SEATED CAT STRETCH

I Pull the chair back from the desk slightly to give yourself more room, then bend forward and clasp your ankles.

2 Carefully arch your back to stretch, then relax back and repeat.

CALF STRETCH

I Sit fairly upright, then lift and straighten each leg alternately. Repeat a few times.

NECK TWISTS

2 Flex the foot to stretch the calf muscle. Repeat a few times.

I Turn your head to one side, feeling the extension in the neck muscles.

2 Repeat, turning the head from side to side. Do both steps quite slowly.

ARM AND CHEST STRETCH

❙ Sitting upright, link your hands together, palms away from your body, and push your arms straight out in front of you. Hold for a couple of seconds, relax and then repeat.

ARM AND BACK STRETCH

❙ Link your hands together behind your back, over the top of the chair, and lift your arms slightly. Do not strain yourself. Push away from your body, hold, then repeat the exercise.

FOREARM STRETCH

❙ Hold your arms straight out to the sides and stretch them. Alternately flex and extend your hands. Feel the pull on the upper and lower sides of your forearms as you do so.

BACK/SHOULDER STRETCH

❙ Stretch your arms up in the air over your head. As you breathe in, arch your back ever so slightly. Relax with the exhalation and repeat the exercise a couple of times.

POSTURE CLASP

❙ Put one arm behind your back and bend it up, with the hand reaching the other shoulder. With your other arm raised and bent down over your shoulder, try to clasp your fingers.

SHOULDER RELEASE

❙ Link your fingers together and stretch your arms high above your head. Repeat several times.

meditation

meditation
meditation

Meditation has been in use from the beginning of time: people have always sought inner quiet and physical relaxation, whether for reasons connected with the spirit, self-realization or health. You do not have to be a physical contortionist to achieve and enjoy the benefits of meditation at both physical and mental levels.

What, then, is meditation? It has been described as just sitting and relaxing. Many people find that their lives are so full of the demands of work, family, friends and organized leisure pursuits that they have no time to "stand and stare". Many are so caught up in planning and working towards the future that they take little pleasure from the here and now. In their bustle to "get on" they miss out on the simple pleasures of life. But beauty and joy are there to be seen and experienced, even in industrial cities.

The benefits of meditation come from regular use. If you are under stress, you may find that meditating twice daily will be effective in restoring composure. Make a time and space you can call your own, and use breathing and relaxation exercises to ease yourself into the meditative state. The more you practise meditation the less time you will need to spend on these, but they remain useful in calming and preparing you. Allow at least 10 minutes, ideally 20, for meditation in each session.

the benefits of meditation
Human beings were never designed to cope with the high-pressure demands of life in the 21st century; life when you are constantly in demand, having to make vital decisions at breakneck speed right through the day, and even during the night. You might say it cannot be done, but it can, with help. Knowing how as well as when to switch off makes all the difference, and even scientists now agree.

PSYCHO-PHYSICAL LINKS

A period of meditation can often lead to a feeling of being refreshed, with a more positive attitude and a general feeling of well-being. Things that had been bothering you may now be seen in a new and more helpful way. You gain a different, wider perspective on things and feel very much more in control.

These beneficial reactions have been well known for years, but only in recent times has anyone found a physiological explanation. Detailed, extensive knowledge of brain scans and even brain wave patterns has given extraordinary new information about what is commonly called the "alpha state".

Mind and body work together in meditation to promote health and well-being in the whole person.

Endorphin Release

When we are truly relaxed, both mentally and physically, there are changes in the brain wave pattern until it is predominantly located and fixed within the alpha state. Within this particular state the brain triggers chemicals known as endorphins. It is in fact this chemical trigger that has the benefits that are experienced as a feeling of well-being. Indeed, endorphins have frequently been called "nature's very own special opiates". Meditation is one of the easiest ways to achieve this, and these good feelings can easily linger for some time after the meditation has ended, the length of time varying considerably. There is also a real physical benefit, as these endorphins boost and recharge the immune system, helping you to fight off all kinds of infections.

Meditation and Work

The tensions of modern working practices often mean that people are so bound up in meeting all the vigorous demands placed upon them that they maintain a high level of mental and physical activity right through the day. This frequently means that they are not only cutting off their extremely important emotional responses and their enjoyment of the simple things in life, but they are also pushing their physical and mental health right to the very limit. Much has now been written about the management of stress, and the significant need for periods of mental and physical relaxation during the working day.

The 20-minute Rule

One writer, Ernest Rossi, has formulated the 20-minute rule which is based on the theory of ultradian rhythms. Ultradian rhythms are biorhythms that the body works through during each day – a little like hyperbolic curves of energy which repeat every 90 to 120 minutes. Naturally, it would be best to work only at peak performance times, but this is just not possible. However, timing work breaks to coincide with the mind/body slow-down pattern every 90 minutes does ensure maximum productivity and restricts the potential build-up of stress.

Rossi suggested the pattern of working for 90 minutes and then taking a brief 20-minute break. He himself usually lies down and meditates during this period because it is the best form of total mental and physical relaxation, and is good preparation for returning to optimum mental processing.

It is important that these breaks take place every 90 minutes or so, and in such a way as to completely change the mind/body state. Ideally, you should stop all work activity and experience a change of physical status (standing rather than sitting, looking into the distance rather than close up, for example) and mental focus. A 20-minute meditation is ideal and the benefits will be felt immediately. On returning to work after the 20 minutes, you will see things afresh and deal with them more efficiently, as you are ready to climb to peak performance on the biorhythmic curve. The feeling of well-being lasts into the next 90-minute period.

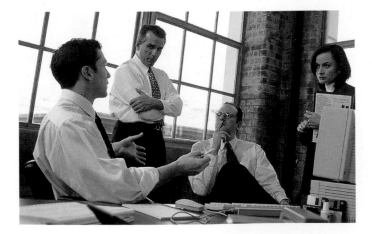

To be at your best for meetings ensure you take regular breaks.

gaining the meditative state

Many religious groups, as well as adherents of Transcendental Meditation, use a sound, or "mantra", to help with meditation. The constant repetition of a phrase, word or sound ("aum" is commonly used in Hinduism) creates the alpha state by an almost hypnotic focus of attention upon that particular sound. In fact chants repeated again and again can lead to its members reaching a "high".

Sound

An effortless sound, repeated with the natural regular rhythm of breathing, can have the same soothing, liberating effect as the constant natural sound of running water, rustling leaves or a beating heart. The single sound, or mantra as it is known, is used to blot out the "chatter" of intrusive thoughts, allowing the mind to find deep repose. Speaking or chanting a mantra as a flowing stream of endless sound is a very old method of heightening a person's awareness by concentrating the senses. The simple gentle sound "om", or "aum", is sometimes known as the first mantra, which is literally an instrument of thought. The curving Sanskrit (the ancient language of Hindus in India) symbol for this primordial word represents the various states of consciousness: waking, dreaming, deep sleep and the transcendental state.

However, the actual sound need not be a special word or incantation; something simple and meaningful will be as effective. The sound of the word "calm" spoken or thought with each exhalation can be very effective, especially while imagining tension leaving your body. Any word that appeals to you will do.

Make sure that you are sitting quite comfortably and then start breathing in the colour of your choice.

Touch

You can use your sense of touch in a lulling, soothing way to induce a state of meditation at times of stress. Young children do this when they adopt a satisfyingly smooth ribbon or piece of fabric to hold and manipulate when they are feeling tense. The same technique is seen all over the Middle East, where strings of worry beads are rhythmically passed through the fingers at difficult moments to focus the mind and calm anxiety. Their uniform size, gentle round shapes, smooth surfaces and rhythmic, orderly clicking as they are passed along their string all assist the meditative state. Use one or two smooth, rounded stones in the same way, passing them slowly from hand to hand.

Colours

Some colours are associated with relaxation and can be a helpful way to clear the mind of tension and allow meditation to start. Sit with your eyes closed, and be aware of the colour that comes into your mind: it may be any colour of the rainbow — red or purple are common. Then slowly and gradually allow that colour to change to a blue or green colour, allowing it to fill the whole of your mind's eye and replacing all other colours. The colour pink is also recommended by colour therapists and this may prove helpful. You will find a feeling of relaxation growing as the new colour builds in your mind, and when the relaxed colour is complete, you will experience feelings of inner peace.

Establish a comfortable rhythm of breathing and then focus on it until your mind is completely still, relaxed and clear. Colours are associated with all kinds of qualities, so choose the best for your own particular moods and needs. Red: vitality, energy, strength and willpower (complementary colour turquoise). Orange: happiness and laughter (complementary colour blue). Yellow: intellect and objectivity (complementary colour violet). Green: cleansing and harmony (complementary colour magenta). Turquoise: boosts and strengthens the immune system, counteracts disease (complementary colour red). Blue: peace and relaxation, restful sleep (complementary colour orange). Violet: beauty, dignity, assured self-respect (complementary colour yellow). Magenta: the liberating release of all obsessional thoughts and memories (complementary colour green).

Repeating a mantra takes you into a world of peace and harmony.

how to use meditation
how to use meditation

how to use meditation

The key to using meditation lies in recognizing that you actually need it. Once you get into the whirlpool of work and stress, they can both all too easily become an integral part of your lifestyle. In fact, they can be such a formidable cornerstone that you cannot imagine what life could possibly be like without them. But once you stand back and see clearly and exactly what is happening to you, what your life has become, then suddenly you see you actually need a way out. One of the best ways involves deep meditation.

Meditation needs to be done like regular exercise. In fact you might say you are exercising the ways in which you relax. The very first step involves switching off, like switching off a light in a room, and concentrating on what could be called the "Inner Other", that is to say the marvellous, relaxed, empty inner spaces inside your head and body. This stage, put crudely, means sweeping out all the noise and mayhem and chaos of everyday life and getting ready to enter another world.

The second stage involves being carried along what one expert teacher calls "a moving but going nowhere sound that coils round and even through itself in a perpetual state of being". Perhaps the best way of evaluating it is by hearing what people have to say after meditation. "As good as a holiday" or "like a wonderful deep refreshing sleep" is what most people say. If you are to get its full, continuous benefits then you really must make sure that meditation is something that you do regularly every day, at certain times, because like almost all forms of exercise the more often you do it, the better you are at it; the quicker you can switch off and tune in, and enter that fantastic deep state of total energizing, refreshing relaxation.

You must use meditation with care though. It is not like switching on and off a tap. It needs to be respected. Few people who meditate try, even if they could, to describe its ultimate power. That would be like divulging a wonderful private secret; to have it is quite enough.

simple meditation techniques If you want to

learn to meditate seriously, you would do well to find an experienced teacher to guide you.

However, there are many simple techniques that you can practise alone, often with quite

powerful effects. Try the ones described here, and see which you feel in tune with. The more

you practise, the easier it will become to reach a deep meditative state.

Introduce a child to meditation by using the Numbers Game.

THE NUMBERS GAME

This is a very simple form of meditation using a blackboard, real or imaginary. It is a good "game" to use with children (or adults), giving them a taste of meditation, and they really enjoy it. It is described here as if you are leading a group, but it can be easily used on one person, and provides an excellent way to clear the mind through concentration, imagination and patterns: all wonderful ways of gaining a real experience of deep meditation.

What you must do is this …

1 Get the children to sit or lie comfortably. Once they have found a really comfortable position ask them to remember it.

2 With chalk on the blackboard, draw a diagram of numbers, making sure that there are no mathematical links, like this:

$$
\begin{array}{ccc}
3 & 1 & 5 \\
8 & 6 & 9 \\
4 & 7 & 2
\end{array}
$$

3 Give the children one minute to memorize this sequence.

4 Ask them to return to their relaxed position, eyes closed, and concentrate on the numbers alone.

5 Rub out the numbers, telling them to do the same in their minds. Do this slowly saying "That leaves just four numbers", etc.

6 Then rub out the last number, saying "Now concentrate on what is left" … Let them remain in silence until you notice a restlessness – this is often three or more minutes.

7 Wake them gently with an instruction to "Sit up". Ask them what the last number was and for their reactions.

THE HAVEN

Once you have managed to achieve complete physical relaxation and calm, gradually allow your mind to enter a place, whether real or imaginary, that is quite special to you. Now you can allow your mind to drift … drift to a pleasant, peaceful place. A place that you know and where you always feel able to relax … completely. A safe … secure … place … where no one … and nothing can ever bother you.

It may be a place you have visited on holiday, a beach or a place in the countryside. Or it may be a room … a room you have had … a room you do have … or a room you would like to have … an imaginary place. But it is a place where you can always feel able to let go … completely … a haven, a haven of tranquillity, unique and special to you.

In order to help you imagine this place … notice first the light: is it bright, natural or dim … is there any particular source of light … natural or man-made? Notice also the temperature level … hot, warm or cool … and any particular source of heat. Be aware of the colours that surround you … shapes … and textures … the familiar objects that make that place special. Begin to see it in all its detail. You can just be there … whether sitting, lying or reclining, enjoying the sounds … the smells … the atmosphere … with nobody wanting anything, nobody needing anything and no one demanding anything from you. Relax.

Everyone has their own haven, a quiet magical place like this.

Try to imagine your perfect country house.

A GUIDED VISIT TO A COUNTRY HOUSE

Imagine that you are visiting a beautiful country house … a really beautiful old country house or a stately home with magnificent sweeping lawns on a warm, sunny, summer's afternoon. You are standing on the staircase that leads into the entrance hall, one of those wide ceremonial types of staircase. And as you look down across the entrance hall you can just glimpse, through the open doors opposite, a gravel drive, and the sunlight on the gravel. It is a beautiful, sunny, summer's afternoon and there is no one around to trouble or bother you as you stand alone on that staircase …

Now you are moving down the last ten steps to the hallway, relaxing more and more with each step down.

10 Taking one step down, relaxing and letting go …
9 Taking another step down, feeling at ease …
8 Becoming more relaxed, letting go even more …
7 Just drifting deeper … and deeper … everything is getting darker and darker, and even deeper down still …

6 Becoming calmer … and calmer … even calmer still …
5 Continuing to relax, continuing to let go and feeling good …
4 Relaxing even more … letting go even more …
3 Sinking deeper … drifting even further into this welcoming, relaxed state …
2 Enjoying those good feelings, all those feelings of inner peace and relaxation …
1 Nearly all the way down now, feeling very good … beautifully relaxed … and **0**.

You are wandering across that hallway now, towards the open doors and the gardens beyond, soaking up the atmosphere of peace and permanence in that lovely old building. You wander out through the doors and down the stone steps outside … and find yourself standing on the gravel drive outside, a wide gravel drive that leads down to the entrance gates.

As you stand there you notice the lush green lawns, so flat and well-clipped … and there are shrubs and trees, different shades of green and brown against a clear, blue sky … and you can feel the warmth of the sun on your head and shoulders as you enjoy this beautiful summer's afternoon in this lovely old garden … There are flowerbeds with their splashes of colour so carefully arranged and neatly tended. And there's no one else about … nobody needing anything, nobody wanting anything and nobody expecting anything from you, so you can enjoy the peace and serenity and solitude of this afternoon in this beautiful garden that's been so well looked after for so many, many years.

A little way down on the right-hand side of the driveway, you notice an ornamental fish pond. So you decide to wander down and have a look at those fish. Sometimes they seem almost to disappear behind the weed and shadows, but always they reappear, with their scales catching the sunlight, red, gold, silver or black. And as you watch those fish your mind becomes even more deeply relaxed …

THE WELL

This continues from the previous visualization of the beautiful country house and is intended to take you to even deeper levels of meditation.

… As you watch those fish you notice that the centre of the pond is very deep. It could be the top of a disused well. You take from your pocket a silver-coloured coin, and toss that coin so that it lands over the centre of the pond, and then you watch as it swings down through the water. The ripples drift to the edges of the pond, but you just watch that coin as it sinks deeper and deeper through that clear water, sometimes it seems to disappear as it turns on edge, at other times a face of the coin catches the sunlight and it flashes through the water … sinking, drifting deeper and deeper, twisting and turning as it makes its way down … Finally it rests at the bottom lying on a cushion of soft brown mud, a silver coin in that still, clean water on its own cushion of mud … And you feel as still as that coin, as still and cool and motionless as that water, enjoying that feeling of inner peace and stillness.

Watch the ripples as the coin lands in the very centre of the pond. Look even more closely as it tumbles down through the water …

personal development
Affirmations are a deceptively simple device that can be used by anyone and they are remarkably effective. Try to use this method while in the meditative state, having planned and memorized the affirmations involved. These powerful, positive phrases will improve communication with all parts of your mind. All you need is a simple phrase summing up how you want to be.

THE POWER OF WORDS
To make affirmations effective, they should
- be made in the present tense
- be positively phrased
- have an emotional reward.

Now contrast the power of such phrases with what happens if you are asked not to do or think of something. The words "no", "not", "never" and so on generally have the opposite effect to that intended, and why? Yours is the most influential voice in your life because you believe it. It comes live, straight out of the personality and intellect, and is fuelled by your dreams and language. The power you have over yourself is extraordinary. That is precisely why you must be careful to avoid any negative or demeaning statements you regularly make about yourself, either to others or to yourself – "I am shy", "I lack confidence", "I cannot", "I get nervous when" and so on – they are self-limiting beliefs that you are reinforcing each time they slip into your conversation or mind. You become what you say.

The point about affirmations is that instead of running yourself down, albeit in a subtle, insidious way, you actually start building yourself up. You start creating the inner psychological scaffolding to support the new you. Such affirmations are best used while in a wonderful state of meditation.

Thinking through what you want to be is the big key to success.

IMPROVED SELF-WORTH
We all have attributes and qualities in which we can take pride and pleasure. This exercise is about emphasizing these positive aspects to allay the doubts that only serve to limit our potential.
- I like my [physical attribute].
- I am proud of my [attitude or achievement].
- I love meeting people – they are fascinating.
- My contribution is valuable to [name person].
- I am lovable and can give love.
- Others appreciate my [opinions, assistance, a personal quality].
- I enjoy being a unique combination of mind and body.

Now imagine yourself speaking to colleagues, boss, employees or friends ... See yourself behaving and looking confident, standing and looking a confident person ... Notice how you stand ... your facial expression ... hear the way that you speak ... slowly, calmly, quietly, clearly and with confidence. You are communicating your needs ... ideas ... opinions in a positive way. Notice how your words flow easily, and how others are listening attentively to you ... valuing what you have to say. Now "climb aboard" ... be there – know how it feels to stand like that ... to speak like that ... and to have that positive reception from others. Get in touch with the stance ... expression ... and feelings ... and know that you can use these any time in the future to gain those same feelings or that inner strength in everything you do. See yourself in different situations: at home, in a social setting, in all the parts of your life, confident and assured, going from strength to strength.

The difference affirmations can make is extraordinary. From shy and introverted to open, confident and winning.

If you want to be No. 1, then take time to concentrate on seeing yourself as the best. Give yourself the power to come out top.

VISUALIZATION

In the same way that you can utilize your voice, so, perhaps more powerfully, you can use your imagination. The imagination can stimulate emotions, and they can register new attitudes in the mind. It can be a direct communication with the deeper levels of the mind, providing a powerful influence for improvements in your attitudes, behaviour patterns and overall confidence.

Visualization requires that you imagine yourself in a situation, behaving, reacting and looking as you would wish to do at an interview, an important meeting, a social gathering, a one-to-one situation, or perhaps a sporting event. Imagine what that will mean for you, your reactions, the reactions of those around you and, importantly, feel all the good feelings that will be there when this happens in reality.

It is like playing a video of the event, on that screen on the inside of the forehead, the mind's eye, from the beginning of the situation through to the perfect outcome. Should any doubts or negative images creep into your "video", push them away and replace them with positive ones. Keep this realistic, and base it upon real information from your past.

CONFIDENCE IN FUTURE SITUATIONS

The meditative state, affirmations and visualization can be a valuable rehearsal and preparation for a future event. Athletes and other sportsmen have proved that it actually does work. We can all use these extraordinary techniques to achieve our own optimum performance during any situation. Now consider the following phrases, and how they relate to you …

* I am quietly confident in meetings.
* I speak slowly, quietly and confidently so that others listen.
* My contribution is wanted and valued by others.
* I enjoy meetings, as they bring forth new ideas and help to renew my enthusiasm.

Imagine an important meeting that is about to happen, and see yourself there, filling in all the details that you know, and the people too; imagine yourself there looking confident and relaxed, concentrating on what is happening. Be aware of the acute interest you are giving to what is happening with complete, concentrated attention, and then imagine yourself speaking, to give information or to ask a question: hear yourself speaking quietly, slowly and calmly …

Notice people listening to what you are saying; they wish you well and support you, as you are expressing your viewpoint or raising a question they may well have wanted to ask, too. Notice how you are sitting or standing, how you lean slightly forward when speaking, that expression of calm confidence on your face. When this is clear in your mind, just like a film playing in your mind's eye, play it back and forth. When you are feeling comfortable with it, get into that imaginary you, "climb aboard" and be there in your mind, seeing things from that perspective, hearing things from that point in the meeting. As you speak, get in touch with those calm feelings, and the attitudes that allow you to feel calm, in control, and quietly confident … It is like a rehearsal; the more you manage to rehearse the better the final performance will be. You will acquire the right attitudes, stance and tone of voice, so that when you are in that situation all of these will be available to you, and it will be just as you imagined, as if you had done it all, successfully, before.

In short, what this technique does is take you step by step through a rehearsal. Imagine every possible scenario, and how you will deal with it. That is the key to a successful outcome.

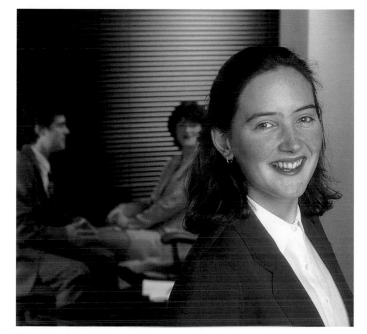

The preparation was worth it; you went into a meeting knowing you could do it, and that is exactly what happened.

enjoyment and achievement The mind and the body
are so completely interlinked that if we keep physically fit we are also mentally alert. The one boosts the other, but it also works the other way around. If we really utilize our mental capacities we can affect and improve our physical health and performance. So it is up to you to make sure that these twin forces keep functioning at full power. Do not let either slip.

A well-tuned lively body keeps you feeling well and alert.

THE BODY/MIND LINK

Regularly say to yourself …
- I feel safe, happy and content in the knowledge that my body is constantly renewing itself. It is alive and well.
- It feels marvellous to know that every damaged cell is replaced by a healthy one.
- My immune system is strong and fights off any infections easily.
- My mind and my body are working in harmony to keep me healthy, well and alert.

Now, imagine yourself lying or sitting comfortably. As you see yourself there you notice a healing glow of coloured light surrounding your body, but not touching it. Let that colour become stronger, until it has a very clear pure colour, which is the colour of healing for you.

Now, as you watch, that healing, coloured light begins to flow into the top of your head. You can see it slowly draining into all parts of the head, face, ears, and starts its journey down through the neck and shoulders, into the tops of the arms … It continues to flow down through the arms and the chest area, that healing, coloured light, penetrating all the muscles and organs … even as you watch you can also feel a healing warmth coming into your body … NOW … as it flows down into the stomach area, the back, right the way down to the base of the spine. Then you can allow the light to disperse again and gradually return to your normal wakeful state, knowing that in those areas that need it, the healing process will continue.

STRESS REDUCTION

Stress is a factor in everyone's life and can even be a major motivator in some circumstances. Meditation can be a great help in coping with it, and combined with visualization, it can change your whole response to stressful demands. Keep saying …
- I enjoy solving problems.
- I work well under pressure.
- I am a calm, methodical and efficient worker.
- I love that feeling of having achieved so much in a day.
- I enjoy being calm when others around me are not.

Imagine yourself in a situation that has in the past caused stress. Picture the situation, and the other people involved … See yourself there … and notice a slight shimmer of light between yourself and those other people … a sort of bubble around you … a protective bubble that reflects any negative feelings back to them … leaving you able to get on with your tasks … your life, with an inner strength and calmness that surprises even you. A protective, invisible bubble surrounds you at all times. It will only allow those feelings that are positive and helpful to you to pass through for you to enjoy and build upon. Others may catch stress from each other … negativity, too, can be infectious … but you are protected … you continue to keep things in perspective … and to deal with things calmly and methodically. You are able to see the way forward clearly … solve problems … find ways around difficulties … by using your own inner resources and strengths, born of experience. In you alone lies the secret of success. You can and you will succeed.

Imagine yourself leading a healthy lifestyle and it will happen.

LIVING NOW

Although we cannot change the past, we can learn from it and build up a range of skills and useful insights from it. The future is that unknown world of possibilities and opportunities before us – but all that we can truly have any effect upon is the present. Keep saying to yourself …

- I have learned a great deal from the past.
- The future is an exciting range of opportunities.
- I enjoy laying good foundations NOW on which to build a better future.

Imagine yourself standing on a pathway. As you look around the left, right and above is brilliantly illuminated, and sounds are amazingly clear. As you check over your shoulder you notice the path behind is unclear. You hear a clock chime in the distance and take a step forward. You notice the slightest of noises, movements or shifts of light, and take pleasure even in the pure sound of silence, too. You can hear that same clock ticking now, and with each tick you can take a small step forward, effortlessly, along the path, and that illumination and awareness moves with you. At any fork in the path you can make decisions easily as you are truly involved in the moment, rather than looking over your shoulder at what might have been, or staring blindly into the future at what might happen. You enjoy being in the brilliantly illuminated, acute awareness of sound, hearing, feeling, taste and smell that is NOW.

For a complete experience, be more acutely aware of shapes and textures as well as sounds, colours and scents.

GOAL ACHIEVEMENT

A goal, in all areas of life, is vitally important in order to focus your attention and inner resources. A goal provides a sense of direction and ultimately the joy of achievement. Without it you might flounder, so keep saying to yourself …

- I direct my energies to achieve my goals.
- I enjoy directing my energies positively.
- I know where I am going and how I am getting there.
- Step by step I am moving in the right direction.
- I have the ability, I have the determination, I shall succeed.

Keep your eyes firmly fixed on your goal and you will achieve it.

Be aware of the different areas of your life: work, social, leisure activities, emotional and spiritual. Select one of these for this exercise … and be aware of what you want to happen in that area of your life, what you want to achieve … Make it realistic and clear in your mind. It may be useful to write it down and describe it fully before beginning this visualization.

While in the meditative state, imagine yourself having achieved that goal, imagine yourself there, in that situation. Surround yourself with all the things or people that indicate that you have achieved that goal. Be as specific as you can … be aware of all the senses … what are you seeing … hearing … touching or sensing … smelling … tasting. Be there … make it real … be specific … about colours … temperatures … lighting, to make it more and more real in your mind.

Now, from where you are at that moment of achieving that goal … look back … as if along a path, a pathway of time … to where you were … and notice the different stages of change … of movement towards achieving that goal … along the way … along that path … the different actions you have taken … the contacts you have made … and the people involved. Be aware of all the stages along the way … and as you return to the here and now … you remain in touch with the feelings that will make it all worthwhile … and you feel more and more determined to take one step at a time … make one change at a time … along that path to the successful achievement of your goal. And as you return from the meditative state so you are more determined to be successful in the achievement of your goal.

FITNESS
AND
EXERCISE

You may use natural remedies and therapies, practise yoga or massage and have a general determination to lead a healthy life-style. But, perhaps you still feel unfit and out of shape. Today, everything is geared to make life as easy as possible. We do not have to walk up stairs because there is usually a lift to carry us, and we do not have to wash clothes by hand because most of us own a washing machine to do the work for us. Those of us who are office workers are amazingly inactive; we sit still all day – in a car, bus, or train, or at a desk – and slump on a favourite chair in the evening. Do you want to improve your fitness but feel it would be too difficult? Getting in trim appears to be hard work and time-consuming, but it does not need to be. So, read on to discover how to get results – and feel like new – in record time.

GENERAL FITNESS

✦━❍━✦

Fitness is the key to a healthy mind and body. It is based on stamina, strength, and suppleness – the three "S"s; better shape and self-esteem are two extra "S" bonuses. Being fit does not merely improve your physical prowess and grace, it also makes you feel better overall. But although we are more health-conscious about our diet nowadays, regular exercise is still not a part of most people's daily lives. Surveys always draw the same conclusion as to the reasons for this: lack of time, energy, interest, and confidence. Becoming fit is neither as difficult nor as time-consuming as it may appear to be: you can get fit – and get a better body into the bargain – more quickly, easily and enjoyably than you may think.

HOW FIT DO YOU NEED TO BE?

There is no such thing as a standard fitness gauge – it all depends on your personal make-up and why you want to be fit: being robust enough to run a marathon, for example, is very different from honing the three "S"s. For exercise to be of any help to you, though, it should boost your metabolism and improve your cardiovascular and respiratory systems.

Swimming is an excellent way of keeping the whole body in good physical condition when done regularly and conscientiously.

WHY BOTHER WITH FITNESS?

Are you tired of running out of puff, being out of shape or always feeling under the weather? Do you often get colds, or suffer from pre-menstrual syndrome (PMS), stress, or sleepless nights? These are just a handful of the signs that could manifest themselves when you are unfit.

So exercise is worth the effort, because when you are fitter, problems such as these may ease or disappear.

Women are increasingly attracted to strenuous sports such as boxing that until recently were considered to be solely a male preserve.

Competitive team sports such as volleyball not only provide an opportunity to improve physical fitness, they are also highly enjoyable.

YOUR GOAL

Finding a goal to inspire you is the secret of success. Set the deadline and stick to it. Depending on what you want to achieve, a three-week plan is ideal because it is not too long and if you persevere (take it week by week or day by day – whichever you find easiest), you will see results. Be realistic: if your goals are too high you are likely to fail: if they are too low, you will not have enough of a challenge.

Goals will inspire you, but speedy results are the key to keeping up regular exercise – it is natural to want to see rewards for all your hard work – although it is advisable to build up a pattern gradually. The minimum amount of exercise you need to do to improve your personal fitness is 20 minutes, three times a week – the "3 × 20" maxim. This means three bouts of exercise vigorous enough to make you fairly breathless (but not gasping for breath). So if you do the general fitness exercises outlined in this book three times a week for 20 minutes you will get fitter. If you want to see fast results, though, you need to add extra activities – such as a couple of games of tennis, swimming, or brisk walking – to your exercise quota, so that you are actually exercising six days a week.

Taking part in a team sport once a week is a good idea: not only will it make you fitter, slimmer, and happier, the competitive spirit will also strengthen your resolve. Some sports need special skills, but you do not have to be an athlete to do most of them.

CAUTION

Before taking up any form of rigorous exercise or training, you should consult your doctor – especially if any of the following conditions apply to you:

- diabetes or epilepsy
- over 35 years of age with a long history of inactivity
- cardiovascular or respiratory problems
- severe illness and ensuing medication
- chronic joint or back problems
- obesity
- pregnancy
- heavy drinking or smoking

WARMING UP AND COOLING DOWN

Warm-up activities are important as they prime you for exercise; they ease your muscles into action so that your muscles react more readily to activity; they also prepare you for a rise in heart rate and body temperature. Warm ups should be done slowly and rhythmically for 5–10 minutes (depending on age and personal fitness).

Be sure also to set time aside to cool down after exercising: keep walking or moving around slowly for 5 minutes. The cool-down period is important because it allows you to decrease gradually the amount of exercise. This avoids feelings of faintness that may be caused by the pooling of blood below the waist that occurs during vigorous exercise.

YOUR PULSE RATE

Monitoring your pulse rate allows you to keep a check on whether you are exercising adequately. The maximum heart rate for an adult is roughly 220 beats per minute minus your age in years. The ideal heart rate during exercise is in a target zone of 65–80 per cent of this figure. The aim of exercise is to get your heart rate to within a certain range. These are the ideal exercise heart rates for the different ages:

Age	Pulse Range
20+	130–160
30+	124–152
40+	117–144

To find out your active pulse rate per minute, rest two fingers lightly on your pulse immediately after exercising, count the beats for 10 seconds and multiply by 6.

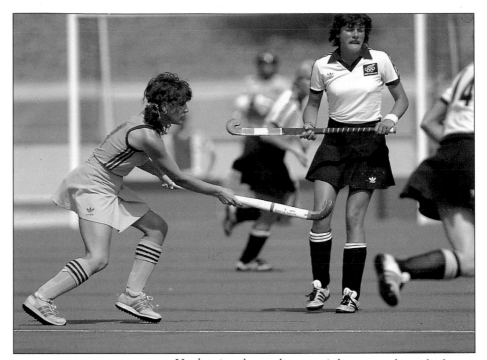

Hockey is a demanding sport that strengthens the legs, is beneficial to the heart and lungs, and significantly improves co-ordination.

A good many water sports demand strength, stamina, and a fine sense of balance. Wind surfing is no exception to the rule.

EXERCISES FOR GENERAL FITNESS

This exercise routine helps to improve over-all fitness and should take you roughly 30 minutes to complete. Aim to do it three times a week and try to do extra aerobic exercise – such as swimming, walking or cycling – on the other days (aerobic exercises include any activity that can be done rhythmically and continually and that boosts the efficient uptake of oxygen). To warm up your muscles before exercising, either spend 2 minutes running up and down the stairs, walking briskly, cycling, or doing the special warm-up exercises outlined below.

WARM-UP EXERCISE A

1 Stand upright with your feet apart and in line with your shoulders, with your arms hanging loosely at your sides and your shoulders down.

2 Bring your shoulders forwards.

❦ If you feel any pain – or experience anything other than the normal sensation of muscle fatigue – stop exercising. Always work out at your own pace; and skip exercise if you are ill.

Toning Exercises	Repeats/Time Allowance
Warm-ups	5 minutes
Press-ups	10 repeats
Lying Flies	10 repeats
Reverse curls	10 repeats
Sit-ups	10 repeats
Squats	10 repeats
Cool Downs	3–5 minutes
Aerobic Exercise	20–30 minutes

The recommended 10 repeats are for beginners – you should aim to repeat each exercise 15 times. Start by doing this set of exercises twice a week, work up to three times a week and combine it with some other form of exercise – ideally aerobics – for the time suggested above.

3 Raise them up high.

4 Move them back as far as possible, then back to the start position.

WARM-UP EXERCISE B

1 Maintain an upright posture as in Exercise A. Tip your head forwards so that your chin is almost resting in your chest.

2 Raise your head, stretching and lengthening your neck as you return to the upright position. Repeat four times.

3 Now tip your head to the left, keeping your shoulders down. Bring it back to the centre and then stretch and lengthen your neck.

4 Repeat step 3 but tip your head to the right side. Repeat four times on each side, remembering not to raise your shoulders.

5 Keep your head upright and turn so that you are looking over your left shoulder. Then face forwards again and stretch and lengthen your neck.

6 Now turn and look over your right shoulder. Face forwards again and stretch and lengthen your neck. Repeat steps 5 and 6 four times, then do the whole sequence again twice.

WARM-UP EXERCISE C

1 Stand with your feet apart; lean forwards from your hips keeping your back straight.

2 Rotate and bend your left leg out from the hip until your knee is over your left foot and pointing in the same direction. Keep your right leg straight and your right foot pressed into the floor. Repeat five times, holding the position for 5 seconds, swap leg positions and repeat.

THE GENERAL EXERCISES

CHEST MUSCLES: PRESS-UPS

1 Place yourself on all fours with your knees directly under your hips, your hands beneath your shoulders with your fingers pointing forwards, your palms flat. Make sure your back is straight – that is, parallel with the ceiling – all the time. Achieve this by pulling your stomach in and tucking your pelvis under.

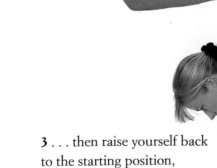

3 . . . then raise yourself back to the starting position, breathing in as you go.

UPPER BACK MUSCLES:
LYING FLIES

1 Lie on your front on the floor with your hips down, and keep your body relaxed. Rest your forehead on the floor, your arms out on each side at right angles to your body, elbows bent.

3 Lower your arms again. Make sure you do not pull your elbows back; keep them in line with your shoulders and keep your hips and feet in contact with the floor all the time.

ABDOMINAL MUSCLES

When you do these exercises, keep your lower back pressed into the floor throughout and work slowly, with total control. In the Upper Abdominals exercise, lift your head and shoulders as one unit, never separately; roll up from the top of your head; imagine you are holding a peach between your chin and your chest and keep this gap constant throughout. Make sure your face muscles are relaxed all the time.

LOWER ABDOMINALS: REVERSE CURLS

1 Lie flat on your back on the floor, arms by your sides, palms flat on the floor beside you.

2 While keeping your arms and hands flat on the floor, bring your knees in towards your chest one at a time, and once there, keep both knees together in the bent position.

3 Breathe in and, keeping your spine pressed into the floor, pull in your abdominal muscles while at the same time curling up your coccyx (tail bone) to bring your knees closer to your chest. Keep your feet relaxed throughout. Lower your body to the starting position, exhaling as you go down.

UPPER ABDOMINALS: SIT UPS

1 Lying flat on the floor with your arms by your side, palms flat on the floor, bend your knees and keep your feet flat on the floor, a little distance apart in line with your hips.

2 Lift your head and shoulders – inhaling as you move up – and push your fingertips towards your knees, keeping your arms straight.

3 Lower your body back to the starting position, exhaling as you go down. Repeat the movement.

LEG MUSCLES: SQUATS

1 Stand up straight with your feet a little wider than shoulder-width apart. If you stand on tiptoe, this exercise tones your calf muscles and your quadriceps, the muscles on the front of your thighs; if you angle your toes slightly outwards while on tiptoe, it benefits your inner thighs.

2 Resting your hands on the front of your thighs and keeping your arms straight, steadily bend your legs until you reach a squatting position, exhaling as you go down.

3 Then, inhale as you rise steadily back to the starting position. When you do this exercise, it is important to keep your back straight and your knees flexible. Do not let your knees bend further forward than your toes.

SPORTS ACTIVITIES

━━◦◦◦━━

Team sports and work-outs at the gym are not only fun, they also give you the chance to add to your exercise quota for the week, and therefore reach your self-improvement goals that much faster. The benefits of taking part in specific sports and of working out are given here.

BADMINTON:

Aerobic; improves joint flexibility, stamina, leg and shoulder tone and strength; 30–40 minutes continuous play burns up around 200–800 calories.

GOLF:

Improves arm, shoulder and leg tone, and strength (you walk four to five miles when you do a round of golf).

JOGGING:

Aerobic, improves stamina, leg strength and tone; an hour's jogging burns up 200–350 calories. If you think that jogging or running will suit your new active way of life, take the standard precautions before you start: check with your doctor and, as with all aerobic exercise, increase the pace gradually; always wear the right trainers (and support bandages if your joints are weak).

TENNIS:

Aerobic; boosts stamina and suppleness; strengthens and tones your shoulders, forearms, calves and thighs; play energetically (ideally twice a week) for an hour and you will burn up around 300–400 calories.

BRISK WALKING:

Aerobic; strengthens and tones your legs.

CYCLING:

Aerobic; builds stamina; tones your legs.

SKIPPING:

Aerobic; boosts stamina, strength and leg tone. Start by doing 3 skipping sets for 30 seconds a time with a 5-minute break after each set; build up to skipping for 2 minutes with a 10-minute break and also increase the repetitions.

Golf is a sport that particularly benefits shoulders, arms, and legs. Playing a round involves a good deal of walking.

Judo is a body contact sport and one of the major martial arts. It requires a good deal of strength, agility, and physical courage.

GYM-BASED BENEFITS
Aerobics: classes combine exercise with constant movement; they arc fast fat-burners and ideal if you are after quick results.
Circuit, cross, resistance, or weight training: aerobic; increase stamina and strength; an hour of circuit training burns up between 350–550 calories.
Step classes: aerobic; improves stamina; tones and strengthens your lower torso; an hour-long class burns up between 500–800 calories.
Yoga: improves posture; tones, strengthens, and relaxes the body; loosens joints; an hour of yoga burns up about 200 calories.

REBOUNDING:
Aerobic; bounding on a mini trampoline is a fun way to get fit at home.

SWIMMING:
Aerobic; swimming is one of the fastest (and best) ways to boost overall fitness, muscle tone, joint flexibility, and relaxation. Do 4 lengths of a 25 m (25 yd) pool, rest for a minute and build endurance by reducing rcst time and increasing swim time; within a fortnight you will bc noticeably fitter; an hour's breaststroke burns 500–800 calories.

FOOTBALL:
Aerobic; improves stamina; strengthens and tones your legs; an hour's play burns up around 250–1000 calories.

HELP FOR PMS
Exercise is the last thing you feel like doing when you are pre-menstrual. But if you do push yourself now, you will relieve the symptoms. If you cannot face an aerobics class, go for a swim; this will ease pre-menstrual cramp and put you in a better mood.

BOXING:
Tones and strengthens your chest, shoulders, and arms; an hour's boxing burns up around 400–600 calories.

VOLLEYBALL:
Aerobic; improves stamina; tones and strengthens the whole body, especially your legs and arms; mobilizes joints; an hour's play burns up 200–600 calories.

SQUASH:
as volleyball; an hour's play burns up 400–1000 calories.

BODY SHAPE

The shape of your body is unique: it is important to remember this because the basic skeletal and muscular form that you inherit is unchangeable. Features such as your height, foot size, shoulder width and the length and shape of your legs, nose, fingers and toes combine to produce a whole. Each person is an individual, with characteristics particular to their genetic make-up.

BODY BRACKETS

Although we come in a variety of shapes and sizes, the human body is cast from three basic moulds. Often, features from two or three of these body types are jumbled with our individual characteristics, but it is the more dominant features that slot us into one of the following groups: ectomorphs; mesomorphs, and endomorphs.

Ectomorphs are usually small- and slender-framed with long limbs, narrow shoulders, hips and joints. They have little muscle or body fat. Mesomorphs have medium to large – but compact – frames with broader shoulders, pelvic girdle and well-developed muscles. Endomorphs are naturally curvaceous, with more body fat than muscle, wider hips, shorter limbs and a lower centre of gravity than the other two body types.

SELF-IMAGE

If you are a bit on the tubby side, it can be annoying to hear someone who you think is poker-thin whining about being overweight. But there is logic behind this that stems from self-image. Very few of us actually see ourselves as we really are. We tend to misjudge our bodies with sweeping claims to fatness, even when we have only a spot of excess flab around our midriff to show for it. And although it sounds amazing, the way we behave in everyday life (and think others see us) often tallies with our self-image. It is a vicious circle: we think that we do not measure up to the standard beauty ideal so our self-esteem dips, often so low that we feel that we will never have a better body. This in turn causes self-confidence to plummet further, we feel even worse, and so the vicious circle continues.

Taking control of your self-image brings enormous bonuses. And the faster you can do this, the greater the rewards, as speedy results boost your confidence more quickly. But before you undertake a scheme to get into better shape, you must work on your positive thinking: realize your potential by deciding on (and accepting) your body model, then use this as your goal. Forget conventional beauty ideals – you do not have to have mile-long legs to have a dynamite figure; what you already have – your basic shape – is great. It just needs perfecting, and that is something that everyone can do with determination.

GOOD POSTURE

Even though it sounds like some pointless exercise from your schooldays, there is real wisdom in the old dictum "head up, shoulders back, bottom in". The difference that good posture makes to the look of our bodies is enormous, mainly because when we are standing properly our abdominal muscles are in their correct supporting role and the whole body is aligned so it looks leaner and taller. Good posture is also helpful to our mental and physical health; some alternative therapies (such as the Alexander Technique) are based on the principle of correct posture because it can ease back pain, stress, and even headaches.

POSTURE EXERCISE

Stand in front of a mirror, try these exercises and see what they do for the shape of your body:

1 Do this exercise facing yourself first, then turn so you are sideways on:

Lift your head up and lengthen your spine.

Tuck in your chin and your bottom.

Bring your shoulders back and down.

2 Now stand with your legs slightly apart.

Check whether your weight is evenly spread.

Keep your shoulders and hips level and your weight balanced between the heel and ball of each foot.

TROUBLE SPOTS

❖⇌∘⇌❖

Very few people are able to say honestly that they are totally happy with their body. Everyone has at least one gripe – if it is not big feet, it is thin hair or knobbly knees. All these perceived "flaws" can be improved or disguised, but as anyone who has ever tried (and failed) to move the fat that sits on strategic points such as hips, thighs, stomachs, and buttocks knows, it is much easier to hide the flaws than to tackle them. But it is possible to alter your outline with a combination of diet and exercise.

The best way to assess your figure is to stand in front of a full-length mirror. Be honest with yourself, and look for areas that need improving.

FINDING AND IMPROVING YOUR TRUE FORM

Step 1: Confront Your Body
Go on, be brave. Strip to your underwear, stand in front of a mirror and have a good look at your body. Take your time and be tough but realistic. You may have disliked your thighs since you were 16 – and they will probably never be those of a super-model – but if you look hard enough you might just find that they are not as bad as you have always thought they were, and that improving them is not going to be that hard after all.

Step 2: Put Your Complaints in Writing
Note down all the things that irk you (and that you can do something about) as well as those that you like or do not mind. Then go through your list of dislikes, ticking the things that you really want to do something about. Also, make a mental note to start appreciating your good points: the more you focus on them the less you will notice the not-so-good zones.

Step 3: Action Checklist
Now, add a set of action points under the problem zones you have listed. If you want to firm up your arms for that sleeveless sundress you have been unable to wear for a decade of summers, make notes like this:
Flabby Upper Arms
❧ *Do Basic Exercises*
❧ *Check Diet*
❧ *Exfoliate/Moisturize*
Finally, add your goal(s) and your deadline to the top of the list and put it somewhere where you are going to see it frequently.

TWO QUICK THIGH-TONERS

If you do not have time to do a full exercise routine, grab 10 minutes in the morning.

Outer Thighs: sit on the floor with your legs straight out in front and hold your arms out to the sides as shown left. Roll sideways on to your bottom – go right over on to your outer thigh and then roll right over on to the other thigh.

Do this twenty times.

Inner Thighs: stand upright and consciously tighten – and hold – your buttock muscles for a slow count of 5. Repeat with your thigh muscles and then your calf muscles.

COMMON PROBLEMS

Any of the following can be discouraging, but remember – each problem has a solution.

SLACK STOMACHS

Our stomachs become flabby when the abdominal muscles slacken; this usually happens through lack of exercise. Your abdomen extends from just under the bustline to the groin, and it is packed with muscles that criss-cross to form a wall to hold the abdominal contents in place – a bit like a corset. Exercise is not the only way to keep your stomach flat: weight is also important and the long-term answer is diet and exercise.

THUNDER THIGHS

Thigh size and tone can certainly be altered with the right diet, correct body care and regular exercise. Sports such as cycling, skiing, tennis, squash, and riding (a great inner-muscle firmer) will tone your thighs, as will weight training for specific areas of the body.

LARGE BOTTOMS

There are three large muscles in our buttocks: *gluteus maximus, medius,* and *minimus.* These create the shape, but not the size, of our rear ends. It is the tone of these muscles and the fatty tissue around them that gives us the bottoms we have. The good news is that buttock muscles respond well to exercise, which means that any effort you put into bottom-toning exercises will be rewarded quite quickly.

ANKLE EXERCISES

Whenever you remember move your ankles around in a clockwise motion ten times, then repeat anti-clockwise.

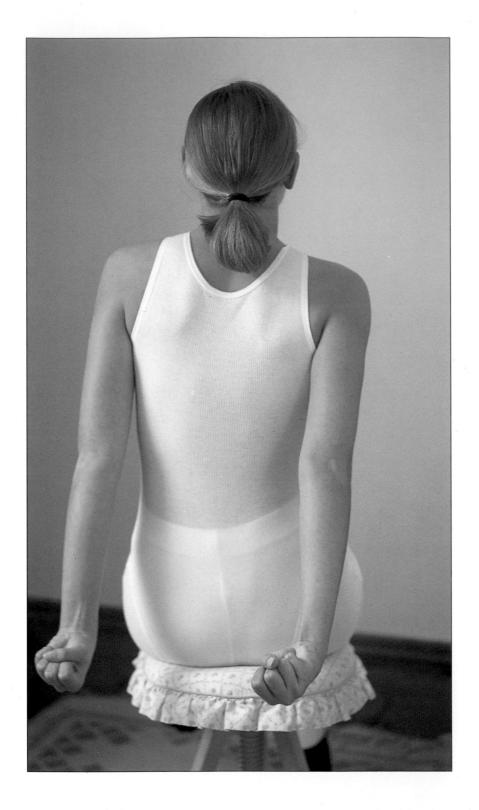

FLABBY ARM FIXER

To firm up flabby arms, add this exercise to your daily exercise routine, or spend five minutes doing it twice a day. Sit on a chair holding your hands in loose fists, and, with your arms extended out behind, make downwards punching movements backwards and forwards.

SLACK UPPER ARMS

Our arms do not really change shape much during our lives, unless we lose or gain a lot of weight. Muscle tone is the main problem, but, as in the case of thighs, exercise and specific weight training will tone up and re-shape flabby arms; very often, any changes in body shape that happen through exercise and diet are noticeable most quickly on your upper arms.

DROOPY BREASTS

Breast shape and size only really change when our weight swings dramatically, or during pregnancy, breast-feeding, menstruation, or if taking oral contraceptives. Gravity is the bust's enemy, especially if the breasts are not given proper support, because it literally drags the breasts down and slackens their tone. Although the breasts are supported by suspension ligaments, they do not contain any muscle (the milk glands are buffered by protective fatty tissue) so you cannot noticeably reverse lost tone. However, if you exercise the pectoral muscles beneath your armpits, you will give your breasts a firmer base and more uplift.

THICK ANKLES

Trim and slender ankles that seem set to snap with every step are a great asset. But if you are not blessed with these, or if your ankles tend to become stiff and puffy from fluid retention, you need to master the art of deception and brush up on some ankle improving exercises.

Assess the flexibility of your ankles by sitting on a chair or stool with your feet on the floor and, while keeping your heel down, pull the rest of your foot up as far as it will go: if the distance between your foot and floor measures 12–15 cm (5–6 in) your joint flexibility is good; if it is between 10–12 cm (4–5 in) it is fair; and if it is less than that, your joint flexibility is poor.

The following exercises will help to improve the muscles that support your breasts.

1 Stand erect and bend your arms at the elbows, holding your arms horizontally in front of your chest, with your fingertips touching. Move your elbows back as far as they will go, with a firm, quick movement. Return to the starting position and repeat as many times as you wish.

2 Resume the position you took in step 1, but this time, as you move your elbows back, straighten your arms, so that you fling them behind you. Repeat several times.

3 Stand erect and hold your arms in front of your chest, with elbows bent. Grasp your left arm just above the wrist with your right hand, and your right arm just above the wrist with your left hand. Now pull on each arm, as if you were trying to pull your hands apart, but maintain a tight grip. Hold for a few seconds. Relax your hands and then repeat several times.

4 Now raise your arms and hold them out in front of your mouth, repeat step 3 in this higher position. If you wish, you can also do the exercise holding your arms just in front of your waistline.

BASIC EXERCISE ROUTINE

Add these basic exercises to your general fitness routine to give special problem areas extra work, or do them on their own as an isolated routine. If you do them on their own, use the abdominal muscle exercises from the general fitness plan for your stomach.

THIGH MUSCLES

EXERCISE A

1 Lie on your back on the floor with your arms resting straight out at right angles to your body and your feet apart, in line with your hips.

2 Hold a cushion between your knees and, keeping your back pressed into the floor, press your knees together ten times quickly, and ten times slowly, keeping the cushion in place throughout.

3 Now repeat the same sequence again, holding a tennis or golf ball between your knees.

EXERCISE B

1 Lie on your back on the floor with your legs straight, and your lower back pressed to the floor. Put your arms along your sides, palms to the floor.

2 Stretch your arms out at right angles to your body. Bend your legs and bring your knees up to your chest.

3 Keeping your legs together, steadily straighten them so that they are pointing up towards the ceiling. Keep your feet relaxed.

4 Slowly open your legs out sideways – as wide as you can – then close them again. Repeat the exercise (steps 2–4) four times. When you get used to the exercise, you can do it with small weights tied to your ankles.

EXERCISE C

1 Stand sideways on to a chair or table (lightly holding the edge to maintain your balance) with your shoulders down and relaxed, and with your knees bent and your feet facing forwards.

2 Lift your left hip slightly and slowly move your leg out and up (no higher than 45°), keeping your foot and knee facing forwards. Make sure you do not let your body tilt – keep it as straight as possible. Carefully lower your leg. Repeat the whole exercise ten times, then turn and repeat with the other leg.

EXERCISE D

1 Lie on your right side on the floor with your legs out straight. Support your head with your right hand.

2 Bend your lower leg behind you to maintain balance and tilt your hips slightly towards the floor; your head, hips, knees, and feet should all be facing forwards. Balance yourself with your left hand on the floor.

3 Slowly lift your upper leg, then bring it down to touch the lower one; raise it again and repeat this action six times. Turn over and repeat steps 1–3 on the other side.

ANKLES AND CALF MUSCLES

EXERCISE A

1 Sit up straight on a chair, with your knees together and heels on the floor and slightly apart, in line with your hips. Bring your big toes up and roll your feet in towards each other.

2 Now tilt and move both feet down and outwards from the ankle, keeping your big toes raised as much as possible as you roll your feet on to their outer edges. Repeat ten times.

EXERCISE B

1 Lie flat on your back on the floor with your legs straight.

2 Bring one leg up and hold it beneath the back of your thigh so that it is pulled towards your chest. Rotate your foot ten times in a clockwise direction and ten times anti-clockwise. Repeat with the other leg. Increase the number of repeats to twenty for each foot, working alternatively in groups of 7.

BUTTOCK MUSCLES

EXERCISE A

1 Stand upright and lightly hold the back of a chair or the edge of a table to maintain your balance. Put your weight on your right leg and turn your left leg out from the hip.

2 Keeping your foot flexed, take your left leg back as far as you can without bending it at the knee, forcing the movement or over-arching your back. Repeat with the other leg. Repeat five times for each leg and gradually build up to twenty repetitions.

EXERCISE B

1 Lie on your back with your knees bent and your feet slightly apart, in line with your hips. Place your arms by your sides, palms flat on the floor.

2 Place your weight on your shoulders and upper back (not your neck), raise your bottom and tighten your buttock muscles, keeping your feet flat on the floor and your arms by your sides. Hold for several seconds. Lower your bottom to the floor. Repeat five times, building up to twenty repetitions.

Exercise C

1 Kneel on all fours with your knees slightly apart, in line with your hips, but keeping them tucked right under your hips. Place your hands in front of you, a shoulder-width apart and facing forwards. Bend your elbows so that you are leaning on your forearms.

2 Keeping your foot flexed, push your left leg out straight behind you, keeping your back and hips parallel.

3 Bring your leg and foot down to the floor, keeping your foot flexed and your leg straight. Repeat steps 2 and 3 twelve times. Return to the original position, then repeat the exercise with your other leg. Build up to twenty repetitions.

GLOSSARY

ACUTE CONDITION: Arising suddenly and with intense severity, but only running a short course. (See chronic condition)

ALLOPATHIC: The conventional method of combating disease by using active ingredients specifically against the disease.

ANAEMIA: A deficiency in red blood cells, or in the haemoglobin carried by them. The resultant lack of oxygen carried around the body produces pallor, breathlessness and no energy.

ANALGESIC: Relieves pain.

APERIENT: A mild laxative.

ATROPHY: The shrinking or wasting away of muscles, glands or tissues due to disease or malnutrition.

BILE: A bitter green to brown alkaline fluid produced by the liver and stored in the gall bladder.

BILIOUS: Any disorder which results in the production of an excess amount of bile.

CHRONIC CONDITION: A disease or ailment that develops slowly and persists over a long period of time. (See acute condition)

DEMULCENT: Oily substance used to soften and soothe damaged surfaces such as the skin, or mucous membranes.

DILUENT: A substance used for dilution, e.g. water, base oil.

DIURETIC: Encourages urination.

DYSPEPSIA: Indigestion.

EMETIC: Causes vomiting.

EMOLLIENT: Softens and soothes the skin.

ENDOGENOUS: Caused or produced by factors within the organism or system.

FEBRIFUGE: Reduces fever.

FEBRILE: Feverish, or relating to a fever.

FIBROIDS: A structure resembling or consisting of fibrous tissue.

FOMENTATION: The act of applying heat and moisture to relieve inflammation and pain.

LEUCORRHEA: White to yellowish vaginal discharge.

MUCOUS MEMBRANE: Soft tissue lining most of the body's cavities and tubes.

PAROXYSMAL: A sudden attack or occurrence of a disease.

PERISTALSIS: Waves of contractions passing along the walls of hollow muscular organs, forcing the contents forwards.

PHARMACOPOEIA: An authoritative written guide to medicinal drugs and their uses.

PROGESTERONE: A natural hormone that prepares the uterus to receive and develop the fertilized egg.

PROPHYLACTIC: Preventing or protecting from disease.

SALICYLATES: Salts of salicylic acid.

SALICYLIC ACID: A white crystalline substance used in the manufacture of aspirin.

SUCCUSS: A special way of shaking a homeopathic remedy in order to extract its medicinal properties.

SUPPURATING: Oozing.

SYNOVIAL MEMBRANE: Soft tissues lining joints and tendon sheaths.

TONIC: Invigorates and tones the body and promotes well-being.

TRIGEMINAL NERVES: Either of the fifth pair of cranial nerves which supply the muscles of the upper and lower jawbone.

WATERBRASH: Gas being brought up into the mouth with acidic fluid.

BIBLIOGRAPHY

Charles, Rachel. *Mind, Body and Immunity,* Methuen, London, England, 1990

Davis, Patricia. *Aromatherapy, An A-Z,* C.W. Daniel, Saffron Walden, England, 1988

Davis, Dr Stephen and Stewart, Dr Alan. *Nutritional Medicine*, Pan Books Ltd, London, England, 1987

Editors of the Prevention Magazine Health Books, *The Doctor's Book of Home Remedies,* Bantam, New York, USA, 1991

Evans, Mark. *A Guide to Herbal Remedies,* C.W. Daniel, Saffron Walden, England, 1990

Evans, Mark. *Instant Aromatherapy for Stress Relief*, Lorenz Books, London, England, 1996

Evans, Mark. *Instant Massage for Stress Relief*, Lorenz Books, London, England, 1996

Evans, Mark. *Instant Stretches for Stress Relief*, Lorenz Books, London, England, 1996

Grieve, Mrs M. *Modern Herbal*, Penguin, London, England, 1984

Hanssen, Maurice. *E For Additives,* Thorsons, London, England, 1990

Hudson, John. *Instant Meditation for Stress Relief*, Lorenz Books, London, England, 1996

Hawkey, Susan. *Herbalism,* Lorenz Books, London, England, 1997

Kusick, James. *A Treasury of Natural First Aid Remedies From A-Z,* Reward Books, Prentice Hall Inc., New York, USA, 1995

Leung, Albert Y. *Encyclopaedia of Common Natural Ingredients used in Food, Drugs and Cosmetics*, John Wiley & Sons, New York, USA, 1980

Maybey, Richard. *The Complete New Herbal*, Elm Tree Books, London, England, 1988

McIntyre, Anne. *Herbs for Common Ailments*, Gaia Books, London, England, 1988

McVica, Jekka. *Jekka's Complete Herb Book,* Kyle Cathie, London, England, 1994

Maxwell-Hudson, Clare. *Aromatherapy Massage Book,* Dorling Kindersley, London, England, 1995

Mellor, Contance. *Natural Remedies for Common Ailments*, Granada Publishing Ltd, London, England, 1975

Mervyn, Leonard. *The Complete Guide to Vitamins and Minerals,* Thorsons, London, England, 1990

Messegne, Maurice. *Health Secrets of Plants and Herbs*, Collins, London, England, 1979

Mills, Simon (ed). *Alternative in Healing,* Macmillan, London, England, 1988

Newman Turner, Roger. *Naturopathic Medicine,* Thorsons, London, England, 1989

Ody, Penelope. *The Herb Society's Complete Medicinal Herbal,* Dorling Kindersley, London, England, 1993

Oxenford, Rosalind. *Reflexology*, Lorenz Books, London, England, 1997

Shepherd, Dr Dorothy. *Magic of the Minimum Dose.* C.W. Daniel, Saffron Walden, England, 1990

Tisserand, Robert. *The Art of Aromatherapy,* C.W. Daniel, Saffron Walden, England, 1977

van Straten, Michael. *The Complete Natural Health Consultant,* Ebury Press, London, England, 1987

various. *Homeopathy, The Family Handbook,* Unwin, London, England, 1987

Worwood, V. *The Fragrant Pharmacy*, Bantam Books, London, England, 1991

PUBLISHER'S ACKNOWLEDGEMENTS

The Publishers would like to thank the following contributors for additional text: John Hudson (Hypnotherapy), Andrew Oldroyd (Moxibustion), Susanne Franzen (Shiatsu), Karine Butchart (Makko Ho), Felicity Roma Bowers (Meditation), Paul Harvey (Yoga), Anne Gains, Nutritionist (Healthy Eating Plan), Clare Harris (Massage).

The Publishers would like to thank Jekka McVica for supplying herbs for photography.

Jekka McVica at
Jekka's Herb Farm, Rose Cottage, Shellards, Aleveston,
Bristol BS12 2SY
Tel: 01454 418878
(mail-order suppliers of herbs)

PHOTOGRAPHY CREDITS
The majority of photographs taken in this book were by Lucy Mason and Don Last.
The publishers would also like to credit the following photographers: Deni Bown; Gary Brettnacher; Jean-Loup Charmet, Paris; Liz Edison; Jacqui Hurst; Michelle Garrett; John Glover; Angela Hampton; Mary Evans Picture Libray; Debbie Patterson; Reflections, Jo Browne; Steve Satushek; Timothy Shonnard; The Image Bank: Chris Close; Tony Stone: Bruce Ayres; Jennie Woodcock; Zefa Norman; Harry Smith.

USEFUL ADDRESSES

UK

AROMATHERAPY
International Society of Professional
Aromatherapists
The Hinckley and District Hospital
The Annex
Mount Road
Hinckley
Leicestershire LE10 1AG
(For information about courses, and
essential oils)

International Federation of
Aromatherapists
4 Eastmearn Road
Dulwich
London SE21 8HA
(Provides a list of professional
aromatherapists)

GENERAL
Natural Childbirth Trust
Alexandra House
Oldham Terrace
Acton
London W3 6NH

Registry of Traditional Chinese
Medicine
19 Trinity Road
London N2 8JJ

Research Council for Complementary
Medicine
60 Great Ormond Street
London WC1N 3JF

Women's Health Concern
83 Earl's Court Road
London W8 6EF

Women's Health Information Centre
52 Featherstone Street
London EC1Y 8RT

HERBALISM
General Council & Register of
Consultant Herbalists
18 Sussex Square
Brighton
East Sussex BN2 5AA

National Institute of Medical
Herbalists
56 Longbrook Street
Exeter
Devon EX4 6AH
(Provides a list of professional
herbalists and information about
training courses)

Natural Medicine Society
Edith Lewis House
Black Lane
Ilkeston
Derbyshire DE7 8EJ

The Herb Society
134 Buckingham Palace Road
London SW1W 9SA
(For information about herbs and
training courses)

The School of Phytotherapy/Herbal
Medicine
Buckstreep Manor
Bodle Street Green
Hailsham
East Sussex, BN27 4RJ
(For information about training
courses)

HOMEOPATHY
The Homeopathic Society
2 Powis Place
Great Ormond Street
London WC1N 3HT
(Provides a list of medically qualified
homeopaths)

*Filling a
herb pillow.*

The Society of Homeopaths
2 Artizan Road
Northampton NN1 4HU

Bach Flower Remedies
Dr. Edward Bach Centre
Mount Vernon Sotwell
Wallingford
Oxon, OX10 0PZ

HYPNOTHERAPY
National Council of Psychotherapists
and Hypnotherapy
Registry
Steam Cottage
98 Wish Hill
Willingdon
East Sussex BM20 9HQ

The School of Meditation
158 Holland Park Avenue
London W11 4UH

NATUROPATHY
British Naturopathic and
Osteopathic Association
6 Netherhall Gardens
London NW3 5RR
(Provides a list of practising
naturopaths)

British Society for Nutritional
Medicine
The Journal of Nutritional Medicine
P.O. Box 3AP
London

Eating Disorder Association
Sackville Place
44-46 Magdalen Street
Norwich
Norfolk NR3 1JE

The Secretary
The Incorporated Society of
Registered Naturopaths
293 Gilmerton Road
Edinburgh EH16 5UQ

Institute for Optimum Nutrition
5 Jerdan Place
London SW6 1BE

The Mc Carrion Society
*Institute of Brain Chemistry and
Human Nutrition*
Queen Elizabeth Hospital for
Children
Hayward Building, 3rd Floor
Hackney Road
London E2 8PS

HERBAL SUPPLIERS
Culpeper Ltd (head office)
Hadstock Road
Linton
Cambridge
CB1 6NJ

East-West Herbs Ltd.
Langston Priory Mews
Kingham
Oxon, OC7 6UW

Gerard House Ltd.
475 Capability Green
Luton LU1 3LU

Midsummer Cottage Clinic
Nether Westcote
Nr Kingham
Oxon OX7 6SD

COUCH GRASS
(Agropyron repens)

Neal's Yard Apothecary
15 Neal's Yard
Covent Garden
London WC2H 9DP

Optimum-Phoenix
The Barn
Higher Trickeys
Morebath
Nr Tiverton
Devon EX16 9AL

The Herbal Apothecary
120 High Street
Syston
Leics IE7 8GC

Fresh herb tea

ESSENTIAL OILS SUPPLIERS
Essence by Empress
P.O. Box 92
Penzance
Cornwall TR18 2XL

Fragrant Earth
P.O. Box 182
Taunton
Somerset TA1 1YR

Hartwood Aromatics
Hartwood House
12 Station Road
Hatton
Warwicks CV35 7LG

Shirley Price Aromatherapy
Wesley House
Stockwell Road
Hinckley
Leics LE10 1RD

SUPPLIERS OF HOMEOPATHIC REMEDIES
Most chemists and health food shops
will stock a limited supply of
homeopathic remedies. The list
below will stock a complete range.

Buxton and Grant
176 Whiteladies Road
Bristol BS8 2XU

Freeman's Pharmacy
7 Eaglesham Road
Clarkston,
Glasgow G76 7BU

Goulds the Chemist
14 Crowndale Road
London NW1 1TT

Helios Pharmacy
97 Camden Road
Tunbridge Wells
Kent TN1 2QR

US

ASSOCIATIONS
American Association of
Naturopathic Physicians (AANP)
2366 Eastlake Avenue
Suite 322
Seattle, WA 98102

American Holistic Medical
Association (AHMA)
4101 Lake Boone Trail
Suite 201
Raleigh, NC 27607

BORAGE *(Borago officinalis)*

American Botanical Council (ABC)
P.O. Box 201660
Austin, TX 78720

College of Maharishi Ayur-Veda
Health Center
P.O. Box 282
Fairfield, IA 52556

American Chiropractic Association
(ACA)
1701 Clarendon Blvd.
Arlington, VA 22209

American Osteopathic Association
(AOA)
142 East Ontario St.
Chicago, IL 60611

Aveda
140 5th Avenue
New York, NY 10011

California School of Herbal Studies
Forestville, CA

Eastern Acupuncture & Natural
Herb Center
8 Spring Street
New York, NY 10009

New Life Resource Center
938 8th Avenue
New York, NY 10019

Tom Thumb Workshops
P.O. Box 357
Mappsville, VA 23407

NEWSLETTERS
Alternatives
Mountain Home Publishing
(210) 367-4492. By David W.
Williams, a chiropractor

Naturally Well
Phillips Publishing Inc.
(301) 424-3700. By Marcus Laux,
M.D., a homeopathic specialist.

*Alternative Medicine: The
Definitive Guide and Alternative
Medicine Yellow Pages.* Compiled
by The Burton Goldberg Group,
Future Medicine Publishing, 1994

OUTLETS FOR HERBS
Cameron Park Botanicals
Highway 64 East
Raleigh, NC 27610

Caprilands Herb Farm
Silver Street
North Coventry, CT 06238

Flower Power Herbs and Roots Inc.
406 East 9th Street
New York, NY 10009

Herb Shoppe
215 West Main Street
Greenwood, IN 46142

San Francisco Herb Co.
250 14th Street
San Francisco, CA 94103

Seeds Blum
Idaho City State
Boise, ID 83706

Richter's Herb Catalog
Goodwood
Ontario
Canada, LOC 1AO

ESSENTIAL OILS SUPPLIERS
Bonny Doon Farm
600 Marin Road
Santa Cruz, CA 95060

Kiehl's
109 Third Avenue
New York, NY 10003

Lorann Oils
4518 Aurelius Road
P.O. Box 22009
Lansing, MI 48909-2009

AUSTRALIA
AROMATHERAPY
International Federation of
Aromatherapists
Information Line: 190 2240 125

HERBALISM
National Herbalist Association
P.O. Box 61
Broadway, NSW 2066

HOMEOPATHY
Australian Institute of Homeopathy
P.O. Box 122
Roseville, NSW 2069

Blackmores Ltd
23 Roseberry Street
Balgowlah, NSW 2093

Newton's Pharmacy
119 York Street
Sydney, NSW 2000

Manuka Pharmacy
Manuka Arcade
Manuka, ACT 2603

Martin and Pleasance
135 Swan Street
Richmond, Vic 3000

Bach Flower Shop
309 Little Collins Street
Melbourne, Vic 3000

Ahimsa
Drivers Court
Samsonvale, Qid 4520

Brauer Biotherapies Pty Ltd
1 Para Road
Tanunda, SA 5352

Fitch's Pharmacy
731 Hay Street
Perth, WA 9000

SAW PALMETTO
(Serenoa serrulata)

INDEX